Mineral Trioxide Aggregate

Mineral Trioxide Aggregate

Properties and Clinical Applications

Edited by

Dr. Mahmoud Torabinejad
Professor of Endodontics
Director of Advanced Education in Endodontics
Department of Endodontics
Loma Linda University School of Dentistry
Loma Linda, California, USA

WILEY Blackwell

Editorial Offices

1606 Golden Aspen Drive, Suites 103 and 104, Ames, Iowa 50010, USA

The Atrium, Southern Gate, Chichester, West Sussex, PO19 8SQ, UK

9600 Garsington Road, Oxford, OX4 2DQ, UK

For details of our global editorial offices, for customer services and for information about how
to apply for permission to reuse the copyright material in this book please see our website at
www.wiley.com/wiley-blackwell.

Library of Congress Cataloging-in-Publication Data

Mineral trioxide aggregate : properties and clinical applications / edited by Dr. Mahmoud Torabinejad.
    p.   cm.
  Includes bibliographical references and index.
  ISBN 978-1-118-40128-6 (cloth)
I. Torabinejad, Mahmoud, editor of compilation. [DNLM: 1. Root Canal Filling Materials.
2. Aluminum Compounds.   3. Biocompatible Materials.   4. Calcium Compounds.
5. Root Canal Therapy–methods.   6. Silicates. WU 190]
  RK351
  617.6′342059–dc23

                                        2014003707

A catalogue record for this book is available from the British Library.

Cover design by Modern Alchemy LLC

Set in 11/13pt Times by SPi Publisher Services, Pondicherry, India
Printed and bound in Malaysia by Vivar Printing Sdn Bhd

1   2014

Contents

Contributors

Seung-Ho Baek, DDS, MSD, PhD
Professor, Department of
Conservative Dentistry
Seoul National University,
School of Dentistry
Jongno-Gu, Seoul, Korea

David W. Berzins, PhD
Graduate Program Director for Dental
Biomaterials
Associate Professor,
General Dental Sciences
Marquette University
Milwaukee, Wisconsin, USA

George Bogen, DDS
Private Practice, Endodontics
Los Angeles, California, USA

Ricardo Caicedo, Dr. Odont,
SE, CSHPE
Associate Professor of Endodontics
Department of Oral Health and
Rehabilitation (Endodontics Division)
University of Louisville,
School of Dentistry
Louisville, Kentucky, USA

Joe H. Camp, DDS, MSD
Private Practice of Endodontics,
Charlotte, North Carolina, USA
and
Adjunct Professor
School of Dentistry,
University of North Carolina,
Chapel Hill, North
Carolina, USA

Nicholas Chandler, BDS,
MSc, PhD
Associate Professor
of Endodontics
Faculty of Dentistry,
University of Otago
Dunedin, New Zealand

Robert P. Corr, DDS, MS
Private Practice, Endodontist
Colorado Springs, Colorado, USA

**Till Dammaschke, Prof. Dr. med.
dent.**
Department of Operative Dentistry,
Westphalian Wilhelms-University
Münster, Germany

Lawrence Gettleman, DMD, MSD
Professor of Prosthodontics &
Biomaterials
Department of Oral Health and
Rehabilitation (Prosthodontics
Division)
University of Louisville,
School of Dentistry
Louisville, Kentucky, USA

George T.-J. Huang, DDS,
MSD, DSc
Professor & Director for Stem Cells
and Regenerative Therapies
College of Dentistry,
Department of Bioscience Research
University of Tennessee Health
Science Center
Memphis, Tennessee, USA

Ron Lemon, DMD
Associate Dean, Advanced Education
Program Director, Endodontics
UNLV, School of Dental Medicine
Las Vegas, Nevada, USA

Ingrid Lawaty, D.M.D.
Private Practice of Endodontics
Santa Barbara, California, USA

Masoud Parirokh, DMD, MS
Professor & Chairman,
Department of Endodontics,
Kerman University of Medical
Sciences School of Dentistry
Kerman, Iran

Shahrokh Shabahang, DDS,
MS, PhD
Associate Professor,
Department of Endodontics
Loma Linda University School of
Dentistry
Loma Linda, California, USA

Su-Jung Shin, DDS, MSD, PhD
Associate Professor, Department of
Conservative Dentistry
Yonsei University,
College of Dentistry,
Gangnam Severance Hospital
Seoul, Korea

Mahmoud Torabinejad, DMD,
MSD, PhD
Professor of Endodontics
Director of Advanced Education in
Endodontics
Department of Endodontics
Loma Linda University School of
Dentistry
Loma Linda, California, USA

David E. Witherspoon, BDSc, MS
Private Practice, Endodontist
North Texas Endodontic Associates
Plano, Texas, USA

Preface

For decades dentists have attempted to preserve the natural dentition by various preventive and treatment modalities. Despite these efforts, many people have developed tooth decay or have suffered traumatic injuries that often require endodontic care. The root canal system and the periodontium communicate through natural and sometimes artificial (iatrogenic) pathways. The pulp tissue is encased in the root canal system, surrounded by dentin, and communicates with the periodontium through the apical foramen and, occasionally, small channels known as accessory or lateral canals. Destruction of enamel and dentin by decay or by traumatic injuries as well as removal of cementum during periodontal treatment can result in communication between the root canal system, its dental pulp, and the periodontium.

Iatrogenic pathways of communication between the root canal system and the periodontium are created during accidental procedures such as perforations during root canal treatment. Exposure of pulp to oral flora via natural or artificial pathways results in the development of pulp and periapical inflammation and eventually destruction of these tissues. Pulpal and periapical diseases do not develop without bacterial contamination. Therefore the main objectives of root endodontic care continue to be prevention of pulpal inflammation and infection, removal of diseased tissue, elimination of microorganisms, and prevention of recontamination after treatment.

Because existing repair or filling materials did not possess adequate biocompatibility and were not able to seal the pathways of communication between the external and internal surfaces of the tooth, an experimental material, mineral trioxide aggregate (MTA), was developed. In a series of tests, our team investigated *in vitro* dye leakage with and without blood contamination, *in vitro* bacterial leakage, scanning electron microscope (SEM) examination of replicas for marginal adaptation, setting time, compressive strength, solubility, cytotoxicity, implantation in bone, and a usage test in animals. Contemporary materials such as amalgam, intermediate restorative material (IRM), or SuperEBA (*O*-ethoxybenzoic acid) were used for comparison. Based on our investigations, we reported that MTA has most of the ideal characteristics of repair materials for pulp capping, pulpotomy, apical plug, root perforation, and root end filling during apical surgery and suggested that MTA should be considered as an alternative material to the currently used root repair materials.

Since MTA's introduction, numerous studies have been published regarding its characteristics. Over 1,000 publications exist regarding the properties and clinical efficacy of MTA. It is one of the most investigated materials in dentistry. Based on the available evidence, it can be concluded that MTA is biocompatible, seals well, and can safely be used for pulp capping, pulpotomy, apical barrier, root perforation, root end filling, root canal filling, and regenerative endodontics. Like any material, MTA has some drawbacks, such as a long setting time and potential for discoloration. A principal objective of this textbook is to incorporate evidence-based information when available and when appropriate. Evidence-based treatment integrates the best clinical evidence with the practitioner's clinical expertise and the patient's treatment needs and preferences.

This textbook is written for dental students, general dentists, and specialists. It contains the information necessary for those who would like to incorporate endodontics into their practices and save natural teeth. It has been systematically organized to provide information regarding pulp and periradicular pathways, methods of their closure, chemical and physical properties of MTA, clinical uses of MTA in vital pulp therapy, use of MTA in teeth with necrotic pulps and open apices, use of MTA in regenerative endodontics, use of MTA as root perforation repair material, root canal obturation, and root end filling material during endodontic surgery. Finally, a chapter is dedicated to a group of materials (calcium silicate–based cements) that have been introduced to the market since the development of MTA approximately 20 years ago. The distinctive features of this textbook are: (1) updated, relevant, and recent information provided by authorities in the field in simple and clear language; and (2) the presentation of many clinical cases in color figures. There is also a DVD with video clips for selected procedures to assist the clinician in performing these procedures. These features provide the reader with a textbook that is concise, current, and easy to follow.

I would like to thank the contributing authors for sharing their materials and expertise with our readers. Their contributions will result in saving millions of teeth that would have been lost otherwise. I also would like to express our appreciation to the editorial staff of John Wiley & Sons and Mohammad Torabinejad, whose collaboration and dedication made this project possible. In addition, we acknowledge our colleagues and students who provided cases and gave us constructive suggestions to improve the quality of this textbook.

Mahmoud Torabinejad

1 Pulp and Periradicular Pathways, Pathosis, and Closure

Mahmoud Torabinejad

Department of Endodontics, Loma Linda University School of Dentistry, USA

Mineral Trioxide Aggregate: Properties and Clinical Applications, First Edition.
Edited by Mahmoud Torabinejad.
© 2014 John Wiley & Sons, Inc. Published 2014 by John Wiley & Sons, Inc.

PULP AND PERIRADICULAR PATHWAYS

The root canal system and the periodontium communicate through natural and artificial (iatrogenic) pathways. The pulp tissue is encased in the root canal system, is surrounded by dentin, and communicates with the periodontium through the apical foramen and occasionally, small channels known as accessory or lateral canals. Iatrogenic pathways of communication between the root canal system and the periodontium are created during accidental procedures such as perforations during root canal treatment. In addition, removal of enamel and dentin by decay or by traumatic injuries as well as removal of cementum during periodontal treatment may result in communication between the root canal system, its dental pulp, and the periodontium.

NATURAL PATHWAYS

The natural pathways of communication between the root canal system and the periodontium include the apical foramen, lateral canals, and dentinal tubules.

Apical foramen

The apical openings of roots are the main pathways between the root canal system, its contents, and the periradicular tissues (cementum, periodontal ligament, and alveolar bone). The apical foramen is initially very large (Fig. 1.1). As tooth eruption and its formation continue, the root canal space is narrowed by apposition of dentin and the apical foramen is modified by cementum

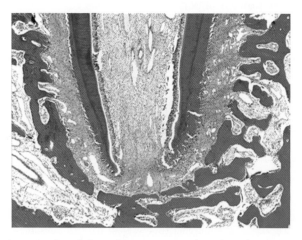

Fig. 1.1 Newly erupted teeth have large root canals with wide-open apices.

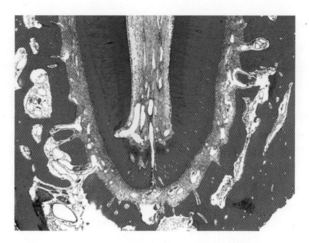

Fig. 1.2 As a tooth erupts, its root canal space is narrowed by apposition of dentin and its apical foramen is modified by cementum apposition.

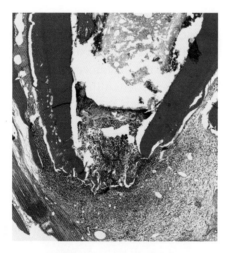

Fig. 1.3 Egress of irritants through the apical foramen into periapical tissues initiates a periapical lesion and destruction of periradicular tissues.

apposition (Fig. 1.2). Continuous passive eruption of the teeth and mesial drifting cause apposition of new layers of cementum at the root apices. As the tooth matures, the apical foramen is reduced in size. Single-rooted teeth usually have a single foramen. However, multi-rooted teeth often contain multiple foramina at each apex (Green 1956, 1960).

Egress of irritants from pathologically involved necrotic pulps via the apical foramen into periapical tissues initiates and perpetuates an inflammatory response and its consequences, such as destruction of apical periodontal ligament and resorption of bone, cementum, and even dentin (Fig. 1.3).

Lateral canals

When the epithelial root sheath breaks down before the root dentin is formed, or the blood vessels that run between the dental papilla and dental sac persist, a direct contact may be established between the periodontal ligament and the dental pulp. This channel of communication is called a lateral or accessory canal. In general, lateral canals occur more frequently in posterior teeth than in anterior teeth and more frequently in the apical portions of roots than in their coronal segments (Hess 1925; Green 1955; Seltzer *et al.*, 1963) (Fig. 1.4). The incidence of lateral canals in the furcation of multi-rooted teeth is reported to be as low as 2 to 3% and as high as 76.8% (Burch & Hulen 1974; De Deus 1975; Vertucci & Anthony 1986). Despite these variations, there is no doubt that a patent lateral canal can contain and carry toxic substances from the root canal system into the periodontium and induce periradicular inflammation.

Dentinal tubules

The dentinal tubules extend from the pulp to the dentinoenamel and cementodentinal junctions. The diameters of these tubules are approximately 2.5 μm near the pulp and about 1 μm at the dentinoenamel and cementodentinal junctions (Garberoglio & Brännström 1976). Although an actual count of the dentinal tubules has not been performed, their numbers are high, with approximately 15,000 dentinal tubules present in a square millimeter of dentin near the cementoenamel junction (Harrington 1979). The dentinal tubules contain tissue fluid,

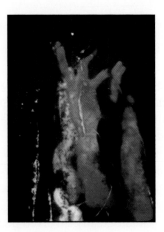

Fig. 1.4 Presence of multiple lateral canals at the end of the mesiobuccal root of a maxillary first molar. Courtesy of Dr. John West.

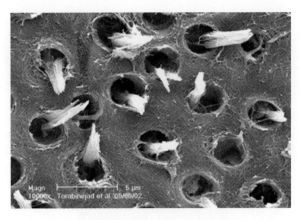

Fig. 1.5   An SEM picture of dentinal tubules containing odontoblastic processes.

odontoblastic processes, and nerve fibers (Fig. 1.5). As the tooth ages or experiences irritation, these tubules tend to reduce in diameter or calcify, thus reducing patency. A continuous layer of cementum on the root surface is an effective barrier for the penetration of bacteria and their byproducts into the root canal system. Congenital absence of cementum, caries, or removal of the cementum during periodontal treatment or vigorous tooth-brushing may result in the opening of numerous patent small channels of communication between the pulp and the periodontium. Theoretically, these tubules could carry the toxic metabolites produced during pulpal or periodontal disease in both directions.

PATHOLOGICAL AND IATROGENIC PATHWAYS

The pathological and iatrogenic pathways of communication between the root canal system and the oral cavity as well as the root canal system and the periodontium include carious pulp exposure, root perforation during access preparation, cleaning and shaping, post preparation and vertical fracture during obturation.

Dental caries

Carious dentin and enamel contain numerous species of bacteria such as *Streptococcus mutans*, lactobacilli, and actinomyces (McKay 1976). The presence of these microbes elicits toxins that penetrate through the dentinal tubules into the pulp. Studies have shown that even small lesions in the enamel are capable

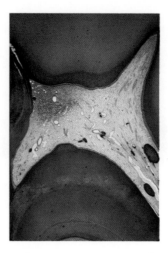

Fig. 1.6 Presence of severe inflammatory response at the site of carious exposure in a human molar.

of attracting inflammatory cells into the pulp tissue (Brännström & Lind 1965; Baume 1970). As a result of the presence of microorganisms and their byproducts in dentin, the pulp tissue is infiltrated locally (at the base of tubules involved in the caries) by chronic inflammatory cells such as macrophages, lymphocytes, and plasma cells. As the decay progresses toward the pulp, the inflammatory process markedly changes in intensity and character (Fig. 1.6). Upon exposure, the pulp is infiltrated predominantly by polymorphonuclear (PMN) leukocytes to form an area of liquefaction necrosis at the site of pulp exposure (Lin & Langeland 1981). Bacteria can colonize in the area of liquefaction necrosis and persist. Pulpal tissue may stay inflamed for long periods before undergoing eventual necrosis, while in other instances the pulp may die quickly. Virulence of bacteria, host resistance, amount of circulation, and most importantly, the amount of drainage play a major role in this process.

Role of microorganisms

As a consequence of pulp exposure to the oral cavity, the root canal system acquires the ability to harbor bacteria and their byproducts. Because of its location, general lack of collateral circulation, and its low compliance (Van Hassel 1971; Heyeraas 1989), the pulp does not have the ability to defend itself against the invading bacteria. Sooner or later the bacterial infection will spread throughout the root canal system and the bacteria and/or bacterial byproducts will diffuse from the root canal into the periradicular tissues with resultant development of a periradicular lesion.

(A)   (B)

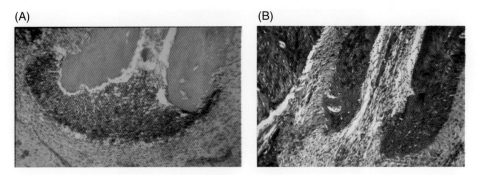

Fig. 1.7 (A) Presence of a periapical lesion in the molar of a rat exposed to bacteria present in its normal micro flora. (B) Absence of pulp and periapical pathosis in a molar of a germ-free rat exposed to its oral cavity. Source: Kakehashi 1965. Reproduced with permission of Elsevier.

To show the importance of bacteria in pathogenesis of pulp and periradicular diseases, Kakehashi *et al.* (1966) exposed the dental pulps of conventional and germ-free rats to their oral flora. Pulpal and periapical lesions were developed in conventional rats. In contrast, they were absent in germ-free rats. (Fig. 1.7). Möller and associates (1981) sealed sterile and contaminated dental pulps in the root canals of monkeys. After 6–7 months, their clinical, radiographic, and histological examinations showed absence of any pathologic changes in the periapical tissues in teeth that had been sealed with sterile amputated pulps. In contrast, teeth sealed with infected pulps had developed inflammatory reactions in their periapical tissues. These studies show the importance of microorganisms in the pathogenesis of pulpal and periapical lesions.

Root perforations

Roots may be perforated during access preparation, cleaning and shaping, or post space preparation.

Root perforations during access preparation

Lateral surface or furcation perforations can occur during access preparations (Fig. 1.8). Lack of attention to the degree of axial inclination of a tooth in relation to its adjacent teeth and failure to parallel the bur with the long axis of a tooth can result in gouging or perforation (see Chapter 7).

Searching for the pulp chamber or the orifices of the root canals through an under-prepared access cavity can also result in accidents. Failing to recognize

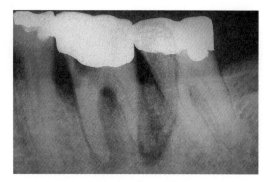

Fig. 1.8   Searching for orifices of the root canals through an under-prepared access cavity can result in lateral root perforation.

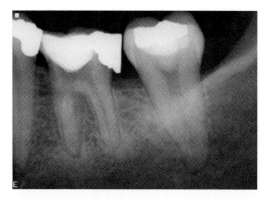

Fig. 1.9   Failure to recognize the depth of bur penetration during an access preparation can cause gouging or furcation perforation.

when the bur passes through a small or flattened calcified pulp chamber in multi-rooted teeth may cause gouging or perforation in the furcation (Fig. 1.9). Furcation perforations can also occur during post space preparation.

Root perforations during cleaning and shaping

Roots may be perforated at different levels during cleaning and shaping. The level of root perforation is critical, that is, whether the perforation is apical, mid-root, or cervical. The level directly affects treatment and prognosis. The further the perforation is from the crestal bone, the better its prognosis. Apical perforations may occur either directly through the apical foramen or through the body of the root itself. Instrumentation of the root canal beyond its anatomic apical foramen results in perforation of the apical foramen. Incorrect working length or inability to maintain proper working length results in apical root perforation.

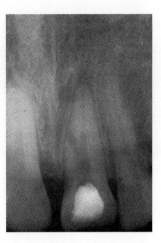

Fig. 1.10 Misdirected pressure and forcing a file during cleaning and shaping can result in a lateral-root perforation.

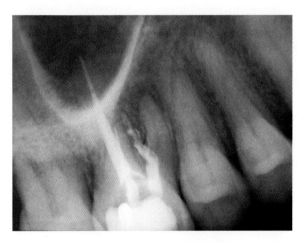

Fig. 1.11 Coronal root perforations can occur by over enlarging canals by files, Gates–Glidden drills, or Peeso reamers. Courtesy of Dr. George Bogen.

Penetration of the last file beyond the radiographic apex is evidence of such a procedural accident. Lateral root perforations are usually a result of the inability of an operator to maintain the curvature of a canal during negotiation of a root canal or after ledge formation. Negotiation of ledged canals is not always possible; misdirected pressure and the forcing of a file may result in the formation of a new canal and eventually a lateral root perforation (Fig. 1.10). Coronal root perforations occur as a result of misdirected burs when the operator is attempting to locate canal orifices. They are also produced by over-enlarging canals by files, Gates-Glidden drills, or Peeso reamers (Fig. 1.11).

Root perforations during post space preparations

Root perforations can occur during post space preparations if the post space is too large or misdirected in the root. Ideally, a post space is a conservative enlargement of the prepared canal space with an optimal length for retention and adequate remaining root canal filling to provide adequate apical seal. The post should be parallel with long access of the root. Its width should not exceed a third of the width of the root and its length should not be more than two-thirds of the working length (Fig. 1.12). Preferably, the preparation should be performed primarily with hand instruments.

Vertical fracture

Although other factors such as post placement and restoration may be co-factors, the principal etiologic factor is associated with root canal treatment procedures (Gher *et al.* 1987). Apparently this results from an overzealous application of condensation forces to obturate an underprepared or over-prepared canal with subsequent vertical root fracture (Holcomb *et al.* 1987). The best means for prevention of vertical root fractures is appropriate canal preparation as well as use of balanced pressure during obturation.

Radiographically, a frank root fracture (Fig. 1.13) or lack of sharp demarcation between an irregular and poorly condensed filling material and the dentinal walls also indicates presence of a vertical root fracture. Long-standing vertical

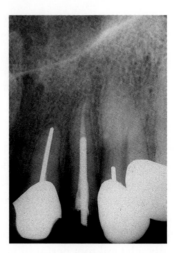

Fig. 1.12 An ideal post should be parallel with the long access of the root, its width should not exceed a third of the width of the root and its length should not be more than two thirds of the working length.

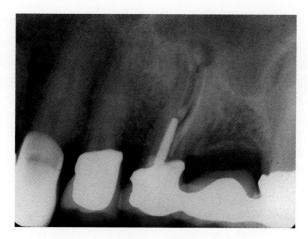

Fig. 1.13   A frank vertical root fracture is usually associated with a narrow periodontal pocket and/or sinus tract stoma and a lateral radiolucency extending to the apical portion of the root.

root fractures often are associated with a narrow periodontal pocket and/or sinus tract stoma and a lateral radiolucency extending to the apical portion of the vertical fracture.

PERIRADICULAR PATHOSIS

In contrast to pulp tissue, periradicular tissues (periodontal ligament and bone) have an almost unlimited source of undifferentiated cells that can participate in the process of inflammation as well as repair. In addition, the periradicular tissues have rich collateral blood supply and lymph drainage. These characteristics enable the periradicular tissues to combat the destructive factors related to the irritants from the root canal system.

Inflammatory process of periradicular lesions

Depending on the severity of irritation, its duration, and host response, periradicular pathosis of pulpal or iatrogenic origin can range from slight inflammation to extensive tissue destruction. Injury to periradicular tissues usually results in cellular damage and the release of nonspecific as well as specific immunologic mediators of inflammatory reactions (Torabinejad *et al.* 1985) (Fig. 1.14). Physical or chemical injury to the periradicular tissues during root canal therapy can cause a release of vasoactive amines such as histamine, activation of the Hageman factor, activation of the kinin system, the clotting cascade, the

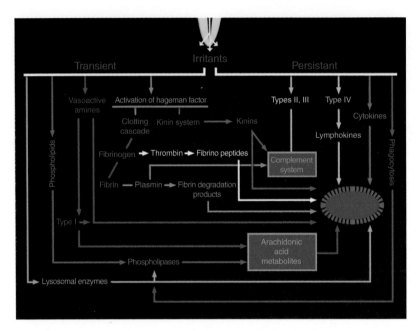

Fig. 1.14 Egress of irritants from an infected root canal into periapical tissues can result in activation of nonspecific as well as specific immunologic mediators of inflammatory reactions.

fibrinolytic system, and the complement system with its release of C3 complement fragments in human periradicular lesions (Pulver *et al.* 1978). Release of these factors can contribute to the inflammatory process in the periradicular tissues and cause inflammation, swelling, pain, and tissue destruction. Inhibition of formation of periapical lesions by systemic administration of indomethacin in cats shows the importance of another group of nonspecific mediators of inflammation (the arachidonic acid metabolites) in the pathogenesis of periradicular lesions (Torabinejad *et al.* 1979).

In addition to the mediators of nonspecific inflammatory reactions, immunologic reactions can also participate in the formation and perpetuation of periapical lesions (Fig. 1.14). Presence of various immunologic *factors* (i.e., antigens, immunoglobulin E (IgE), mast cells in pathologically involved dental pulps and periapical lesions) indicates that a type I immunologic reaction can occur in periapical tissues. Various *classes* of immunoglobulins and different types of immunocompetent cells, such as PMN leukocytes, macrophages, B and T cells, C3 complement fragments, and immune complexes, have been found in human periapical lesions (Torabinejad & Kettering 1985). Presence of these components in periapical lesions indicates that types II, III, and IV immunologic reactions can also participate in the genesis of these lesions.

MATERIALS TO SEAL THE PATHWAYS TO THE ROOT CANAL SYSTEM AND THE PERIODONTIUM

Numerous materials have been suggested to seal off the communication between the root canal system and external surfaces of the tooth. They include: gutta-percha, amalgam, polycarboxylate cements, zinc phosphate cements, zinc oxide eugenol paste, IRM cement, EBA cement, Cavit, glass ionomers, composite resins, and other materials such as gold foil and leaf, silver points, cyanoacrylates, polyHEMA and hydron, Diaket root canal sealer, titanium screws, and Teflon. For years, existing materials did not possess the "ideal" characteristics of a repair material, and therefore an experimental material, mineral trioxide aggregate (MTA), was developed in 1993.

In a series of tests, Torabinejad and associates investigated *in vitro* dye leakage with and without blood contamination, *in vitro* bacterial leakage, scanning electron microscope (SEM) examination of replicas for marginal adaptation, setting time, compressive strength, solubility, cytotoxicity, implantation in bone, and a usage test in animals (Torabinejad *et al.* 1993; Higa *et al.* 1994; Pitt Ford *et al.* 1995; Torabinejad *et al.* 1995a, b, c, d, e, f, g; Tang *et al.* 2001). Existing materials, such as amalgam, Intermediate Restorative material (IRM), or SuperEBA (*O*-ethoxybenzoic acid) were used for comparison. The sealing ability of MTA was superior to that of amalgam and SuperEBA in both dye, bacterial, and endotoxin leakage methods and was not adversely affected by blood contamination (Torabinejad *et al.* 1993, 1995a; Higa *et al.* 1994; Tang *et al.* 2001). The marginal adaptation of MTA was better than that of amalgam, IRM, and SuperEBA (Torabinejad *et al.* 1995 g). The setting time of MTA was found to be less than three hours, which is much longer than that of amalgam and IRM. Compressive strength and solubility of MTA were similar to that of IRM and SuperEBA, respectively (Torabinejad *et al.* 1995c). It also has some antibacterial effects on some of the bacterial species in the oral cavity (Torabinejad *et al.* 1995e).

The cytotoxicity of MTA was investigated by two methods, agar overlay and radiochromium release. MTA was ranked less cytotoxic than IRM and SuperEBA, but more cytotoxic than amalgam in the agar overlay method. It was found to be less cytotoxic than amalgam, IRM, and SuperEBA when the radiochromium release method was used (Torabinejad *et al.* 1995f). With implantation of materials in guinea pig mandibles and tibias, MTA was more biocompatible than other test materials (Torabinejad *et al.* 1995d). Root-end fillings or furcation perforations repaired with MTA or amalgam placed in the teeth of dogs and root-end filling in monkeys were examined histologically (Pitt Ford *et al.* 1995; Torabinejad *et al.* 1995b, 1997). There was less inflammation around the root ends filled with MTA, with the evidence of healing in the surrounding tissues. In

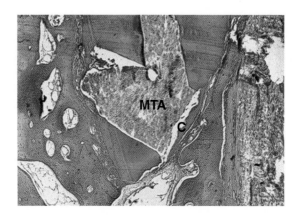

Fig. 1.15 Cementum (C) formation was found on the surface MTA when it was used as a root-end filling in dogs.

addition, with the longer-term teeth filled with MTA new cementum was found on the surface of the material when used as a root-end filling or furcation perforation material; this was not the case with amalgam (Fig. 1.15). Based on these studies, it appears that MTA is an alternative material to be used for root-end fillings.

Since its introduction, numerous studies have been published regarding various aspects of this material. Parirokh and Torabinejad (2010a) conducted a search (electronically and manually) of the literature regarding the chemical and physical properties and antibacterial activity of MTA from November 1993 to September 2009. Their search showed that there are many published reports regarding the properties of MTA and a material composed of calcium, silica, and bismuth. It has a long setting time, high pH, and low compressive strength. It possesses some antibacterial and antifungal properties depending on its powder-to-liquid ratio. Based on their search, they concluded that MTA is a bioactive material that influences its surrounding environment. In the second part of their review, Torabinejad and Parirokh (2010) conducted a comprehensive literature search using electronic and manual methods for the sealing ability and biocompatibility of MTA from November 1993 to September 2009. Their review showed the presence of numerous studies regarding these properties of MTA. Based on the available evidence, they concluded that MTA seals well and is a biocompatible material. In the third part of their literature review Parirokh and Torabinejad (2010b) conducted a comprehensive review of the literature regarding the clinical applications of MTA in experimental animals and humans, as well as its drawbacks and mechanism of action from November 1993 to September 2009. Their search of the literature shows that MTA is a promising material for root-end filling, perforation repair, vital pulp therapy, and apical barrier formation for teeth with necrotic pulps and open apices. Furthermore, they reported that MTA has some known drawbacks such as a long setting time, high cost, and potential for discoloration. Regarding its mode of action, it appears that hydroxyapatite crystals form over MTA when it comes in contact with tissue synthetic fluid. This can act as a nidus for the formation of calcified structures, following the use of this material in endodontic treatments.

Based on the available information, they concluded that MTA is the material of choice for sealing the pathways of communication between the root canal system and its external surfaces.

REFERENCES

Baume, L.J. (1970) Dental pulp conditions in relation to carious lesions. *International Dental Journal* **20**, 309–37.

Brännström, M., Lind, P.O. (1965) Pulpal response to early dental caries. *Journal of Dental Research* **44**, 1045–50.

Burch, J.G., Hulen, S. (1974) A study of the presence of accessory foramina and the topography of molar furcations. *Oral Surgery, Oral Medicine, Oral Pathology* **38**, 451–5.

De Deus, Q.D. (1975) Frequency, location, and direction of the lateral, secondary, and accessory canals. *Journal of Endodontics* **1**, 361–6.

Garberoglio, R., Brännström, M. (1976) Scanning electron microscopic investigation of human dentinal tubules. *Archives of Oral Biology* **21**, 355–62.

Gher, M.E. Jr, Dunlap, R.M., Anderson, M.H., *et al.* (1987) Clinical survey of fractured teeth. *Journal of the American Dental Association* **114**, 174–7.

Green, D. (1955) Morphology of the pulp cavity of the permanent teeth. *Oral Surgery, Oral Medicine, Oral Pathology* **8**, 743–59.

Green, D. (1956) A stereomicroscopic study of the root apices of 400 maxillary and mandibular anterior teeth. *Oral Surgery, Oral Medicine, Oral Pathology* **9**, 1224–32.

Green, D. (1960) Stereomicroscopic study of 700 root apices of maxillary and mandibular posterior teeth. *Oral Surgery, Oral Medicine, Oral Pathology* **13**, 728–33.

Harrington, G.W. (1979) The perio-endo question: differential diagnosis. *Dental Clinics of North America* **23**, 673–90.

Hess, W. (1925) *The Anatomy of the Root-Canals of the Teeth of the Permanent Dentition.* John Bale Sons, and Danielsson, Ltd, London.

Heyeraas, K.J. (1989) Pulpal hemodynamics and interstitial fluid pressure: balance of transmicrovascular fluid transport. *Journal of Endodontics* **15**, 468–72.

Higa, R.K., Torabinejad, M., McKendry, D.J., *et al.* (1994) The effect of storage time on the degree of dye leakage of root-end filling materials. *International Endodontics Journal* **27**, 252–56.

Holcomb, J.Q., Pitts, D.L., Nicholls, J.I. (1987) Further investigation of spreader loads required to cause vertical root fracture during lateral condensation. *Journal of Endodontics* **13**, 277–84.

Kakehashi, S., Stanley, H.R., Fitzgerald, R.J. (1965) The effects of surgical exposures of dental pulps in germfree and conventional laboratory rats. *Oral Surgery, Oral Medicine, Oral Pathology* **20**, 340.

Lin, L., Langeland, K. (1981) Light and electron microscopic study of teeth with carious pulp exposures. *Oral Surgery, Oral Medicine, Oral Pathology* **51**, 292–316.

McKay, G.S. (1976) The histology and microbiology of acute occlusal dentine lesions in human permanent molar teeth. *Archives of Oral Biology* **21**, 51–8.

Möller, A.J., Fabricius, L., Dahlén, G., *et al.* (1981) Influence on periapical tissues of indigenous oral bacteria and necrotic pulp tissue in monkeys. *Scandinavian Journal of Dental Research* **89**, 475–84.

Parirokh, M., Torabinejad, M. (2010a) Mineral trioxide aggregate: a comprehensive literature review – Part I: chemical, physical, and antibacterial properties. *Journal of Endodontics* **36**(1), 16–27.

Parirokh, M., Torabinejad, M. (2010b) Mineral trioxide aggregate: a comprehensive literature review – Part III: Clinical applications, drawbacks, and mechanism of action. *Journal of Endodontics* **36**(3), 400–13.

Pitt Ford, T.R., Torabinejad, M., Hong, C.U., *et al.* (1995) Use of mineral trioxide aggregate for repair of furcal perforations. *Oral Surgery* **79**, 756–63.

Pulver, W.H., Taubman, M.A., Smith, D.J. (1978) Immune components in human dental periapical lesions. *Archives of Oral Biology* **23**, 435–43.

Seltzer, S., Bender, I.B., Ziontz, M. (1963) The interrelationship of pulp and periodontal disease. *Oral Surgery, Oral Medicine, Oral Pathology* **16**, 1474–90.

Tang, H.M., Torabinejad, M., Kettering, J.D. (2001) Leakage evaluation of root end filling materials using endotoxin. *Journal of Endodontics* **28**(1), 5–7.

Torabinejad, M., Kettering, J.D. (1985) Identification and relative concentration of B and T lymphocytes in human chronic periapical lesions. *Journal of Endodontics* **11**, 122–5.

Torabinejad, M., Parirokh, M. (2010) Mineral trioxide aggregate: a comprehensive literature review – part II: leakage and biocompatibility investigations. *Journal of Endodontics* **36**(2), 190–202.

Torabinejad, M., Clagett, J., Engel, D. (1979) A cat model for the evaluation of mechanisms of bone resorption: induction of bone loss by simulated immune complexes and inhibition by indomethacin. *Calcified Tissue International* **29**, 207–14.

Torabinejad, M., Eby, W.C., Naidorf, I.J. (1985) Inflammatory and immunological aspects of the pathogenesis of human periapical lesions. *Journal of Endodontics* **11**, 479–88.

Torabinejad, M., Watson, T.F., Pitt Ford, T.R. (1993) The sealing ability of a mineral trioxide aggregate as a retrograde root filling material. *Journal of Endodontics* **19**, 591–5.

Torabinejad, M., Falah, R., Kettering, J.D., *et al.* (1995a) Bacterial leakage of mineral trioxide aggregate as a root end filling material. *Journal of Endodontics* **21**, 109–21.

Torabinejad, M., Hong, C.U., Lee, S.J., *et al.* (1995b) Investigation of mineral trioxide aggregate for root end filling in dogs. *Journal of Endodontics* **21**, 603–8.

Torabinejad, M., Hong, C.U., Pitt Ford, T.R. (1995c) Physical properties of a new root end filling material. *Journal of Endodontics* **21**, 349–53.

Torabinejad, M., Hong, C.U., Pitt Ford, T.R. (1995d) Tissue reaction to implanted SuperEBA and mineral trioxide aggregate in the mandibles of guinea pigs: A preliminary report. *Journal of Endodontics* **21**, 569–71.

Torabinejad, M., Hong, C.U., Pitt Ford, T.R., *et al.* (1995e) Antibacterial effects of some root end filling materials. *Journal of Endodontics* **21**, 403–6.

Torabinejad, M., Hong, C.U., Pitt Ford, T.R., *et al.* (1995f) Cytotoxicity of four root end filling materials. *Journal of Endodontics* **21**, 489–92.

Torabinejad, M., Wilder Smith, P., Pitt Ford, T.R. (1995g) Comparative investigation of marginal adaptation of mineral trioxide aggregate and other commonly used root end filling materials. *Journal of Endodontics* **21**, 295–99.

Torabinejad, M., Pitt Ford, T.R., McKendry, D.J., *et al.* (1997) Histologic assessment of MTA as root end filling in monkeys. *Journal of Endodontics* **23**, 225–28.

Van Hassel, H.J. (1971) Physiology of the human dental pulp. *Oral Surgery, Oral Medicine, Oral Pathology* **32**, 126–34.

Vertucci, F.J., Anthony, R.L. (1986) A scanning electron microscopic investigation of accessory foramina in the furcation and pulp chamber floor of molar teeth. *Oral Surgery, Oral Medicine, Oral Pathology* **62**, 319–26.

2 Chemical Properties of MTA

David W. Berzins

General Dental Sciences, Marquette University, USA

INTRODUCTION

Mineral trioxide aggregate (MTA) was first described in the scientific literature in 1993 (Lee *et al.* 1993) as an aggregate of mineral oxides added to "trioxides" of tricalcium silicate, tricalcium aluminate, and tricalcium oxide silicate oxide.

Mineral Trioxide Aggregate: Properties and Clinical Applications, First Edition.
Edited by Mahmoud Torabinejad.
© 2014 John Wiley & Sons, Inc. Published 2014 by John Wiley & Sons, Inc.

The initial patent (United States Patent #5,415,547, continued to #5,769,638) on what would become known as MTA was filed the preceding April by Mahmoud Torabinejad and Dean White, and described the tooth filling material as being comprised of Portland cement. In 1997, Tulsa Dental Products (now Dentsply Tulsa Dental Specialties) received a decision from the US Food and Drug Administration (FDA) that MTA was substantially equivalent in intended use and technological characteristics to similar products on the market for repairing pulpal tissues. With its designation as a Class II medical device for root canal filling from the FDA, MTA was subsequently marketed as ProRoot MTA. The commercial product was first available as a gray variety, and a tooth-colored version commonly referred to as "white MTA" was introduced in 2002 (Figs 2.1 and 2.2). Since the first research reports, further studies, numbering in the hundreds, were conducted on the initial experimental cement and the commercial ProRoot MTA products (as well as individual constituents and/or similar products). Despite some differences between the experimental and commercial materials, except when noted, no delineation will be made in this chapter between the varieties of MTA.

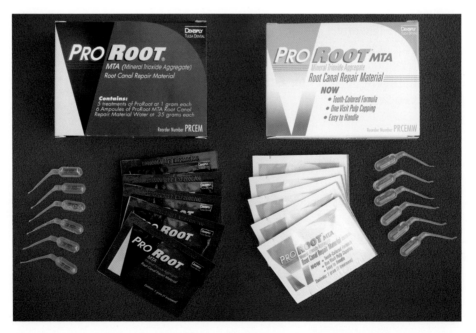

Fig. 2.1 Gray and tooth-colored ProRoot MTA. Courtesy of James Brozek.

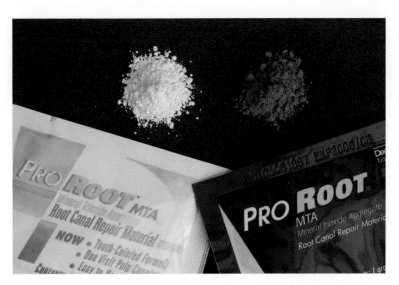

Fig. 2.2   Gray and white ProRoot MTA powder. Courtesy of James Brozek.

MTA COMPOSITION

As stated in the patent, MTA is comprised primarily of Portland cement. The Material Safety Data Sheet (MSDS) of ProRoot MTA states that it is approximately 75 wt% Portland cement, 20 wt% bismuth oxide (Bi_2O_3), and 5 wt% calcium sulfate dihydrate or gypsum ($CaSO_4 \cdot 2H_2O$). Additional minor trace elements may also be present as stated in the MSDS.

Portland cement

The origins of Portland cement date back to the early to mid-1800s in Britain where the Aspdin family was involved in its development. Its name is derived from its similarity to a type of limestone quarried on the Isle of Portland in the county of Dorset in southwest England. Today, it is a very common hydraulic cement due to its inclusion in concrete, stucco, and mortar. The ASTM International (formerly the American Society for Testing and Materials) recognizes 10 types of Portland cement (ASTM Standard C150/C150M – 12 2012), but the Portland cement in MTA is restricted to Type I Portland cement. From ASTM C150/C150M, it is apparent that a strict, fixed composition for Portland cement is not set and a range of constituent component concentrations is tolerable. Additionally, variability in raw sources and manufacturing processes among different cement producers is to be expected; therefore, interpretation of research reports that compare MTA to Portland cement should be mindful of this.

Ordinary Portland cement is manufactured by first obtaining the raw materials (typically limestone or calcium carbonate, clay, and/or other materials), crushing the individual raw materials to acquire a smaller particle size, and proportioning them to create a specific composition. Next, the mixture is ground and blended together and introduced into a rotary, cylindrical kiln where it is heated to 1430–1650 °C. This fuses the materials together after a series of reactions which include evaporation of water, dehydration of the clays, and decarbonation of the calcium carbonate (loss of carbon dioxide to yield calcium oxide). At this point, the mixture is called clinker. Once the clinker cools, it is ground to a fine powder size and is now considered Portland cement.

The Portland cement component in MTA consists of tricalcium silicate ($3CaO \cdot SiO_2$ or Ca_3SiO_5, also known as alite), dicalcium silicate ($2CaO \cdot SiO_2$ or Ca_2SiO_4, also known as belite), and tricalcium aluminate ($3CaO \cdot Al_2O_3$ or $Ca_3Al_2O_6$). Less of the latter component is contained in white MTA versus gray MTA, but it is still present (Asgary *et al.* 2005). Tetracalcium aluminoferrite ($4CaO \cdot Al_2O_3 \cdot Fe_2O_3$), on the other hand, is considered present in gray MTA but not in white MTA. Alternatively, the Portland cement fraction in MTA may also be thought of as mixtures of CaO (lime), SiO_2 (silica), and Al_2O_3 (alumina) – as well as Fe_2O_3 (iron oxide) for gray MTA. In a typical Portland cement powder, tricalcium silicate and dicalcium silicate are in greatest proportion and are estimated to be roughly 75–80% of the cement, with tricalcium aluminate and tetracalcium aluminoferrite at approximately 10% each (Ramachandran *et al.* 2003). However, MTA has lower amounts of tricalcium aluminate compared with ordinary Portland cement, and it has been determined that the content of Ca_3SiO_5, Ca_2SiO_4, $Ca_3Al_2O_6$, $CaSO_4$, and Bi_2O_3 in white MTA is 51.9, 23.2, 3.8, 1.3, and 19.8 wt%, respectively (Belío-Reyes *et al.* 2009). This leads to the suggestion that MTA powder is not produced in a kiln but in a laboratory (Camilleri 2007, 2008), although others have said it is manufactured the same way as Portland cement (Darvell & Wu 2011). Alternatively, the amounts of CaO, SiO_2, Al_2O_3, and Fe_2O_3 may be considered to be approximately 50–75, 15–25, <2, and 0–0.5 wt%, respectively (Darvell & Wu 2011).

Role of bismuth oxide and gypsum

Bismuth oxide is included in MTA to serve as a radiopaque agent because Portland cement is not sufficiently radiopaque for dental purposes. Although generally considered insoluble in water, speculation exists that it is not totally inert and plays a limited role in the setting of MTA as some bismuth oxide has been shown to form part of the calcium silicate hydrate structure (described below) and leach out over time (Camilleri 2007, 2008). However, others debate this (Darvell & Wu 2011). Regardless, it appears that the addition of bismuth oxide to Portland cement decreases its compressive strength and increases porosity (Coomaraswamy *et al.* 2007), suggesting that bismuth oxide has effects other than radiopacity as well.

Gypsum is added to Portland cement/MTA to alter the setting time and does so primarily by influencing the reactions of the tricalcium aluminate. Some conflicting reports exist as to whether it is truly calcium sulfate dihydrate in MTA, with other possibilities being calcium sulfate hemihydrate ($CaSO_4 \cdot \frac{1}{2}H_2O$) or the anhydrous form ($CaSO_4$) (Camilleri 2007, 2008; Belío-Reyes *et al.* 2009; Gandolfi *et al.* 2010b; Darvell & Wu 2011). Comparatively, ordinary Portland cement contains approximately double the amount of calcium sulfate species as found in MTA.

MTA powder morphology

The size and shape of the powder fraction of MTA has been examined by several researchers (Fig. 2.3). The size of Portland cement particles in the powder of white MTA generally range from <1 μm to 30–50 μm, and the bismuth oxide particles are approximately 10–30 μm (Camilleri 2007). Between MTA products, it appears the particles are more homogeneously sized in white MTA compared with gray MTA (Komabayashi & Spångberg 2008) and have fewer larger particles (Camilleri *et al.* 2005), which may explain the better handling properties of white versus gray MTA. In terms of shape, many of the particles are rather irregular, with some appearing needle-like (Camilleri *et al.* 2005). As mentioned above, comparison to ordinary Portland cement is problematic due to variations in Portland cement commercial products, but using microscopy, Dammaschke and associates observed white MTA powder to have a more uniform and smaller particle size compared with Portland cement powder (Fig. 2.4) (Dammaschke *et al.* 2005), but few differences have been noted as to the shape of particles between MTA and Portland cement (Komabayashi & Spångberg 2008). As would stand to reason, if the initial powder particles in MTA are smaller than those in Portland cement, the particles contained in set (hydrated) MTA are, similarly, smaller than in ordinary Portland cement (Asgary *et al.* 2004). This also holds true for white MTA versus gray MTA (Asgary *et al.* 2005, 2006). Overall, the Portland cement fraction of MTA appears to be more refined than industrial ordinary Portland cement.

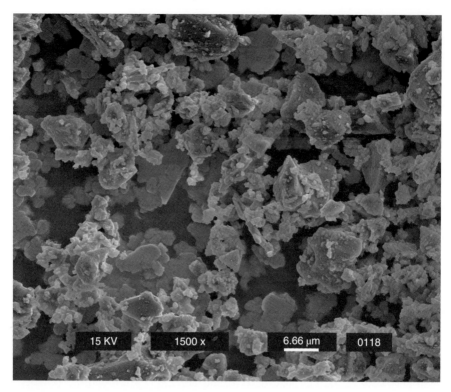

Fig. 2.3 Scanning electron micrograph of MTA powder. Source: Lee *et al.* 2004. Reproduced with permission of Elsevier.

(A)   (B)

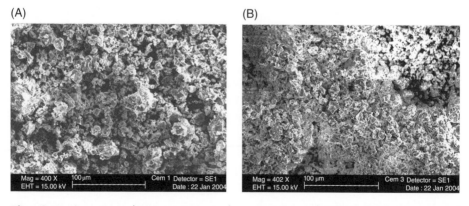

Fig. 2.4 Scanning electron micrograph comparison of (A) Portland cement and (B) MTA powders. Source: Dammaschke *et al.* 2005. Reproduced with permission of Elsevier.

Trace elements and compounds

Several researchers have noted the absence of iron in white MTA in contrast to its presence in gray MTA (Camilleri *et al.* 2005; Song *et al.* 2006). However, others have observed trace amounts of iron in white MTA (Belío-Reyes *et al.* 2009). Additionally, magnesium (or a magnesium oxide form) is also frequently observed in greater proportion in gray MTA than in white MTA (Song *et al.* 2006), and also accounts for some of the color difference. Other elements and compounds observed in MTA have been: As, Ba, Cd, Cl, Cr, Cu, Ga, In, K, Li, Mn, Mo, Ni, P_2O_5, Pb, Sr, TiO_2, Tl, V, and Zn (Funteas *et al.* 2003; Dammaschke *et al.* 2005; Monteiro Bramante *et al.* 2008; Comin-Chiaramonti *et al.* 2009; Chang *et al.* 2010; Schembri *et al.* 2010). While some of these elements would generally be of concern from a toxicological point of view, given their low concentration in MTA and MTA's excellent biocompatibility, they likely have no impact on health. Although calcium hydroxide is a reaction product, as mentioned below, some does appear in MTA powder, possibly due to reaction with ambient humidity (Camilleri 2008; Chedella & Berzins 2010). Compared with Portland cement, MTA typically has less heavy metal content (Cu, Mn, Sr) (Dammaschke *et al.* 2005) but greater amounts of bismuth (as Bi_2O_3 for radiopacity), and, therefore, its Portland cement component is of purer form. Although it has been debated in the literature whether a clinician could use Portland cement in place of MTA due to its general similarities, it should be pointed out again that MTA is approved for use in patients by the FDA and is sterilized. Thus, substituting Portland cement for MTA is not advised in clinical procedures.

SETTING REACTIONS

MTA is a hydraulic type of cement, meaning that it sets by reacting with water, and is then stable in water. When mixed with water, it forms via an exothermic reaction. The setting reactions in MTA are approximated to be similar to those in Portland cement, which are best studied by analyzing the hydration of its individual components. The two most important hydration reactions are those of the greatest constituents, tricalcium silicate and dicalcium silicate. Tricalcium silicate sets via the following reaction (Bhatty 1991; Ramachandran *et al.* 2003):

$$2(3CaO \cdot SiO_2) + 6H_2O \rightarrow 3CaO \cdot 2SiO_2 \cdot 3H_2O + 3Ca(OH)_2$$

The setting of dicalcium silicate is similarly given by the following reaction (Bhatty 1991; Ramachandran *et al.* 2003):

$$2(2CaO \cdot SiO_2) + 4H_2O \rightarrow 3CaO \cdot 2SiO_2 \cdot 3H_2O + Ca(OH)_2$$

The principal products are calcium silicate hydrates and calcium hydroxide (also known as Portlandite). While the calcium hydroxide is mostly crystalline and able to be detected using X-ray diffraction (XRD; Camilleri 2008), the calcium silicate hydrates are primarily amorphous and may exhibit a range of compositions. Thus, water is both a reactant and is contained in the reaction products of MTA. This is important for understanding the effects of water on properties as discussed below. The calcium silicate hydrate may be considered a gel that forms on the calcium silicate particles and hardens with time to form a solid network with the calcium hydroxide nucleated within the pore and void space (Gandolfi *et al.* 2010b). The amount of calcium hydroxide produced in MTA has been found to be approximately 10–15% of the hydrated material (Camilleri 2008; Chedella & Berzins 2010), which is below that expected for Portland cement (20–25%; Ramachandran *et al.* 2003). Furthermore, exposure of the calcium hydroxide to carbon dioxide contained in physiological fluids is expected to convert some of it to calcium carbonate (Chedella & Berzins 2010; Darvell & Wu 2011).

The hydration reactions of the two minor components of Portland cement are influenced by gypsum. In the presence of gypsum and water, tricalcium aluminate forms ettringite $[Ca_6(AlO_3)_2(SO_4)_3 \cdot 32H_2O]$ according to the following reaction:

$$Ca_3(AlO_3)_2 + 3CaSO_4 + 32H_2O \rightarrow Ca_6(AlO_3)_2(SO_4)_3 \cdot 32H_2O$$

Ettringite has been observed as small needle-like crystals in set MTA (Gandolfi *et al.* 2010a). After all of the gypsum is consumed, the tricalcium aluminate reacts with ettringite to form monosulfates according to the following reaction (Bhatty 1991; Ramachandran *et al.* 2003):

$$Ca_6(AlO_3)_2(SO_4)_3 \cdot 32H_2O + Ca_3(AlO_3)_2 + 4H_2O \rightarrow 3Ca_4(AlO_3)_{22}(SO_4) \cdot 12H_2O$$

Without gypsum, the tricalcium aluminate may form hexagonal and/or cubic calcium aluminate hydrates ($4CaO \cdot Al_2O_3 \cdot 13H_2O$ and $3CaO \cdot Al_2O_3 \cdot 6H_2O$, respectively). These aluminates may also appear intermediate to the formation of ettringite when gypsum is present. Finally, tetracalcium aluminoferrite hydration in the presence of gypsum is given by the following reaction (Bhatty 1991; Ramachandran *et al.* 2003):

$$2Ca_2AlFeO_5 + CaSO_4 + 16H_2O \rightarrow Ca_4(AlO_3/FeO_3)_2(SO_4) \cdot$$
$$12H_2O + 2Al/Fe(OH)_3$$

(A)

(B)

(C)

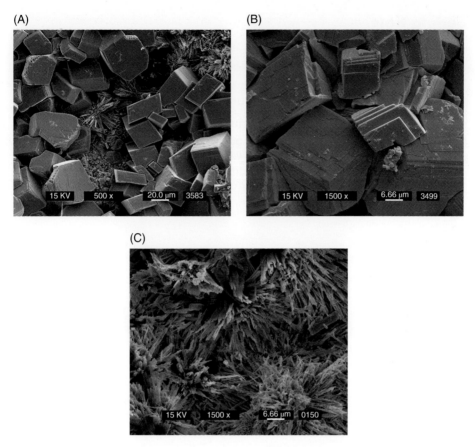

Fig. 2.5 Scanning electron micrograph of set MTA showing different reaction particle morphologies (A). Higher magnification of cubic (B) and needle-like (C) particles. Source: Lee *et al.* 2004. Reproduced with permission of Elsevier.

Of the three main reactants, it is considered that the calcium aluminate phase would react first, followed by the tricalcium silicate and then dicalcium silicate phases. Although multiple analytical techniques generally support that the above setting reactions do indeed occur in MTA, it should be realized that MTA is a mixture of these components and, therefore, complex interactions between them are possible, as is influence from minor constituents. Furthermore, not all powder particles may be fully reacted as some calcium silicate powder phases are still present at seven (Lee *et al.* 2004) and 30 days (Camilleri 2008) and have been observed in set MTA with microscopy (Camilleri 2007). Figure 2.5 displays scanning electron micrographs of set MTA.

Setting time

Directions for use of MTA specify a working time of 5 minutes and state that it will "set over a period of 4 hours". Alternatively, the setting time of MTA has been quoted by different researchers as 165 minutes (Torabinejad *et al*. 1995), 45–140 minutes for initial and final setting (Chng *et al*. 2005), 40–140 minutes for initial and final setting (Islam *et al*. 2006), 50 minutes (Kogan *et al*. 2006), 220–250 minutes (Ding *et al*. 2008), 151 minutes (Huang *et al*. 2008), and 150 minutes (Porter *et al*. 2010). The variations in setting time may be ascribed to the different experimental methods used for determination, as they involve penetration of the cement by needles of various dimension and/or weight.

Maturation

Like other dental materials such as glass ionomers and amalgam, MTA continues to mature over time. Although determined to be "set" by rudimentary measures as mentioned above, calorimetric data has shown maximum development of calcium hydroxide at 7 days (Chedella & Berzins 2010) and continued refinement of the amorphous calcium silicate hydrates for longer periods. Similarly, several researchers have observed temporal developments in strength indicative of continued reaction. Sluyk and associates observed a significant increase in furcal repair strength at 72 hours from 24 hours (Sluyk *et al*. 1998). VanderWeele and associates found progressively greater resistance to displacement of furcal repairs from 24 hours to 72 hours and then 7 days (VanderWeele *et al*. 2006). Torabinejad and associates found the compressive strength of MTA to increase from 40 MPa at 24 hours to 67 MPa at 21 days (Torabinejad *et al*. 1995).

Factors that affect setting: additives and accelerants

Various additives have been suggested to improve the handling properties and long setting time of MTA. Among the additives that have been mixed with MTA (or Portland cement and similar products) have been calcium chloride ($CaCl_2$), sodium hypochlorite (NaOCl), chlorhexidine gluconate, K-Y jelly, lidocaine HCl, saline, calcium lactate gluconate, sodium fluorosilicate (Na_2SiF_6), disodium hydrogen orthophosphate (Na_2HPO_4), sodium fluoride (NaF), strontium chloride ($SrCl_2$), hydroxyapatite [$Ca_{10}(PO_4)_6(OH)_2$], tricalcium phosphate [$Ca_3(PO_4)_2$], citric acid ($C_6H_8O_7$), calcium formate, calcium nitrite/nitrate, methylcellulose, methylhydroxyethyl cellulose, and water-soluble polymers (Ridi *et al*. 2005; Bortoluzzi *et al*. 2006a, b, 2009; Kogan *et al*. 2006; Ber *et al*. 2007; Wiltbank *et al*. 2007; Ding *et al*. 2008; Hong *et al*. 2008; Huang *et al*. 2008; Camilleri, 2009; Gandolfi *et al*. 2009; Hsieh *et al*. 2009; AlAnezi *et al*. 2011;

Ji *et al.* 2011; Lee *et al.* 2011; Appelbaum *et al.* 2012). While many additives were successful in improving setting time, handling properties, or other properties, their clinical and bioactive equivalence has largely been undemonstrated. Thus, caution is advised when selecting material preparations other than the original MTA until equivalence has been demonstrated.

Effect of water and moisture

Being a hydraulic cement, water/moisture is a critical component for the setting of MTA and also for establishing optimal properties. However, deficient or excessive moisture will affect setting and properties in a detrimental way. Excess moisture may cause increased porosity and washout of the MTA during setting or cause material degradation with a decrease in strength in set MTA (Walker *et al.* 2006). On the other hand, although water is used during mixing, it should be realized that moisture from the tooth or surrounding tissues may aid the setting of MTA in clinical applications. For instance, even dry MTA powder packed into a canal may eventually set if given enough time for moisture to diffuse through cementum or travel through accessory canals (Budig & Eleazer 2008). Nevertheless, MTA in a relatively dry environment does not perform as well as MTA in a relatively moist environment (Gancedo-Caravia & Garcia-Barbero 2006). Availability of water will also dictate other properties such as expansion, where the primary mechanism is via water sorption prior to setting (Gandolfi *et al.* 2009).

Interaction with environment

In various clinical applications, MTA may encounter different physiological fluids as well as those introduced during endodontic procedures. Whether during setting or after setting, these solutions may impact the chemistry and properties of MTA.

During setting, exposure of MTA to acidic environments, like those possible in inflamed pulpal or periapical tissues, will affect reaction product development. Lee and associates observed a reduction of calcium hydroxide formation when MTA (two minutes after mixing) was exposed to a pH 5 solution (Lee *et al.* 2004). Furthermore, surface dissolution of reaction product particles was evident, leading to weakening of the material manifested as reduced microhardness. This was also supported by another study (Namazikhah *et al.* 2008). Others, however, found no difference in compressive strength when MTA was mixed with water and exposed to phosphate-buffered saline (PBS) at pH 5.0 or 7.4 (Watts *et al.* 2007). Exposure to serum has also been shown to detrimentally affect the setting of MTA as displayed by a difference in surface morphology and chemical distribution (Tingey *et al.* 2008) as well as hardness (Kang *et al.* 2012; Kim *et al.* 2012). Furcal perforations repaired with MTA contaminated with blood have been shown to have less resistance than noncontaminated MTA repairs (VanderWeele *et al.* 2006), and MTA exposed to blood has compromised compressive strength (Nekoofar *et al.* 2010) and microhardness (Nekoofar *et al.* 2011).

Similarly, during setting, exposure of MTA to calcium-chelating agents such as ethylenediaminetetraacetic acid (EDTA) irrigating solution is especially problematic for MTA, which again contains roughly 50–75 wt% calcium oxide. As outlined above, the setting of the calcium silicates relies on dissolution in water followed by precipitation of the reaction products. The EDTA irrigating solution effectively chelates the released calcium. Therefore, disrupts the hydration of MTA with no formation of calcium hydroxide (Lee *et al.* 2007) and hinders formation of the calcium silicate hydrates. In terms of properties, MTA exposed to irrigating solutions (sodium hypochlorite, chlorhexidine gluconate, EDTA, and BioPure MTAD) during setting exhibits lower microhardness and flexural strength after seven days than when it sets in distilled water (Aggarwal *et al.* 2011). Of these, EDTA and BioPure MTAD had the greatest detrimental effect; the latter is both acidic (pH 2) and depletes calcium. Although it is likely that contact with irrigating solution for more clinically relevant times would have a lesser effect, if an area where MTA will be applied has previously contacted irrigating solutions (especially EDTA and BioPure MTAD), it should be sufficiently flushed with distilled water to remove any trace chemical residue.

With regard to set MTA, BioPure MTAD and, to a lesser extent, EDTA have both been shown to roughen its surface (72 hours post mixing), extract calcium, and cause dissolution of the surface (Smith *et al.* 2007) with just 5 minutes of exposure. However, it should be kept in mind that contact with these solutions would be short-lived, not to mention that other materials such as dentin are similarly affected. Thus, the clinical significance of set MTA contacting irrigation solutions is likely not of great concern.

DEVELOPMENT OF REACTION ZONES

Since its introduction, numerous studies have appeared in the literature showing MTA to have excellent biocompatibility and to have better sealing ability than other dental materials used in similar applications. Coincidentally, other research has shown that MTA stored in a phosphate solution presented with crystals on its surface, whereas MTA stored in water did not (Camilleri *et al.* 2005). Sarkar and associates were the first to propose the bioactive nature of MTA that explains these phenomena (Sarkar *et al.* 2005). They examined the composition of the

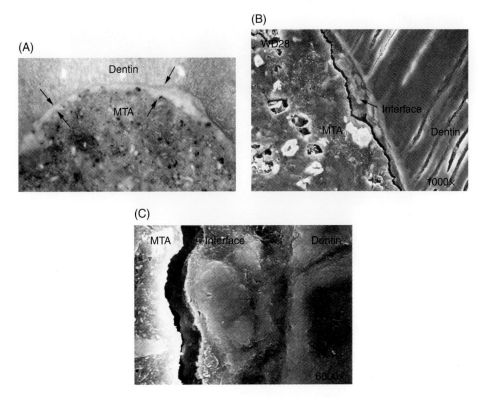

Fig. 2.6 (A) Optical micrograph of the MTA-dentin interface, (B) Scanning electron micrograph of the MTA-dentin interface cross-section, (C) area identified by box in (B) at a higher magnification. Source: Sarkar *et al.* 2005. Reproduced with permission of Elsevier.

globular precipitates that form on MTA when exposed to a PBS solution and reported them to be similar to hydroxyapatite. Additionally, they observed that an interfacial layer formed between MTA and surrounding dentin (Fig. 2.6). From this, they suggested MTA's bioactive nature is brought about by dissolution of calcium, which then complexes with phosphate to form hydroxyapatite crystals that grow and fill the space between MTA and dentin. Over time, this mechanical layer transforms to a chemically-bonded seal. Subsequent research confirmed this reaction layer to be similar to hydroxyapatite (Bozeman *et al.* 2006), although others characterize it as just apatitic in nature. Nevertheless, the bioactivity of MTA as outlined above is largely responsible for its better sealing ability compared with many other dental materials and also its greater bond in physiological solutions compared with distilled water (Reyes-Carmona *et al.* 2010). Further understanding of the apatite reaction layer formation has been explored by several researchers. It appears the initial nucleus is of an amorphous calcium phosphate, which acts as a precursor to the formation of carbonated apatite (Tay *et al.* 2007;

(A)

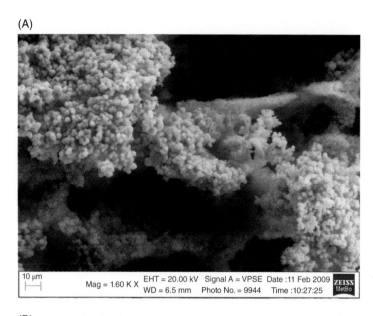

(B)

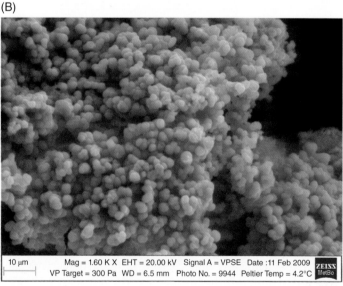

Fig. 2.7 MTA after 7 days of storage in a phosphate buffered saline solution. Apatite-like precipitates appear on the surface. (A) 1600X, (B) 3200X. Source: Gandolfi *et al.* 2010. Reproduced with permission of John Wiley & Sons, Inc.

Reyes-Carmona *et al.* 2009; Han *et al.* 2010). The formation of the precipitate on the surface begins rather quickly, occurring after only five hours, with progressive development over time and a uniform thickness appearing within seven days (Fig. 2.7) (Gandolfi *et al.* 2010).

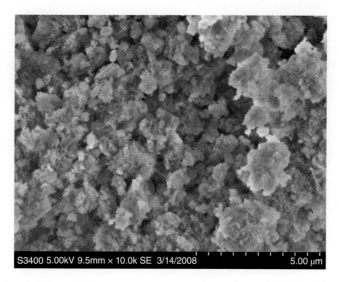

S3400 5.00kV 9.5mm × 10.0k SE 3/14/2008   5.00 μm

Fig. 2.8 Apatite-like precipitates appearing on the surface of calcium silicate hydrate. Courtesy of Dr. Nikhil Sarkar.

Due to the production of calcium hydroxide from hydration of the calcium silicates in MTA and the similarities in biological response between calcium hydroxide and MTA (Pitt Ford *et al.* 1996; Faraco & Holland 2001), early research focused on calcium hydroxide as the bioactive product of MTA. However, there is evidence that the calcium silicate hydrate also is bioactive (Theriot *et al.* 2008) and, since it is in greater proportion, may be the more significant reaction product with regard to the biocompatibility of MTA. While the conversion to carbonated apatite associated with calcium hydroxide is thought to be predominantly through a dissolution-precipitation reaction, anion exchange processes and surface nucleation have been proposed for the same apatite appearing on calcium silicate hydrate (Fig. 2.8) (Theriot *et al.* 2008).

REFERENCES

Aggarwal, V., Jain, A., Kabi, D. (2011) In vitro evaluation of effect of various endodontic solutions on selected physical properties of white mineral trioxide aggregate. *Australian Endodontics Journal* **37**, 61–4.

Alanezi, A. Z., Zhu, Q., Wang, Y. H., *et al.* (2011) Effect of selected accelerants on setting time and biocompatibility of mineral trioxide aggregate (MTA). *Oral Surgery, Oral Medicine, Oral Pathology, Oral Radiology, and Endodontics* **111**, 122–7.

Appelbaum, K. S., Stewart, J. T., Hartwell, G. R. (2012) Effect of sodium fluorosilicate on the properties of Portland cement. *Journal of Endodontics* **38**, 1001–3.

Asgary, S., Parirokh, M., Eghbal, M. J., *et al.* (2004) A comparative study of white mineral trioxide aggregate and white Portland cements using X–ray microanalysis. *Aust Endod J*, **30**, 89–92.

Asgary, S., Parirokh, M., Eghbal, M. J., *et al.* (2005) Chemical differences between white and gray mineral trioxide aggregate. *Journal of Endodontics* **31**, 101–3.

Asgary, S., Parirokh, M., Eghbal, M. J., *et al.* (2006) A qualitative X–ray analysis of white and grey mineral trioxide aggregate using compositional imaging. *Journal of Materials Sciience: Materials in Medicine* **17**, 187–91.

ASTM Standard C150/C150M – 12, 2012, "Standard Specification for Portland Cement", ASTM International, West Conshohocken, PA.

Belío-Reyes, I. A., Bucio, L., Cruz-Chavez, E. (2009) Phase composition of ProRoot mineral trioxide aggregate by X-ray powder diffraction. *Journal of Endodontics* **35**, 875–8.

Ber, B. S., Hatton, J. F., Stewart, G. P. (2007) Chemical modification of ProRoot MTA to improve handling characteristics and decrease setting time. *Journal of Endodontics* **33**, 1231–4.

Bhatty, J. I. (1991) A review of the application of thermal analysis to cement-admixture systems. *Thermochimica Acta* **189**, 313–50.

Bortoluzzi, E. A., Broon, N. J., Bramante, C. M., *et al.* (2006a) Sealing ability of MTA and radiopaque Portland cement with or without calcium chloride for root-end filling. *Journal of Endodontics* **32**, 897–900.

Bortoluzzi, E.A., Juárez Broon, N., Antonio Hungaro Duarte M., *et al.* (2006b) The use of a setting accelerator and its effect on pH and calcium ion release of mineral trioxide aggregate and white Portland cement. *Journal of Endodontics* **32**, 1194–7.

Bortoluzzi, E. A., Broon, N. J., Bramante, C. M., *et al.* (2009) The influence of calcium chloride on the setting time, solubility, disintegration, and pH of mineral trioxide aggregate and white Portland cement with a radiopacifier. *Journal of Endodontics* **35**, 550–4.

Bozeman, T. B., Lemon, R. R., Eleazer, P. D. (2006) Elemental analysis of crystal precipitate from gray and white MTA. *Journal of Endodontics* **32**, 425–8.

Budig, C. G., Eleazer, P. D. (2008) In vitro comparison of the setting of dry ProRoot MTA by moisture absorbed through the root. *Journal of Endodontics*, **34**, 712–4.

Camilleri, J. (2007) Hydration mechanisms of mineral trioxide aggregate. *International Endodontics Journal* **40**, 462–70.

Camilleri, J. (2008) Characterization of hydration products of mineral trioxide aggregate. *International Endodontics Journal* **41**, 408–17.

Camilleri, J. (2009) Evaluation of selected properties of mineral trioxide aggregate sealer cement. *Journal of Endodontics* **35**, 1412–7.

Camilleri, J., Montesin, F. E., Brady, K., *et al.* (2005) The constitution of mineral trioxide aggregate. *Dental Materials* **21**, 297–303.

Chang, S. W., Shon, W. J., Lee, W., *et al.* (2010) Analysis of heavy metal contents in gray and white MTA and 2 kinds of Portland cement: a preliminary study. *Oral Surgery, Oral Medicine, Oral Pathology, Oral Radiology, and Endodontics* **109**, 642–6.

Chedella, S. C., Berzins, D. W. (2010) A differential scanning calorimetry study of the setting reaction of MTA. *International Endodontics Journal* **43**, 509–18.

Chng, H. K., Islam, I., Yap, A. U., *et al.* (2005) Properties of a new root–end filling material. *Journal of Endodontics* **31**, 665–8.

Comin-Chiaramonti, L., Cavalleri, G., Sbaizero, O., *et al.* (2009) Crystallochemical comparison between Portland cements and mineral trioxide aggregate (MTA). *Journal of Applied Biomaterials and Biomechanics* **7**, 171–8.

Coomaraswamy, K. S., Lumley, P. J., Hofmann, M. P. (2007) Effect of bismuth oxide radioopacifier content on the material properties of an endodontic Portland cement-based (MTA-like) system. *Journal of Endodontics* **33**, 295–8.

Dammaschke, T., Gerth, H. U., Züchner, H., *et al.* (2005) Chemical and physical surface and bulk material characterization of white ProRoot MTA and two Portland cements. *Dental Materials* **21**, 731–8.

Darvell, B. W., Wu, R. C. (2011) "MTA" – an hydraulic silicate cement: review update and setting reaction. *Dental Materials* **27**, 407–22.

Ding, S. J., Kao, C. T., Shie, M. Y., *et al.* (2008) The physical and cytological properties of white MTA mixed with Na_2HPO_4 as an accelerant. *Journal of Endodontics* **34**, 748–51.

Faraco, I. M., Holland, R. (2001) Response of the pulp of dogs to capping with mineral trioxide aggregate or a calcium hydroxide cement. *Dental Traumatology* **17**, 163–6.

Funteas, U. R., Wallace, J. A., Fochtman, E. W. 2003. A comparative analysis of mineral trioxide aggregate and Portland cement. *Australian Endodontics Journal* **29**, 43–4.

Gancedo-Caravia, L., Garcia-Barbero, E. (2006) Influence of humidity and setting time on the push–out strength of mineral trioxide aggregate obturations. *Journal of Endodontics* **32**, 894–6.

Gandolfi, M. G., Iacono, F., Agee, K., *et al.* (2009) Setting time and expansion in different soaking media of experimental accelerated calcium-silicate cements and ProRoot MTA. *Oral Surgery, Oral Medicine, Oral Pathology, Oral Radiology, and Endodontics* **108**, e39–45.

Gandolfi, M. G., Taddei, P., Tinti, A., *et al.* (2010a) Apatite-forming ability (bioactivity) of ProRoot MTA. *International Endodontics Journal* **43**, 917–29.

Gandolfi, M. G., Van Landuyt, K., Taddei, P., *et al.* (2010b) Environmental scanning electron microscopy connected with energy dispersive x–ray analysis and Raman techniques to study ProRoot mineral trioxide aggregate and calcium silicate cements in wet conditions and in real time. *Journal of Endodontics* **36**, 851–7.

Han, L., Okiji, T., Okawa, S. (2010) Morphological and chemical analysis of different precipitates on mineral trioxide aggregate immersed in different fluids. *Dental Materials Journal* **29**, 512–7.

Hong, S. T., Bae, K. S., Baek, S. H., *et al.* (2008) Microleakage of accelerated mineral trioxide aggregate and Portland cement in an in vitro apexification model. *Journal of Endodontics* **34**, 56–8.

Hsieh, S. C., Teng, N. C., Lin, Y. C., *et al.* 2009. A novel accelerator for improving the handling properties of dental filling materials. *Journal of Endodontics* **35**, 1292–5.

Huang, T. H., Shie, M. Y., Kao, C. T., *et al.* (2008) The effect of setting accelerator on properties of mineral trioxide aggregate. *Journal of Endodontics* **34**, 590–3.

Islam, I., Chng, H. K., Yap, A. U. (2006) Comparison of the physical and mechanical properties of MTA and portland cement. *Journal of Endodontics*, **32**, 193–7.

Ji, B. (1991) A review of the application of thermal analysis to cement–admixture systems. *Thermochimica Acta* **189**, 313–350.

Ji, D. Y., Wu, H. D., Hsieh, S. C., *et al.* (2011) Effects of a novel hydration accelerant on the biological and mechanical properties of white mineral trioxide aggregate. *Journal of Endodontics* **37**, 851–5.

Kang, J. S., Rhim, E. M., Huh, S. Y., *et al.* (2012) The effects of humidity and serum on the surface microhardness and morphology of five retrograde filling materials. *Scanning* **34**, 207–14.

Kim, Y., Kim, S., Shin, Y. S., *et al.* (2012) Failure of setting of mineral trioxide aggregate in the presence of fetal bovine serum and its prevention. *Journal of Endodontics* **38**, 536–40.

Kogan, P., He, J., Glickman, G. N., *et al.* (2006) The effects of various additives on setting properties of MTA. *Journal of Endodontics* **32**, 569–72.

Komabayashi, T., Spångberg, L. S. (2008) Comparative analysis of the particle size and shape of commercially available mineral trioxide aggregates and Portland cement: a study with a flow particle image analyzer. *Journal of Endodontics* **34**, 94–8.

Lee, B. N., Hwang, Y. C., Jang, J. H., *et al.* (2011) Improvement of the properties of mineral trioxide aggregate by mixing with hydration accelerators. *Journal of Endodontics* **37**, 1433–6.

Lee, S. J., Monsef, M., Torabinejad, M. (1993) Sealing ability of a mineral trioxide aggregate for repair of lateral root perforations. *Journal of Endodontics* **19**, 541–4.

Lee, Y. L., Lee, B. S., Lin, F. H., *et al.* (2004) Effects of physiological environments on the hydration behavior of mineral trioxide aggregate. *Biomaterials* **25**, 787–93.

Lee, Y. L., Lin, F. H., Wang, W. H., *et al.* (2007) Effects of EDTA on the hydration mechanism of mineral trioxide aggregate. *Journal of Dental Research* **86**, 534–8.

Monteiro Bramante, C., Demarchi, A. C., De Moraes, I. G., *et al.* (2008) Presence of arsenic in different types of MTA and white and gray Portland cement. *Oral Surgery, Oral Medicine, Oral Pathology, Oral Radiology, and Endodontics* **106**, 909–13.

Namazikhah, M. S., Nekoofar, M. H., Sheykhrezae, M. S., *et al.* (2008) The effect of pH on surface hardness and microstructure of mineral trioxide aggregate. *International Endodontics Journal* **41**, 108–16.

Nekoofar, M. H., Stone, D. F., Dummer, P. M. (2010) The effect of blood contamination on the compressive strength and surface microstructure of mineral trioxide aggregate. *International Endodontics Journal* **43**, 782–91.

Nekoofar, M. H., Davies, T. E., Stone, D., *et al.* (2011) Microstructure and chemical analysis of blood-contaminated mineral trioxide aggregate. *International Endodontics Journal* **44**, 1011–8.

Pitt Ford, T. R., Torabinejad, M., Abedi, H. R., *et al.* (1996) Using mineral trioxide aggregate as a pulp-capping material. *Journal of the American Dental Association* **127**, 1491–4.

Porter, M. L., Bertó, A., Primus, C. M., *et al.* (2010) Physical and chemical properties of new-generation endodontic materials. *Journal of Endodontics* **36**, 524–8.

Ramachandran, V. S., Paroli, R. M., Beaudoin J. J., *et al.* (2003) *Handbook of Thermal Analysis of Construction Materials.* Noyes Publication/William Andrew Publishing, New York.

Reyes-Carmona, J. F., Felippe, M. S., Felippe, W. T. (2009) Biomineralization ability and interaction of mineral trioxide aggregate and white portland cement with dentin in a phosphate-containing fluid. *Journal of Endodontics* **35**, 731–6.

Reyes-Carmona, J. F., Felippe, M. S., Felippe, W. T. (2010) The biomineralization ability of mineral trioxide aggregate and Portland cement on dentin enhances the push-out strength. *Journal of Endodontics* **36**, 286–91.

Ridi, F., Fratini, E., Mannelli, F., *et al.* (2005) Hydration process of cement in the presence of a cellulosic additive. *A calorimetric investigation. Journal of Physical Chemistry B* **109**, 14727–34.

Sarkar, N. K., Caicedo, R., Ritwik, P., *et al.* (2005) Physicochemical basis of the biologic properties of mineral trioxide aggregate. *Journal of Endodontics* **31**, 97–100.

Schembri, M., Peplow, G., Camilleri, J. (2010) Analyses of heavy metals in mineral trioxide aggregate and Portland cement. *Journal of Endodontics* **36**, 1210–5.

Sluyk, S. R., Moon, P. C., Hartwell, G. R. (1998) Evaluation of setting properties and retention characteristics of mineral trioxide aggregate when used as a furcation perforation repair material. *Journal of Endodontics* **24**, 768–71.

Smith, J. B., Loushine, R. J., Weller, R. N., *et al.* (2007) Metrologic evaluation of the surface of white MTA after the use of two endodontic irrigants. *Journal of Endodontics* **33**, 463–7.

Song, J. S., Mante, F. K., Romanow, W. J., *et al.* (2006) Chemical analysis of powder and set forms of Portland cement, gray ProRoot MTA, white ProRoot MTA, and gray MTA-Angelus. *Oral Surgery, Oral Medicine, Oral Pathology, Oral Radiology, and Endodontics* **102**, 809–15.

Tay, F. R., Pashley, D. H., Rueggeberg, F. A., *et al.* (2007) Calcium phosphate phase transformation produced by the interaction of the portland cement component of white mineral trioxide aggregate with a phosphate-containing fluid. *Journal of Endodontics* **33**, 1347–51.

Theriot, S. T., Chowdhury, S., Sarkar, N. K. (2008) Reaction between CSH and phosphate buffered saline solution. *Journal of Dental Research* **87**, Special issue A. Abstract #1068.

Tingey, M. C., Bush, P., Levine, M. S. (2008) Analysis of mineral trioxide aggregate surface when set in the presence of fetal bovine serum. *Journal of Endodontics* **34**, 45–9.

Torabinejad, M., Hong, C. U., McDonald, F., *et al.* (1995) Physical and chemical properties of a new root-end filling material. *Journal of Endodontics* **21**, 349–53.

VanderWeele, R. A., Schwartz, S. A., Beeson, T. J. (2006) Effect of blood contamination on retention characteristics of MTA when mixed with different liquids. *Journal of Endodontics* **32**, 421–4.

Walker, M. P., Diliberto, A., Lee, C. (2006) Effect of setting conditions on mineral trioxide aggregate flexural strength. *Journal of Endodontics* **32**, 334–6.

Watts, J. D., Holt, D. M., Beeson, T. J., *et al.* (2007) Effects of pH and mixing agents on the temporal setting of tooth–colored and gray mineral trioxide aggregate. *Journal of Endodontics* **33**, 970–3.

Wiltbank, K. B., Schwartz, S. A., Schindler, W. G. (2007) Effect of selected accelerants on the physical properties of mineral trioxide aggregate and Portland cement. *Journal of Endodontics* **33**, 1235–8.

3 Physical Properties of MTA

Ricardo Caicedo[1] and Lawrence Gettleman[2]

[1]Department of Oral Health and Rehabilitation (Endodontics Division),
University of Louisville, School of Dentistry, USA
[2]Department of Oral Health and Rehabilitation (Prosthodontics Division),
University of Louisville, School of Dentistry, USA

Mineral Trioxide Aggregate: Properties and Clinical Applications, First Edition.
Edited by Mahmoud Torabinejad.
© 2014 John Wiley & Sons, Inc. Published 2014 by John Wiley & Sons, Inc.

INTRODUCTION

The two versions of mineral trioxide aggregate (MTA; gray and white) have enjoyed clinical success in endodontics since 1995. The grayness of GMTA arises from the presence of an iron-containing compound, tetracalcium-aluminoferrite ($4CaO\text{-}Al_2O_3\text{-}Fe_2O_3$) in Portland cement (ProRoot® MTA product literature). In 2002, a white formula of MTA was introduced, achieved by eliminating iron oxide from the formulation. To distinguish between the two materials in this chapter, we will refer to the gray and white versions of MTA as GMTA and WMTA, respectively. Values in tables preceded by "~" were read from figures in the reference articles rather than from tables or text.

pH

In chemistry, pH is the measure of the solvated hydrogen ion. By definition, pure water has a pH close to 7.0. Solutions with a pH lower than 7.0 are acidic and those with a higher value are called basic or alkaline. The pH of a solution is measured with an electronic glass electrode or chemical indicators. Several studies have evaluated the pH value of MTA, which is ~10.2 immediately after mixing, and rises to 12.5 and remains constant after 3 hours (Torabinejad *et al*. 1995). When comparing pH values of GMTA with WMTA, the white material has been reported to display significantly higher pH values over an extended period of time following mixing (Chng *et al*. 2005; Islam *et al*. 2006). The pH of GMTA and WMTA were compared with ordinary and white Portland cement over 60 min. The pH values of all four products rise within 20 min after initial mixing and plateau by 60 min. White Portland and ordinary Portland cement also reached their peak pH values earlier than GMTA and WMTA (Table 3.1) (Islam *et al*. 2006).

Mineral Trioxide Aggregate reportedly kept its high pH value throughout the course of a long-term study performed over a 78-day period (Fridland & Rosado 2005).

Table 3.1 pH of two MTA products and two Portland cement products at two time periods. Source: Islam *et al*. 2006. Reproduced with permission of Elsevier Publishing.

Material	Initial pH	60 min pH
Ordinary Portland cement	~12.3	~13.0
White Portland cement	~11.9	~13.1
Gray PMTA	~11.3	~12.8
White WMTA	~11.9	~13.0

Table 3.2 Changes in pH of a Brazilian MTA product and an experimental cement up to 15.4 days. Source: Santos *et al.* 2005. Reproduced with permission of John Wiley & Sons, Inc.

Time in hours	0	25	50	100	200	250	370
MTA-S (Angelus)	~6.0	~10.4	~9.5	~7.2	~9.4	~7.5	~7.6
Expt'l. cement	~6.0	~10.3	~9.8	~7.2	~9.4	~7.6	~7.6

Table 3.3 Immediate pH of WMTA and three experimental MTA formulations. Source: Porter *et al.* 2010. Reproduced with permission of Elsevier Publishing.

	Immediate pH
White ProRoot MTA	12.6
Capasio 150	10.3
Ceramicrete-D	2.2
Generex-A	10.8

Table 3.4 pH of WMTA and WMTA modified with Na_2HPO_4 buffer. Source: Ding *et al.* 2008. Reproduced with permission of Elsevier Publishing.

WMTA mixed with	Initial pH	6 h
Distilled water	~11.0	~13.5
15% Na_2HPO_4 buffer	~11.1	~13.3

A Brazilian experimental formulation was measured for various properties and for pH compared with a commercial MTA product for up to 15 days. There were very few differences noted over this time period, but the pH values were much lower than reported in other studies (Table 3.2) (Santos *et al.* 2005).

White MTA and three experimental MTA formulations were tested for pH and other properties by Porter and associates (Porter *et al.* 2010). The pH of Ceramicrete-D was very acidic, measuring 2.2. The others were typically basic (Table 3.3).

As part of a larger study of WMTA, pH measurements were made at intervals of up to 6 hours. There were no differences between WMTA mixed with distilled water and WMTA mixed with 15% Na_2HPO_4 buffer solution (Table 3.4) (Ding *et al.* 2008).

White MTA Angelus, an experimental MTA, white Portland cement, and AH Plus epoxy sealer were placed in 1.5 mm tubes and immersed in 10 mL flasks for varying times up to 28 days, followed by pH measurements of the liquid. Modest changes in pH were observed, probably due to the small size of the

Table 3.5   pH of an experimental MTA, Portland cement, WMTA, and an epoxy sealant up to 28 days. Source: Massi *et al*. 2011. Reproduced with permission of Elsevier Publishing.

pH	MTAS	White Portland cement	WMTA Angelus	AH Plus
3 h	9.83	8.46	7.66	6.14
6 h	8.18	7.79	8.06	5.77
12 h	9.49	7.96	7.64	6.06
24 h	8.76	7.62	7.62	5.88
48 h	8.16	7.67	7.66	6.04
7 days	7.97	7.82	8.00	4.97
14 days	7.90	7.82	8.00	4.96
28 days	8.08	8.03	8.10	6.75

cement samples, but the measured pH values were much lower than others reported in the literature. The pH of the three cement-based materials rose, but fell for the AH Plus sealer (Table 3.5) (Massi *et al*. 2011).

Most references report pH values from 10 to 13, except the studies by Santos *et al*. (2005) and Massi *et al*. (2011). In general, pH rises after mixing and mimics the alkalinity of calcium hydroxide used in endodontics in the past, which may help to account for its favorable biological response.

SOLUBILITY

The solubility of a substance fundamentally depends on the solvent as well as on temperature and pressure. The extent of the solubility of a substance in a specific solvent is measured as the saturation concentration, after which adding more solute does not increase its concentration in the solution. The degree of solubility of MTA was assessed according to a modified American Dental Association specification (ANSI/ADA 1991). While the majority of studies have reported low or no solubility for MTA (Torabinejad *et al*. 1995; Danesh *et al*. 2006; Poggio *et al*. 2007; Shie *et al*. 2009), partial solubility with a decreasing rate over time was reported in a long-term study over a 78-day period (Fridland & Rosado 2005).

The water-to-powder ratio influences the amount of solubility, with higher water-to-powder ratios increasing MTA solubility and porosity (Fridland & Rosado 2005).

The release of calcium ions from MTA has been reported by several investigators (Sarkar *et al*. 2005; Bortoluzzi *et al*. 2006; Bozeman *et al*. 2006; Ozdemir *et al*. 2008). Despite the fact that the formation of apical barriers is highly successful using calcium hydroxide, this material is quickly reabsorbed when in

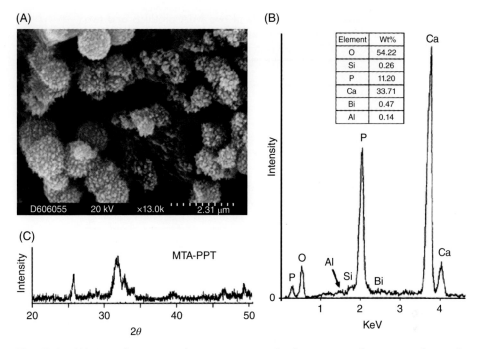

Fig. 3.1 (A) Typical scanning electron micrograph of precipitates from mineral trioxide aggregate – synthetic tissue fluid interaction (×13,000). (B) Energy dispersive X-ray analysis spectrum from precipitates in A (above) and their semi-quantitative chemical composition (below). (C) X-ray diffraction pattern of mineral trioxide aggregate – synthetic tissue fluid precipitates. Source: Sarkar *et al.* 2005. Reproduced with permission of Elsevier Publishing.

contact with the apical tissues, making it necessary to follow the clinical case long-term to confirm the formation of the barrier. With the MTA, this formation is predictable and it is not necessary to monitor. MTA offers a barrier with excellent sealing properties and a high degree of biocompatibility (Linsuwanont 2003). Addition of $CaCl_2$ to WMTA revealed a significant increase in calcium release during the first 24 hours (Bortoluzzi *et al.* 2006). Interestingly, high levels of calcium in a cell culture environment decreased cell proliferation (Midy *et al.* 2001), suggesting that released calcium ions from MTA may interact with phosphorus in tissue fluid to yield hydroxylapatite, which helps to explain the physicochemical basis for MTA's successful clinical applications (Fig. 3.1) (Sarkar *et al.* 2005). Calcium release from MTA might be influenced by certain clinical conditions. Islam and associates found that the percent solubility of WMTA was greater than that of white Portland cement, ordinary Portland cement, and, especially, GMTA (Islam *et al.* 2006). Solubility in this case may be beneficial to the success of the product in that it allows for

Table 3.6 Percent solubility of two MTA products and two Portland cement products at an unspecified time. Source: Islam *et al.* 2006. Reproduced with permission of Elsevier Publishing.

	Solubility in % ± SD
White WMTA	1.28 ± 0.02
Gray PMTA	0.97 ± 0.02
White Portland cement	1.05 ± 0.02
Ordinary Portland cement	1.06 ± 0.07

Table 3.7 Percent solubility and porosity at 24 hours of WMTA as a function of water-to-powder ratios. Source: Fridland & Rosado 2003. Reproduced with permission of Elsevier Publishing.

Water/powder ratio WMTA	W/W % Solubility	% Porosity
0.26	1.76	30.25
0.28	2.25	35.72
0.30	2.57	35.19
0.33	2.83	38.39

the dissolution of components, which leads to the formation of reaction products at the interface between the material and the tooth, generating a biologic seal mostly of calcium hydroxide (Table 3.6).

Fridland & Rosado (2003) found that the higher the water-to-powder ratio for WMTA, the lower the degree of solubility and porosity at 24 hours (Fridland & Rosado 2003). This is in accord with the notion that the chemical reaction may be extended and incomplete using a wetter mix, accounting for the greater clinical success of WMTA (Table 3.7).

In a later study, Fridland & Rosado (2005) found that the solubility of WMTA at 0.33 water-to-powder ratio decreased over nine days from 0.37% to 0.02%, and that the calculated cumulative solubility was a remarkable 24.02% at 80 days. The solubility was considerably less for the 0.28 water-powder-ratio mix (Table 3.8).

Poggio and associates measured the percent solubility of four retrograde filling materials as weight loss after one day and two months and found no significant difference between them. ProRoot WMTA displayed 0.91% solubility after two months (Table 3.9) (Poggio *et al.* 2007).

Solubility was tested for white Portland cement and WMTA, both modified with added $CaCl_2$. Setting time was greatly reduced and WMTA gained weight

Table 3.8 Daily and cumulative percent solubility of WMTA up to 80 days. Source: Fridland & Rosado 2003. Reproduced with permission of Elsevier Publishing.

	Water/powder ratio	Tested W/W % daily solubility
1 day	0.28	~2.9
	0.33	~3.7
2 days	0.28	~1.2
	0.33	~1.8
9 days	0.28	~0.1
	0.33	~0.2
80 days	0.28	Calculated cumulative solubility 16.13
	0.33	Calculated cumulative solubility 24.02

Table 3.9 Weight loss of four root sealant materials for up to 2 months. Source: Poggio *et al.* 2007. Reproduced with permission of Elsevier Publishing.

Material (*n* = 6)	% Weight loss after 24 h (SD)%	Weight loss after 2 months (SD)
IRM	0.65 (0.19)	1.01 (0.22)
ProRoot MTA	0.70 (0.26)	0.91 (0.29)
Superseal	0.23 (0.25)	0.40 (0.24)
Argoseal	0.97 (0.33)	1.50 (0.35)

by 72 hours. Solubility was reduced for the white Portland cement and both products increased in pH (Table 3.10) (Bortoluzzi *et al.* 2009).

In general, the tests show low solubility of MTA products in most cases. However, there is enough solubility in the early stages to begin the formation of a calcium-rich and highly basic environment, which is thought to stimulate the formation of calcium hydroxide, a precursor of biologically formed hydroxylapatite.

Silver zeolite is a crystalline aluminosilicate material that releases silver ions, which are antimicrobial against most microbes. Silver ions were added to sodium zeolite ($Na_2O:Al_2O_3:2SiO_2:XH_2O$) with sodium nitrate by an ion exchange mechanism. MTA powder (Dentsply, DeTrey, Germany) received the activated zeolite at 0.2% or 2.0% mass fraction. The control material was unmodified MTA. Calcium release, setting times, water solubility and absorption were measured at 7 days (Cinar *et al.* 2013).

Table 3.10 Composition of modifications of WMTA and two Portland cements, with solubility values up to 28 days. Source: Bortoluzzi et al. 2009. Reproduced with permission of Elsevier Publishers.

WMTA (1.0 g)	1.0 g WMTA + 0.26 mL H_2O
WMTA + $CaCl_2$	1.0 g WMTA + 0.1 g $CaCl_2$ + 0.18 mL H_2O
White Portland cement	0.8 g white Portland cement + 0.2 g Bi_2O_3 + 0.26 mL H_2O
White Portland cement + $CaCl_2$	0.8 g white Portland cement + 0.2 g Bi_2O_3 + 1 g $CaCl_2$ + 1 g WPC with 0.1 g $CaCl_2$ + 0.18 mL H_2O

	24 h		72 h		7 days		14 days		28 days	
	M	MP	M	MP	M	MP	M	MP	M	MP
WMTA	−0.468	15.50	−0.659	15.50	−0.331	15.5	−0.721	15.5	−0.499	15.5
WMTA+$CaCl_2$	−0.593	9.333	3.462	18.66	3.875	19.00	3.991	19.16	4.112	19.50
WPC	−0.199	19.00	−4.696	6.333	−5.064	6.00	−5.863	6.000	−6.777	6.00
WPC+$CaCl_2$	−0.878	6.166	−1.267	9.500	−1.920	9.500	−2.646	9.333	−2.809	9.00

Negative values indicate weight loss.
M, median, MP, mean posts of solubility (%) of hydrated cements in each period.

There were no differences in calcium release, with the highest value for 2.0% at 24 hours. Water absorption and solubility for the 0.2% sodium zeolite MTA was 8.59% and 1.38%, respectively. For the 2.0% sodium zeolite MTA it was 6.79% and −7.09%, respectively, c.f. 8.98% and 1.01%, respectively. The 2.0% addition significantly reduced setting time and was significantly more soluble than 0.2% zeolite MTA and plain MTA. These mineral additions to MTA have not been shown to be advantageous (Cinar *et al.* 2013).

SETTING EXPANSION

One reason for the sealing ability of MTA is its slight expansion upon setting. Both GMTA and WMTA are composed of approximately 75% Portland cement. White MTA differs from GMTA in its lower content of tetracalcium aluminoferrite. This difference in composition may affect setting expansion. Researchers have measured the setting expansion of several versions of MTA and found that GMTA expanded much more than WMTA or Portland cement, and that the water-to-powder ratio had little effect on expansion (Tables 3.11 and 3.12) (Storm *et al.* 2008; Hawley *et al.* 2010).

Table 3.11 Percent expansion of MTA as a function of water-to-powder ratios after 25 hours. Source: Hawley *et al.* 2010. Reproduced with permission of Elsevier Publishing.

Water/powder ratio	WMTA	GMTA
0.26	0.084 ± 0.012	2.42 ± 0.324
0.28	0.058 ± 0.044	2.38 ± 0.034
0.30	0.093 ± 0.013	2.56 ± 0.393
0.35	0.086 ± 0.029	2.15 ± 0.337

Table 3.12 Mean percentage of linear setting expansion of GMTA and WMTA submerged in distilled water or Hank's buffered salt solution and Portland cement submerged in water. Source: Storm *et al.* 2008. Reproduced with permission of Elsevier Publishing.

Groups	5 h (SD) (*n*)	7.7 h (SD) (*n*)	24 h (SD) (*n*)
GMTA/water	0.47 (0.09) (5)	0.74 (0.15) (3)	1.02 (0.19) (3)
GMTA/HBSS	0.34 (0.04) (3)	0.45 (0.06) (3)	0.68 (0.12) (3)
WMTA/water	0.04 (0.01) (5)	0.06 (0.01) (5)	0.08 (0.01) (3)
WMTA/HBSS	0.09 (0.03) (3)	0.10 (0.03) (3)	0.11 (0.03) (3)
PC/water	0.24 (0.05) (5)	0.26 (0.04) (5)	0.29 (0.04) (5)

RADIOPACITY

The radiopacity of MTA is determined using the method described by ISO 6876, section 7.7. The thickness of an aluminum step wedge is plotted against the logarithm of the corresponding densitometer values to calculate relative radiopacity, expressed as the equivalence of aluminum (International Organization for Standardization 2001). Due to the additions of Bi_2O_3 as a radiopacifier, WMTA and GMTA were found to have more than six times the radiopacity of modified and unmodified Portland cement (Islam *et al.* 2006). Conversely, Porter and associates found a higher level using the same methods and looked at the relative radiopacity of other dental sealants as well (Table 3.13) (Porter *et al.* 2010).

Húngaro Duarte and associates examined the relative radiopacities of various heavy metals and other oxides at 20% concentration as possible radiopaquing additions to Portland cement (Húngaro Duarte *et al.* 2009). Bismuth oxide was found to be the most radiopaque of the additions, almost six times as radiodense as pure Portland cement (Table 3.14).

Radiopacity should be a fundamental characteristic of all materials and devices used in dentistry and medicine because, if these materials become embedded in the tissues of the body and are swallowed or inhaled, they must be identifiable in the case of trauma or other untoward events. Heavy metal powders, metal oxides and compounds, metallic glasses, and polymeric additives containing heavy metals all have advantages and disadvantages. Bismuth oxide has been used to successfully increase the radiopacity of MTA. Other substituents may be used in future studies that satisfy all requirements.

Cytotoxicity, radiopacity, pH, and flow of a calcium silicate-based (MTA Fillapex (Angelus, Brazil) and an epoxy resin-based (AH Plus, Dentsply, Germany) endodontic sealer were measured at 3, 24, 72, and 168 h. Cytotoxicity was evaluated by the MTT assay to check the viability of BALB/c 3T3 cells up to 4 weeks (Silva *et al.* 2013).

Table 3.13 Radiopacity equivalent of pure aluminum

Islam *et al.* (2006)	
WMTA	6.74 mm
PMTA	6.47 mm
White Portland cement	0.95 mm
Ordinary Portland cement	0.93 mm
Porter *et al.* (2010)	
ProRoot WMTA	8.5 mm
Capasio 150	4.2 mm
Ceramicrete-D	3.2 mm
Generex-A	6.8 mm

Table 3.14 Radiopacity of Portland cement, human dentin, and various additives to Portland cement. Source: Húngaro Duarte *et al.* 2009. Reproduced with permission of Elsevier Publishing.

	Equivalent mm Al (±SD)
Pure Portland cement	1.01 ± 0.01
Portland cement + 20% bismuth carbonate	3.25 ± 0.38
Portland cement + 20% iodoform	4.24 ± 0.32
Portland cement + 20% bismuth oxide	5.93 ± 0.34
Portland cement + 20% lead oxide	5.74 ± 0.66
Portland cement + 20% zinc oxide	2.64 ± 0.02
Portland cement + 20% zirconium oxide	3.41 ± 0.19
Portland cement + 20% barium sulfate	2.80 ± 0.18
Portland cement + 20% bismuth subnitrate	4.66 ± 0.42
Portland cement + 20% calcium tungstate	3.11 ± 0.25
Dentin	1.74 ± 0.02

Table 3.15 Mean pH values and per cent cytotoxicity at different time periods. Silva *et al.* 2013.

	pH					Cytotoxicity (% of control)				
Time in hours 3	24	48	72	168		Time in weeks 0	1	2	3	4
AH Plus	7.08[a]	6.93[a]	6.78[a]	6.90[a]	6.92[a]	37[c]	70[c]	92[c]	100[c]	98[c]
MTA Fillapex	9.68[b]	9.34[b]	8.25[b]	8.02[b]	7.76[b]	4[d]	15[d]	13[d]	23[d]	30[d]
Control	6.50	6.50	6.50	6.50	6.50					

Superscripts indicate significant differences ($p < 0.05$).

Radiopacity (mm Al) of the sealers were 8.59 for AH Plus and 7.06 for MTA Fillapex. Although significantly different, both sealers were sufficiently radiopaque, compared to 3 mm Al (Table 3.15). One gram of mixed sealer was pressed between glass plates under a 120 g load for 180 s. MTA Fillapex (31.09±0.67 mm) flowed significantly more than AH Plus (25.80±0.83 mm).

There were significant differences in pH and cytotoxicity between brands at all time periods. AH Plus was more cytotoxic than MTA Fillaplex, but both are adequate as an endodontic sealer.

Portland cement was modified with additions of 10, 20, and 30 wt. % Bi_2O_3, ZrO_2 or YbF_3. Controls were ProRoot MTA (Dentsply, Tulsa, USA) and pure Portland cement. An aluminum step wedge on occlusal dental films was radiographed next to tooth slices to measure radiopacity. Compressive strength, mercury intrusion porosimetry, and setting time were measured. The morphology was examined by scanning electron microscopy (Antonijevic *et al.* 2013).

Significant increases in porosity were observed in all experimental cements. Bi_2O_3 extended the setting time significantly, from 90 to 115 minutes; ZrO_2

Table 3.16 Mean (±SD) for various properties. Cavenago *et al.* 2014.

p/l ratio	Mean radiopacity (mm Al)	Mean solubility (%)	Setting time Initial (minutes)	Setting time Final (hours)	pH 3	pH 24	pH 72	pH 168	Calcium release (mg/L) (hours) 3	24	72	168
4:1	6.94[a]	1.62 (1.27)[e]	57.0 (2.0)[g]	112 (2.0)[g]	7.75[i]	7.84[i]	7.31[i]	7.71[i]	5.29[n]	4.46[n]	2.15[n]	5.48[n]
3:1	5.70[b]	1.83 (0.77)[e]	105 (1.52)[h]	135 (2.0)[h]	7.87[i]	7.89[i]	7.34[i]	7.78[i]	6.33[n]	4.70[n]	3.16[np]	6.20[n]
2:1	5.31[c]	6.46 (1.83)[f]	120 (2.51)[i]	321 (2.0)[i]	9.47[k]	8.00[i]	7.59[i]	8.43[i]	9.21[p]	6.73[p]	3.92[p]	9.72[p]
Dentin	0.79[d]											

Different letters in each group and column indicate statistical differences ($p < 0.05$).

and YbF_3 had no effect on setting time. Additions of at least 10 wt. % Bi_2O_3 and 20 wt. % ZrO_2 or 20 wt. % YbF_3 increased radiopacity above 3 mm Al. Compressive strength of Portland cement was increased by adding ZrO_2 and YbF_3, but not significantly; Bi_2O_3 significantly decreased it. No degradation of physical properties was observed by adding ZrO_2 and YbF_3, which may be used to replace Bi_2O_3 in MTA (Antonijevic *et al.* 2013).

White MTA Angelus (Angelus, Brazil) with powder-to-water ratios of 4:1, 3:1 and 2:1 were tested for radiographic density and compared to cylinders of dentin and an aluminum step wedge. Mean solubility, setting time, pH, and calcium ion release (measured using atomic absorption spectrophotometry) were carried out at 3, 24, 72 and 168 h (Table 3.16). Root-end fillings of 30 acrylic teeth were scanned twice by micro-CT before and after immersion in ultrapure water for 168 hours (Cavenago *et al.* 2014).

Higher radiopacity was seen with a powder/liquid ratio of 4:1. More water in the mix lengthens the setting time and the pH and calcium ion release are higher ($p < 0.05$). The more dilute group (2:1) was significantly more soluble (6.46%) compared to the other groups. The powder/water ratio significantly affected the physical and chemical properties of white MTA Angelus (Cavenago *et al.* 2014 and Table 3.16).

VARIOUS TYPES OF STRENGTH

Compressive strength

The *compressive strengths* of dental materials are determined according to the method recommended by ISO 6876. Using a mechanical testing machine, the compressive strength is calculated in pascals (Pa = N/m^2), where the maximum applied load in newtons (kg m/s^2) is divided by the diameter of the specimen in square meters. Since this is usually a small number for most properties, this unit is expressed as MPa or megapascals and is used for compressive, tensile, push-out, and shear strength (the latter two using the circumference of the interface being sheared divided by the height or cross-section).

Compressive strength up to 7 days was used as a measure of performance of two experimental Portland cements, compared with commercial MTA and ordinary Portland cement. MTA and ordinary Portland cement displayed the highest values, especially at 3 days (Hwang *et al.* 2011). It was also used to test four commercial MTA products (Porter *et al.* 2010). Islam and associates also measured compressive strength and found much higher values at three days and 28 days (Table 3.17) (Islam *et al.* 2006).

Table 3.17 Compressive strength of various commercial and experimental products at one, three, seven, and 28 days.

Compressive strength (MPa)	1 days	3 days	7 days
Portland cement	28.06 ± 4.31[b]	43.36 ± 4.39[b]	32.10 ± 1.01[b]
Expt'l Portland cement	5.81 ± 1.17[a]	10.47 ± 1.54[a]	14.88 ± 1.13[a]
Expt'l Portland cement + CaSO$_4$	8.51 ± 0.55[a]	9.66 ± 0.76[a]	13.82 ± 2.99[a]
MTA	27.41 ± 3.83[b]	43.65 ± 8.35[b]	30.77 ± 0.51[b]
Hwang et al. (2011)			

Compressive strength (MPa)	7 days
ProRoot WMTA	27.0 ± 7.0
Capasio 150	30.7 ± 5.1
Ceramicrete-D	6.60 ± 3.5
Generex-A	38.9 ± 10.9
Porter et al. (2010)	

Compressive strength (MPa)	3 days	28 days
Ordinary Portland cement	48.06 ± 6.14	50.66 ± 1.37
White Portland cement	40.39 ± 2.86	48.53 ± 1.37
WMTA	45.84 ± 1.32	86.02 ± 10.32
PMTA	50.43 ± 1.30	98.62 ± 5.74
6 mm × 12 mm specimens. Load rate not specified.		

Kogan and associates added various components to WMTA and measured the compressive strength (Kogan et al. 2006). When mixed with saline, the highest values were 39.2 MPa, compared with 32.6 MPa (with 2% lidocaine) and 28.4 MPa (with sterile water). Other additives displayed much lower compressive strength values (Table 3.18) (Kogan et al. 2006).

In a 2×2×2 study, GMTA was (a) mixed with either 2% lidocaine HCl (1:100 000 epinephrine) or sterile water; (b) mixed at pH 5.0 or 7.4; and (c) measured in compression at either 7 or 28 days. Interactions were noted in the comparisons between mixing liquids, but it appears that sterile water strength is higher than that of 2% lidocaine. White MTA had higher values than GMTA at both pH values. Overall, the values at pH 7.4 were higher than those at pH 5.0 (Table 3.19 and Fig. 3.2) (Watts et al. 2007). These values are considerably higher than those found by Kogan and associates (Kogan et al. 2006).

Hwang and associates worked with an experimental cement formulation with added CaSO$_4$, and compared it with WMTA and Portland cement (Hwang et al.

Table 3.18 Compressive strength in MPa of WMTA with various additives. Source: Kogan *et al.* 2006. Reproduced with permission of Elsevier Publishing.

Additives to WMTA	Compressive strength (MPa) at 7 days
Sterile water	28.4
Sodium hypochlorite gel (NaOCl gel, ChlorCid V)	17.1
K-Y Jelly	18.3
2% lidocaine HCl with 1:100 000 epinephrine	32.6
Saline	39.2
3% $CaCl_2$	19.3
5% $CaCl_2$	19.6
6 × 14 mm specimen	

Table 3.19 Compressive strength of GMTA and WMTA at two pH levels, using sterile water or 2% lidocaine, over 7 days and 28 days. Source: Watts *et al.* 2007. Reproduced with permission of Elsevier Publishing.

	pH	Time in days	Compressive strength (MPa ± SD)
GMTA lidocaine	5.0	7	38.2 ± 19.51
GMTA sterile water	5.0	7	47.8 ± 25.54
GMTA lidocaine	7.4	7	55.9 ± 25.08
GMTA sterile water	7.4	7	66.6 ± 27.10
WMTA lidocaine	5.0	7	62.3 ± 19.04
WMTA sterile water	5.0	7	92.3 ± 22.69
WMTA lidocaine	7.4	7	74.3 ± 23.87
WMTA sterile water	7.4	7	81.8 ± 25.48
GMTA lidocaine	5.0	28	23.3 ± 18.02
GMTA sterile water	5.0	28	65.5 ± 18.59
GMTA lidocaine	7.4	28	46.3 ± 20.62
GMTA sterile water	7.4	28	57.4 ± 17.99
WMTA lidocaine	5.0	28	51.3 ± 19.24
WMTA sterile water	5.0	28	70.8 ± 26.21
WMTA lidocaine	7.4	28	60.0 ± 20.88
WMTA sterile water	7.4	28	76.3 ± 19.24

2011). The compressive strength values of the latter two products were considerably higher than the experimental material up to 7 days, but they reached peaks as soon as 3 days (Table 3.20).

Appelbaum and associates added sodium fluorosilicate to Portland cement to accelerate its set (as used with concrete), since MTA is ~75% Portland cement. Na_2SiF6 in concentrations of 1–15% weight/weight was mixed with sterile water and

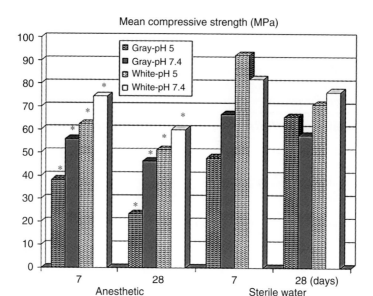

Fig. 3.2 The compressive strength of GMTA and WMTA with different mixing agents, pH, and time from initial mixing until compression test. *When mixed with local anesthetic, WMTA was significantly stronger than GMTA ($p < 0.0001$), pH 7.4 was significantly stronger than pH 5.0 ($p < 0.0001$), and 7-day samples were significantly stronger than 28-day samples ($p < 0.001$). Source: Watts et al. 2007. Reproduced with permission of Elsevier Publishing.

Table 3.20 Compressive strength of experimental Portland cement and MTA up to 7 days. Source: Hwang et al. 2011. Reproduced with permission of Elsevier Publishing.

Compressive strength (MPa) (n = 6)	1 day	3 days	7days
Portland cement	28.06 ± 4.31	43.36 ± 4.39	32.10 ± 1.01
Expt'l Portland cement	5.81 ± 1.17	10.47 ± 1.54	14.88 ± 1.13
Expt'l Portland cement + CaSO$_4$	8.51 ± 0.55	9.66 ± 0.76	13.82 ± 2.99
MTA	27.41 ± 3.83	43.65 ± 8.35	30.77 ± 0.51

Table 3.21 Effect of sodium fluorosilicate on the properties of Portland cement. Source: Appelbaum et al. 2012. Reproduced with permission of Elsevier Publishing.

Group	n	24-h (mean)	n	3-week (mean)
PC	6	23.4	8	42.1
1% SF in PC	9	18.9	8	41.6
2% SF in PC	7	10.7	8	40.9
3% SF in PC	8	10.0	9	38.7
4% SF in PC	8	15.6	7	35.1
5% SF in PC	6	17.9	–	–
10% SF in PC	6	2.00	–	–
15% SF in PC	6	1.80	–	–

Table 3.22 The effect of various mixing and placement techniques on the compressive strength of mineral trioxide aggregate. Source: Basturk *et al.* 2013. Reproduced with permission of Elsevier Publishing.

MTA type	Mixing/placement technique	Mean (MPa)	SD (MPa)
ProRoot	MM + US	101.7	18.64
ProRoot	MM	90.85	25.25
ProRoot	Man M + US	90.78	33.60
ProRoot	Man M	90.77	27.21
Angelus	MM + US	81.36	24.94
Angelus	MM	74.14	28.43
Angelus	Man M + US	54.96	17.47
Angelus	Man M	53.47	22.31

Man M, manual mixing; MM, mechanical mixing; US, ultrasonic agitation.

Table 3.23 Setting time, compressive and flexural strength (in MPa) of modified MTA formulations mixed with water ($n = 3$). Akbari *et al.* 2013.

Group	Setting time in minutes (SD)	Compressive strength (SD)		Flexural strength (SD)
	1 day	1 week	3-point bending @ 1 day	
MTA	229.66 (0.31[a])	1.16 (0.31[a])	2.19 (0.87[a])	0.93 (0.65[b])
MTA+8% nano-SiO_2	202.33 (0.31[b])	2.7 (0.66[a])	2.75 (0.81[a])	1.96 (0.33[b])
MTA+10% nano-SiO_2	199.33 (0.31[b])	1.92 (1.29[a])	2.39 (0.52[a])	1.99 (0.73[b])

Same superscript letters within the same column indicate no significant difference between groups ($p > 0.05$).

tested for compressive strength (in MPa), and setting time (only 1% w/w). It was found that Na_2SiF_6 additions had no effect on setting time but directly reduced compressive strength. Its use is contraindicated. (Appelbaum *et al.* 2012) (Table 3.21).

Basturk and colleagues (2014) measured compressive strength of tooth-colored ProRoot MTA (Dentsply Maillefer, Switzerland) and white MTA Angelus (Brazil). They where mixed mechanically (30 s @ 4,500 rpm) by a saturation technique condensed at 3.22 MPa for 1 min or by agitation using indirect ultrasonic activation. Compressive strength was tested after 4 days. (Table 3.22)

ProRoot MTA had significantly greater compressive strength than MTA Angelus. Mechanical mixing of encapsulated MTA resulted in higher strength values than when mixed manually. Regardless of the mixing techniques, ultrasonic agitation improved compressive strength (Basturk *et al.* 2014).

Nano-SiO_2 (8% and 10%) was added to white MTA powder and mixed with water. The setting time, compressive strength, and flexural strength were measured and compared with pure MTA (Akbari *et al.* 2013 and Table 3.23). Additions

Table 3.24 Compressive strength of materials (Mean ± SD). Basturk *et al.* 2013.

MTA type	Mixing/placement technique	Compressive strength (MPa)
ProRoot	MechM + US	101.71 ± 18.64
ProRoot	MechM	90.85 ± 25.25
ProRoot	ManM + US	90.78 ± 33.60
ProRoot	ManM	77.27 ± 21.58
Angelus	MechM + US	81.36 ± 24.94
Angelus	MechM	74.14 ± 28.43
Angelus	ManM + US	54.96 ± 17.47
Angelus	ManM	53.47 ± 22.31

ManM ≡ manual mixing; MechM ≡ mechanical mixing; US ≡ ultrasonication.

of nano-SiO$_2$ significantly reduced setting time (from 230 min to as low as 199 min) but had no effect on compressive or flexural strength.

Compressive strength of ProRoot MTA (Dentsply, Switzerland) and white MTA Angelus (Angelus, Brazil) were evaluated either by (a) mechanical mixing in capsules (30 s at 4500 rpm), or (b) hand mixing, and both slurries were packed into a mold and compressed at 3.22 MPa for 1 min (Basturk *et al.* 2013). Both mixes (0.34 g H$_2$O/1 g powder) were also molded in 6×4 mm cylindrical specimens while ultrasonic energy was applied to the mold periphery for 30 s, and all specimens were incubated in water for 4 days.

ProRoot MTA displayed significantly greater compressive strength than MTA Angelus (Table 3.24; $p < 0.05$). Ultrasonically agitated groups were stronger in compressive strength than either mechanical mixes alone ($p < 0.001$). Mechanical mixing yielded higher values compared to specimens mixed manually ($p < 0.05$).

Flexural strength

Because MTA sets so slowly and in a moist clinical environment, Walker and associates used *flexural strength* as a measure of the setting of WMTA when exposed to moisture on one or two sides of the specimen after 24 or 72 h (Walker *et al.* 2006). Clinically, the pulpal surface is moistened with a cotton pellet before closing the tooth, the tissue side being wet from exposure to blood and tissue fluids (Torabinejad & Chivian 1999). In the test, the flexural specimen is a slab of material, which is easily kept wet or dry on one or both sides. In this study, it is unclear whether the tension or compression side was moistened, which might affect properties. The highest values were recorded at 24 h when both sides of the flexural specimen were exposed to moisture (Table 3.25).

Table 3.25   Three-point flexural strength in MPa ± SD of WMTA when wetted on various sides at 24 and 72 hours ($n = 10$). Source: Walker *et al.* 2006. Reproduced with permission of Elsevier Publishing.

24h/moist/2-sided	14.27 ± 1.96^{sd}
24h/moist/1-sided	10.77 ± 1.44^{nsd}
72h/moist/2-sided	11.16 ± 0.96^{nsd}
72h/moist/1-sided	11.18 ± 0.99^{nsd}

sd ≡ significant difference.
nsd ≡ no significant difference.

Table 3.26   Flexural strength and porosity of materials (mean ± SD). Basturk *et al.* 2014.

MTA type	Mixing/placement technique	Flexural strength (MPa)	Porosity (%)
ProRoot	MechM + US	10.5 ± 1.82	1.81 ± 1.25
ProRoot	MechM	9.99 ± 1.36	1.29 ± 1.34
ProRoot	ManM + US	11.3 ± 1.71	1.11 ± 0.46
ProRoot	ManM	10.5 ± 2.14	1.58 ± 1.62
Angelus	MechM + US	8.73 ± 2.11	1.85 ± 1.37
Angelus	MechM	8.91 ± 1.99	1.11 ± 0.33
Angelus	ManM + US	8.96 ± 1.45	1.44 ± 0.28
Angelus	ManM	9.52 ± 2.12	1.48 ± 0.42

ManM, manual mixing; MechM, mechanical mixing; US, ultrasonication.

The 3-point flexural strength and micro CT porosity of ProRoot MTA (Dentsply, Switzerland) and white MTA Angelus (Angelus, Brazil) were evaluated either by (a) mechanical mixing in capsules (30 s at 4500 rpm), or (b) hand mixing, and both slurries were packed into a mold and compressed at 3.22 MPa for 1 min. Both mixes (0.34 g H_2O/1 g powder) were also molded while ultrasonic energy was applied to the mold periphery for 30 s, and all specimens were incubated in water for 4 days (Basturk *et al.* 2014).

No statistical differences were found for all groups for flexural strength or porosity (Table 3.26). Mechanical mixing saves time, but imparts no mechanical advantage to the MTA material over hand mixing.

Shear strength

Shear strength was measured between a resin-based composite and MTA, a calcium-enriched MTA, and resin-reinforced glass ionomer cement. Although no data is given, shear bond strength was greatest for the glass ionomer cement, and there was no difference between the regular MTA and calcium-enriched

MTA. Acid etching also had no effect on the MTA versions. All failures were cohesive (Oskoee *et al.* 2011).

Push-out strength

Push-out strength was used by Loxley and associates to determine the effect of MTA, SuperEBA, and IRM against bovine dentin after immersion in NaOCl, 35% H_2O_2 (Superoxol), $NaBO_3 \cdot H_2O$, and various combinations for 7 days (Loxley *et al.* 2003). MTA push-out values were highest against saline-immersed dentin and lowest when immersed in $NaBO_3 \cdot H_2O$ + saline. Values for SuperEBA were highest against dry dentin and lowest against $NaBO_3 \cdot H_2O$ + saline. Values for IRM were highest when exposed to 35% H_2O_2 (Loxley *et al.* 2003).

Yan and associates soaked MTA-filled dentin discs in full-strength NaOCL, 2% chlorhexidine, Glyde™ File Prep (EDTA/carbamide peroxide gel), and saline for two hours and measured the push-out strength. Glyde File Prep values were significantly lower than those of the other agents tested (Yan *et al.* 2006).

Shear bond strength

Shear bond strength using two different bonding agents was measured between a resin-based composite (Dyract), a polyacid modified composite ("compomer" Z250), and WMTA. One bonding agent was significantly stronger than the other, and the bond to the compomer was stronger than the resin-based composite (Table 3.27) (Tunç *et al.* 2008).

Tanomaru-Filho and associates measured the setting time and compressive strength at 24 h and 21 days of white Portland cement (to which 20% W/W of four radiopaquing agents was added) and compared them with the strength of MTA-Angelus. There were small but significant strength differences when compared with unmodified Portland cement ($41.2^a \pm 3.4$ MPa @ 21 days). Addition of bismuth oxide resulted in the weakest composition ($22.9^c \pm 4.8$ MPa) when tested at 21 days. Zirconium oxide ($37.1^a \pm 7.4$ MPa) and calcium tungstate

Table 3.27 Mean shear bond strength in MPa ± SD of two bonding agents and two resin-based restorative materials to WMTA. Source: Tunç *et al.* 2008. Reproduced with permission of Elsevier Publishing.

	3M/ESPE single bond	3M/ESPE Prompt L-Pop (*n* = 10)
Z250	13.22 ± 1.22^a	10.73 ± 1.67^b
Dyract	15.09 ± 2.74^a	5.44 ± 0.86^c

Equivalent superscript letters ≡ no significant difference.

$(36.6^a \pm 8.3$ MPa) displayed compressive strength similar to that of MTA-Angelus $(43.4^a \pm 6.5$ MPa) and unmodified Portland cement (Tanomaru-Filho *et al.* 2012). (Equivalent superscript letters indicate no significant differences.)

Overview

Using compressive strength as a measure, MTA products are very weak, but gain strength over time. It is fortunate that these products are not used in stress-bearing structures, at least not initially. Constant exposure to water and the temperature of the mouth can be expected to drive the chemical reaction to completion. Coupling MTA to structurally rigid restorative materials using modern bonding agents provides adequate strength to withstand occlusal forces in most situations, but the final restoration should be placed at a subsequent appointment, at least a few days later. Current studies indicate that more time between the use of MTA and the final restoration is beneficial.

Dental impact injuries in younger patients often lead to pulpal necrosis, which usually results in the cessation of formation in developing roots. The open apex and thin dentinal walls of the immature roots create endodontic and restorative challenges for the dental practitioner. Push-out and shear fracture tests are relatively easy to fabricate and perform and are often used to measure MTA properties of importance, as described below for research papers from the recent literature.

Push-out strength was used as a measure of early bond strength of ProRoot MTA to dentin after setting for 48 h. The MTA was then modified with $CaCl_2$ as an accelerator in the mix. Both groups were then irrigated for 30 min with either 3.5% NaOCl or 2% chlorhexidine. Accelerated MTA with the NaOCl and chlorhexidine rinses were significantly stronger than unaltered MTA with the same rinses. Accelerated MTA with the NaOCl rinse registered the highest values; unaltered MTA with the chlorhexidine rinse was weaker than the control group, which only had a wet cotton pellet placed over the MTA (Table 3.28) (Hong *et al.* 2010).

Biopure® MTAD® antibacterial root cleanser was paired with a diode laser and both were used alone and with a negative control to prepare simulated drilled pulp chamber walls against WMTA for push-out retention measurements in human teeth. The no-treatment control values were significantly higher $(7.88 \pm 0.37$ MPa), followed by values for pulp chambers treated with the diode laser $(6.74 \pm 0.48$ MPa) or the root cleanser alone $(6.86 \pm 0.66$ MPa). The combined diode laser treatment plus cleanser displayed the lowest values $(5.95 \pm 0.40$ MPa) and are not recommended (Saghiri *et al.* 2012).

White MTA was placed in human root sections and tested for push-out strength after 72 h. The material was mixed using ultrasonic, mechanical trituration, or

Table 3.28 Push-out values of MTA and accelerated MTA with two different rinses at 48 hours (in MPa). Source: Hong *et al.* 2010. Reproduced with permission of Elsevier Publishing.

Groups	Rinse	Push-out value
MTA (1.0g MTA + 0.3mL H_2O)	3.5% NaOCl	63.13 ± 18.03[b]
MTA (1.0g MTA + 0.3mL H_2O)	2% chlorhexidine	31.33 ± 13.40[c]
Accelerated MTA (1g MTA+0.1g $CaCl_2$+0.25mL H_2O)	3.5% NaOCl	98.06 ± 9.18[a]
Accelerated MTA (1g MTA+0.1g $CaCl_2$+0.25mL H_2O)	2% chlorhexidine	82.18 ±13.68[ad]
Control (wet cotton pellet)		66.34 ± 6.74[bd]

Means ± standard deviations. Equivalent superscript letter ≡ no significant difference. ($p > 0.05$).

Table 3.29 Push-out bond strength of MTA using three mixing methods at 3 days (in MPa). Source: Shahi *et al.* 2012. Reproduced with permission of Elsevier Publishing.

Ultrasonic	105.67 ± 12.79
Conventional	118.95 ± 12.76
Trituration	99.60 ± 14.27

conventional hand mixing (Table 3.29). No significant differences were found (Shahi *et al.* 2012).

MTA and BioAggregate cements were placed in artificial furcation perforations in extracted human molars, stored for 4 days, and measured by a push-out test at pH 7.4 or pH 5.4, with both groups then stored at pH 7.4 for 30 more days. MTA displayed significantly higher push-out values than BioAggregate, but MTA values were significantly lower after low pH exposure at 4 days. After 34 days, MTA gained strength after exposure to low pH and exceeded BioAggregate (Table 3.30) (Hashem & Wanees Amin 2012).

Twenty slices of extracted human root chambers were filled with ProRoot WMTA for 4 days and exposed to solutions at pH 7.4, 6.4, 5.4, and 4.4, followed by push-out tests. Strength decreased significantly and progressively as pH was lowered, down to 2.47 MPa at pH 4.4 (Table 3.31) (Shokouhinejad *et al.* 2010).

In a similar study to the one above, the pH was adjusted above 20 slices of extracted human roots by exposing filled root lumen with ProRoot WMTA, but this time for 3 days. Significant differences were noted between pH values of 7.4, 8.4, 9.4, and 10.4, with the highest push-out strength at pH 8.4 and the lowest at pH 10.4. Adhesive failure was noted for all specimens under light-microscopic examination (Table 3.32) (Shahi *et al.* 2012).

Gancedo-Caravia & Garcia-Barbero measured the push-out strength of MTA when stored dry and wet for up to 28 days. Values up to 5.0 MPa were shown for dry specimens versus up to 10.4 MPa for specimens stored wet. External

Table 3.30 Push-out strength of MTA and BioAggregate products in MPA at two pH levels up to 34 days. Source: Hashem *et al.* 2012. Reproduced with permission of Elsevier Publishing.

	MTA			**BioAggregate**	
pH 7.4*	pH 5.4**	pH 7.4*	pH 5.4**		
4 days	8.49		5.36	4.66	4.72
34 days	7.56		10.12	7.83	6.71

*Acetic acid pH 5.4 for 4 days + **phosphate-buffered saline (PBS) pH 7.4 for 30 days.

Table 3.31 Push-out strength as a function of pH at 4 days. Source: Shokouhinejad *et al.* 2010. Reproduced with permission of Elsevier Publishing.

	Push-out strength at 4 days in MPa
pH 7.4	~7.28
pH 6.4	~5.80
pH 5.4	~3.60
pH 4.4	~2.47

1 mm/min crosshead speed; predominantly adhesive failures.

Table 3.32 Push-out strength of WMTA at 3 days (in MPa). Source: Shahi *et al.* 2012. Reproduced with permission of Elsevier Publishing.

pH 7.4	7.68
pH 8.4	9.46
pH 9.4	7.10
pH 10.4	5.68

moisture is needed by MTA to complete its curing process (Gancedo-Caravia & Garcia-Barbero 2006).

Atabek and associates studied the shear bond strength against one resin-based composite of three bonding agents from the same manufacturer, and found that a two-step product (One-Step Plus) was significantly stronger at 96 h (18.4 MPa) than a one-step (All-Bond SE, 15.1 MPa) and a three-step product (All-Step 3, 14.9 MPa) (Atabek *et al.* 2012).

MICROHARDNESS

Hardness is a composite property related to the indentation resistance of a material and is a very easily measured property. It is expressed as a number using the area of the indentation and its relationship to the applied load (gf/m^2 or $178F/d^2$, where F is the load in kg and d is the diameter in mm). It is also related to a material's compressive, tensile, and flexural strength. In dentistry, microhardness is usually used where the indenter is a cut diamond with shallow face angles and the size of the indentation is measured with a metallurgical microscope.

Microhardness is a convenient and even more easily measured property than compressive, push-out, or shear bond strength. For accurate comparison with other materials, specimens at least 6 mm thick and 12 mm wide are required, and specimens should be polished, conditions that are excluded in clinical endodontics. Thus, tests in this field are mainly comparative for use within each study.

Open tooth apices were simulated using 44 human tooth roots, which were then sealed with either ProRoot GMTA or ProRoot WMTA at either 2 mm or 5 mm from the apex, immediately in one step or in a second step after 24 h. After 48 h of storage in methylene blue, samples were sectioned and examined for microleakage, and microhardness (HV_{100}) measurements were made. Gray MTA leaked less (~30%) than WMTA (95%), and the 1-step leaked more (~73%) than the 2-step (~55%) procedure. The authors state that the 5 mm samples were significantly harder than the 2 mm, but no data are given. They recommend GMTA, 5 mm long fills, and a 2-step procedure with final endodontic filling after 24 h (Matt *et al.* 2004).

Sixty-four specimens of ProRoot WMTA and Aureoseal were packed in stainless steel molds and stored in solutions at pH 4.4 and 7.4 for 7 days. Microhardness was significantly higher at pH 7.4 for both products (Table 3.33). Analysis with SEM showed more unhydrated structures at pH 4.4 than 7.4 for WMTA, and amorphous structures at both pH values for Aureoseal (Giuliani *et al.* 2010).

White MTA was packed into 60 glass tubes and exposed to neutral and alkaline solutions at a pH of 7.4, 8.4, 9.4, and 10.4 for 3 days. Significant differences in microhardness were observed, with harder surfaces at pH exposures at 8.4 and 9.4. Imaging with SEM showed greater porosity and unhydrated structures at pH 7.4 and 10.4, with needle-like structures at pH 9.4 and amorphous structures at 10.4 (Table 3.34) (Saghiri *et al.* 2009).

Namazikhah and associates noted significantly lower microhardness of WMTA as the pH was lowered (Table 3.35) (Namazikhah *et al.* 2008).

Table 3.33 Vickers microhardness of two MTA products (HV_{50}, 50 gf load, 10 s dwell) at 7 days (SD). Source: Giuliani *et al.* 2010. Reproduced with permission of Elsevier Publishing.

	pH 4.4	**pH 7.2**
ProRoot WMTA	30.24 ± 1.47	37.54 ± 1.52
Aureoseal	28.67 ± 1.07	40.63 ± 1.35

Table 3.34 Vickers microhardness of WMTA at four pH levels at 3 days (HV$_{50}$) ± SD. Source: Shahi *et al.* 2009. Reproduced with permission of Elsevier Publishing.

pH 7.4	58.28 ± 8.21
pH 8.4	68.84 ± 7.19
pH 9.4	67.32 ± 7.22
pH 10.4	59.22 ± 9.14

Table 3.35 Vickers microhardness of WMTA at four pH levels (HV$_{50}$) at 4 days ± SD. Source: Namazikhah *et al.* 2008. Used with permission of John Wiley & Sons, Inc.

pH 4.4	14.34 ± 6.48
pH 5.4	37.75 ± 1.75
pH 6.4	40.73 ± 3.15
pH 7.4	53.19 ± 4.124

COLOR AND AESTHETICS

Discoloration of MTA material and surrounding tooth structure remains a challenge for clinicians, as do manipulation problems (sandy texture), extended setting time, and difficulty to re-enter due to the hardness of the material (Watts *et al.* 2007; Boutsioukis *et al.* 2008). Dentsply Tulsa Dental Specialties introduced a tooth-colored version referred to as WMTA (Glickman & Koch 2000). Discoloration of teeth with MTA used as a pulpotomy material was reported in three cases (Maroto *et al.* 2005; Naik & Hegde 2005; Percinoto *et al.* 2006). White MTA was immersed in phosphate-buffered saline and was observed to discolor after 3 days (Watts *et al.* 2007). Dark discolorations were observed from most WMTA root canal fillings after re-opening extracted teeth after 10 days in water (Boutsioukis *et al.* 2008). These authors also noted difficulty re-entering WMTA fillings with rotary instruments. Salts of iron and manganese were thought to be responsible for discoloration (Asgary *et al.* 2005; Dammaschke *et al.* 2005; Bortoluzzi *et al.* 2007).

One case report described a maxillary central incisor root perforation on the facial side, treated with GMTA. After 6 months, graying of the gingiva was noted, followed by retreatment with WMTA and sealer to correct the discoloration (Bortoluzzi *et al.* 2007). Another case report describes discoloration in a WMTA-filled vital partial pulpotomy in a maxillary central incisor that returned 17 months after treatment. Upon re-entry, a dentin bridge was noted. At this point, some of the outermost WMTA was removed, which, with bleaching, improved discoloration (Belobrov & Parashos 2011).

Discoloration of even the newer version of ProRoot MTA still seems to be a problem in some clinical cases. The material should therefore be used in aesthetic areas (coronal portions of anterior teeth) with caution. Clinicians are advised to warn patients that some discoloration may occur, which is a small disadvantage when considering the many other benefits of this material.

PHYSICOCHEMICAL PROPERTIES

In spite of the minor differences between GMTA and WMTA materials noted above, calcium, which triggers the chain of physicochemical reactions in biological environments, is released in quantities significantly larger than those of any other cation from WMTA. The consequence is the formation of hydroxylapatite in a diffusion-controlled physicochemical reaction between hydroxylapatite and dentin, leading to a tenacious chemical bond between the dentin and WMTA, filling any gap between the two (Table 3.36 and Fig. 3.3) (Sarkar *et al.* 2005).

These structural characteristics, as well as the dominance of released calcium ions, are identical to those displayed by both GMTA and WMTA. It therefore appears that the alteration in composition and manufacturing process that has been used to whiten MTA exerts little or no influence on the nature of its *in vitro* physicochemical activities. We consider this activity to be the fundamental basis of the reported favorable sealing ability, biocompatibility, and dentinogenic activity of GMTA (Sarkar *et al.* 2005). The indistinguishable *in vivo* physicochemical response of the two materials led these authors to conclude that the clinical performance of WMTA is not any different from that of GMTA. This conclusion is bolstered by two studies that show that the two materials are equally effective in canine pulpotomies (Menezes *et al.* 2004), and demonstrate similar mechanisms of mineralization in rat connective tissues (Holland *et al.* 2002).

Table 3.36 Semi-quantitative elemental composition (wt. %) of areas identified as M, I, and D in Fig. 3.3C. Source: Sarkar *et al.* 2005. Reproduced with permission of Elsevier Publishing.

	Ca	Al	Si	Bi	Fe	Mg	O	S	C	P
GMTA (M)	1.1	2.6	11.8	7.8	7.5	1.4	41.5	1.3	5.0	–
Interfacial layer (I)	21.5	0.6	3.0	5.6	–	0.1	60.6	–	4.9	3.7
Dentin (D)	31.7	–	–	–	–	0.4	50.8	–	6.0	11.1

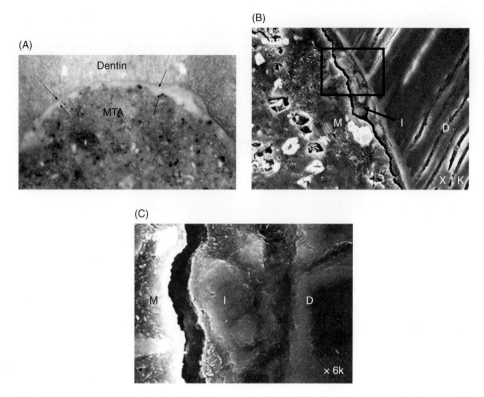

Fig. 3.3 (A) Typical optical photomicrograph of an MTA–dentin cross-section in a tooth furcation (orig. mag. 200×). (B) Typical scanning electron micrograph of a GMTA-dentin cross-section (1000×). M, MTA; I, interface; D, dentin. (C) Area identified by box in B at a higher magnification (6000×). Source: Sarkar *et al.* 2005. Reproduced with permission of Elsevier Publishing.

The "self-sealing" property of MTA from the secondary formation of hydroxylapatite is similar to the "self-sealing" ability of conventional dental amalgam, which forms tin-rich compounds over time at the interface between the tooth and the filling material. This phenomenon requires more research.

The bond strength of two MTA sealers (Endo-CPM sealer, EGEO SRL, Argentina) and MTA Fillapex (Angelus, Brazil), and an epoxy resin-based sealer (AH Plus sealer, Dentsply–De Trey, Germany) was tested on extracted human teeth after lateral condensation with gutta-percha (Assmann *et al.* 2012). After rinsing with 2.5% NaOCl and 17% EDTA and distilled water, the roots were sectioned and push-out strength of the root canal contents determined (Table 3.37).

A two- to three-fold advantage in push-out strength was seen for Endo-CPM sealer (almost the same composition as original MTA formulations) compared

Table 3.37   Dentin bond strength for samples filled with Endo-CPM Sealer (CPM), MTA Fillapex (FLX), and AH Plus Sealer (AHP). Assmann et al. 2012.

	N	**Median resistance**	**25%**	**75%**
CPM	15	8.265[b]	6.143	9.687
FLX	15	2.041[a]	1.490	3.039
AHP	15	3.034[a]	2.358	3.634

Push-out test medians and percentile values (MPa).
Different superscript letters show statistical difference ($p < 0.05$).

to FLX and AHP; MTA Fillapex contains other resins, silica, and MTA. Sites of failure for FLX and AHP were at the sealer-dentin interface, but were mixed for CPM. Voids were observed in radiographs of the teeth before sectioning for CPM but not for the other two.

Push-out bond strength was measured by Nagas et al. (2012) as a function of moisture within the canals after rinsing with (a) 95% ethanol (dry), (b) drying with paper points, (c) moist (canals were dried with low vacuum followed by 1 paper point for 1 second), and (d) wet (the canals remained totally flooded). Four sealers were used: (1) AH Plus (Dentsply-Tulsa, USA, (2) iRoot SP (Innovative BioCeramix, Canada), (3) MTA Fillapex (Angelus, Brazil), and (4) Epiphany (Pentron, USA).

iRoot SP had significantly more bond strength to root dentin, followed by AH Plus, Epiphany+Resilon, and MTA Fillapex. Moist and wet conditions yielded the highest values. Canals should be left slightly moist before applying sealer (Table 3.38).

Four endodontic sealers, subjected to the System B heat source continuous-wave plugger (Analytic Technology, Redmond, Washington, USA) were evaluated for heat transfer to the root surface (Viapiana et al. 2014). AH Plus (Dentsply, UK), Pulp Canal Sealer (Kerr, Orange, California), MTA Fillapex (Angelus, Brazil) and a prototype Portland cement sealer were assessed for heat generation or transmission at the apical, middle, and cervical positions of the root surface, using thermocouples with the tooth suspended in air, in Hank's balanced salt solution, or gelatinized Hank's balanced salt solution. Chemical changes in the sealers were monitored by FTIR spectroscopy. Heat changes to the compressive strength and setting time were also measured.

The heated plugger was warmed to 80°C at the shank, and it took up to 1.5 min for heat to peak at the mid-root surface, returning to body temperature at 6 min. Heat dissipated for all the sealers in the mid-root and cervix, with the greatest increase (60°C) recorded in air. Temperature rise at the apex was unaffected by any of the four sealers, but a larger temperature rise was noted for AH

Table 3.38 Distribution of push-out bond strength (in MPa) and failure modes. Nagas et al. 2012.

Moisture	Dry					Normal moisture					Moist					Wet				
Root filling	MPa	A1	A2	C	M	MPa	A1	A2	C	M	MPa	A1	A2	C	M	MPa	A1	A2	C	M
AH Plus+GP	**1.0**	15	2	8	0	**1.7**	3	12	7	3	**1.8**	1	14	6	4	**0.4**	14	0	11	0
iRoot SP+GP	**2.5**	13	3	8	1	**2.9**	2	15	6	2	**3.1**	0	16	7	2	**1.7**	16	1	8	0
MTA Fillapex+GP	**0.25**	13	0	12	0	**0.5**	1	11	11	2	**1.2**	2	12	9	2	**0**	23	0	2	0
Epiphany+Resilon	**0.70**	15	2	7	1	**0.8**	3	10	10	2	**1.1**	3	10	9	3	**0.3**	13	0	12	0

A ≡ adhesive (A1 ≡ sealer/dentin interface; A2 ≡ sealer/core material interface); C ≡ cohesive; M ≡ mixed.

Plus, reducing its setting time and strength; the chemical composition of AH Plus was changed by high temperature. Temperature and humidity also influenced heat dissipation during the condensation obturation technique, and root canal sealers presented different conductive/isolating properties (Viapiana *et al*. 2014).

ACKNOWLEDGMENT

The authors thank Nikhil Sarkar, PhD (Louisiana State University, School of Dentistry), who collaborated on the early stages of this chapter.

REFERENCES

Akbari, M., Zebarjad, S. M., Nategh, B., *et al*. (2013) Effect of nano silica on setting time and physical properties of mineral trioxide aggregate. *Journal of Endodontics* **39**, 1448–51.

Antonijevic D., Medigovic, I., Zrilic, M., *et al*. (2013) The influence of different radiopacifying agents on the radiopacity, compressive strength, setting time, and porosity of Portland cement. *Clinical Oral Investigations*. DOI 10.1007/s00784-013-1130-0. Published online 15 November 2013.American National Standards Institute/American Dental Association. (1991) Revised American National Standard/American Dental Association Specification N° 30 for dental zinc oxide eugenol cements and zinc oxide noneugenol cements 7.5. Chicago, IL.

Asgary, S., Parirokh, M., Eghbal, M. J., *et al*. (2005) Chemical differences between white and gray mineral trioxide aggregate. *Journal of Endodontics* **31**(2), 101–3.

Assmann, E., Scarparo, R. K., Böttcher, D. E., *et al*. (2012) Dentin bond strength of two mineral trioxide aggregate–based and one epoxy resin–based sealers. *Journal of Endodontics* **38**(2), 219–21.

Atabek, D., Sillelioğlu, H., Olmez, A. (2012) Bond strength of adhesive systems to mineral trioxide aggregate with different time intervals. *Journal of Endodontics* **38**(9), 1288–92. doi: 10.1016/j.joen.2012.06.004

Appelbaum, K.S., Stewart, J.T., Hartwell, G.R. (2012) Effect of sodium fluorosilicate on the properties of Portland cement. *Journal of Endodontics* **38**(7), 1001–3.

Basturk, F.B, Nekoofar, F.M., Günday, M., *et al*. (2013) The effect of various mixing and placement techniques on the compressive strength of mineral trioxide aggregate. *Journal of Endodontics* **39**, 111–14.

Basturk, F. B., Nekoofar, M. H., Günday, M., *et al*. (2014). Effect of various mixing and placement techniques on the flexural strength and porosity of mineral trioxide aggregate. *Journal of Endodontics in press*.

Belobrov, I., Parashos, P. (2011) Treatment of tooth discoloration after the use of white mineral trioxide aggregate. *Journal of Endodontics* **37**(7), 1017–20. doi: 10.1016/j.joen.2011.04.003

Bortoluzzi, E. A., Broon, N. J., Bramante, C. M., *et al*. (2006) Sealing ability of MTA and radiopaque Portland cement with or without calcium chloride for root-end filling. *Journal of Endodontics* **32**(9), 897–900. doi: 10.1016/j.joen.2006.04.006

Bortoluzzi, E. A. S., Araújo G., Guerreiro Tanomaru, J. M., *et al.* (2007) Marginal gingiva discoloration by gray MTA: a case report. *Journal of Endodontics* **33**(3), 325–7. doi: 10.1016/j.joen.2006.09.012

Bortoluzzi, E. A., Broon, N. J., Bramante, C. M., *et al.* (2009) The influence of calcium chloride on the setting time, solubility, disintegration, and pH of mineral trioxide aggregate and white Portland cement with a radiopacifier. *Journal of Endodontics* **35**(4), 550–4. doi: 10.1016/j.joen.2008.12.018

Boutsioukis, C., Noula, G., Lambrianidis, T. (2008) Ex vivo study of the efficiency of two techniques for the removal of mineral trioxide aggregate used as a root canal filling material. *Journal of Endodontics* **34**(10), 1239–42. doi: 10.1016/j.joen.2008.07.018

Bozeman, T. B., Lemon, R. R., Eleazer, P. D. (2006) Elemental analysis of crystal precipitate from gray and white MTA. *Journal of Endodontics* **32**(5), 425–8. doi: 10.1016/j.joen.2005.08.009

Cavenago, B. C., Pereira, T. C., Duarte, M. A. H., *et al.* (2014) Influence of powder-to-water ratio on radiopacity, setting time, pH, calcium ion release and a micro-CT volumetric solubility of white mineral trioxide aggregate. *International Endodontic Journal* **47**, 120–6.

Chng, H. K., Islam, I., Yap, A. U., *et al.* (2005) Properties of a new root-end filling material. *Journal of Endodontics* **31**(9), 665–8.

Çinar, Ç., Odabaş, M., Gürel,, M. A., *et al.* (2013) The effects of incorporation of silver-zeolite on selected properties of mineral trioxide aggregate. *Dental Materials Journal* **32**(6), 872–6.

Dammaschke, T., Gerth, H. U., Züchner, H., *et al.* (2005). Chemical and physical surface and bulk material characterization of white ProRoot MTA and two Portland cements. *Dental Materials* **21**(8), 731–8. doi: 10.1016/j.dental.2005.01.019

Danesh, G., Dammaschke, T., Gerth, H. U., *et al.* (2006). A comparative study of selected properties of ProRoot mineral trioxide aggregate and two Portland cements. *International Endodontics Journal* **39**(3), 213–19. doi: 10.1111/j.1365-2591.2006.01076.x

Ding, S. J., Kao, C. T., Shie, M. Y., *et al.* (2008) The physical and cytological properties of white MTA mixed with Na2HPO4 as an accelerant. *Journal of Endodontics* **34**(6), 748–51. doi: 10.1016/j.joen.2008.02.041

Fridland, M., Rosado, R. (2003). Mineral trioxide aggregate (MTA) solubility and porosity with different water-to-powder ratios. *Journal of Endodontics* **29**(12), 814–17. doi: 10.1097/00004770-200312000-00007

Fridland, M., Rosado, R. (2005). MTA solubility: a long term study. *Journal of Endodontics* **31**(5), 376–9.

Gancedo-Caravia, L., Garcia-Barbero, E. (2006). Influence of humidity and setting time on the push-out strength of mineral trioxide aggregate obturations. *Journal of Endodontics* **32**(9), 894–6. doi: 10.1016/j.joen.2006.03.004

Giuliani, V., Nieri, M., Pace, R., *et al.* (2010). Effects of pH on surface hardness and microstructure of mineral trioxide aggregate and Aureoseal: an in vitro study. *Journal of Endodontics* **36**(11), 1883–6. doi: 10.1016/j.joen.2010.08.015

Glickman, G. N., Koch, K. A. (2000). 21st-century endodontics. *Journal of the American Dental Association* **131 Suppl**, 39S–46S.

Hashem, A. A., Wanees Amin, S. A. (2012). The effect of acidity on dislodgment resistance of mineral trioxide aggregate and bioaggregate in furcation perforations: an in vitro comparative study. *Journal of Endodontics* **38**(2), 245–9. doi: 10.1016/j.joen.2011.09.013

Hawley, M., Webb, T. D., Goodell, G. G. (2010) Effect of varying water-to-powder ratios on the setting expansion of white and gray mineral trioxide aggregate. *Journal of Endodontics* **36**(8), 1377–9. doi: 10.1016/j.joen.2010.03.010

Holland, R., Souza, V., Nery, M. J., *et al.* (2002) Reaction of rat connective tissue to implanted dentin tubes filled with a white mineral trioxide aggregate. *Brazilian Dental Journal* **13**(1), 23–6.

Hong, S. T., Bae, K. S., Baek, S. H., *et al.* (2010) Effects of root canal irrigants on the push-out strength and hydration behavior of accelerated mineral trioxide aggregate in its early setting phase. *Journal of Endodontics* **36**(12), 1995–9. doi: 10.1016/j.joen.2010.08.039

Húngaro Duarte, M. A., de Oliveira El Kadre, G. D., Vivan, R. R., *et al.* (2009) Radiopacity of portland cement associated with different radiopacifying agents. *Journal of Endodontics* **35**(5), 737–40. doi: 10.1016/j.joen.2009.02.006

Hwang, Y. C., Kim, D. H., Hwang, I. N., *et al.* (2011) Chemical constitution, physical properties, and biocompatibility of experimentally manufactured Portland cement. *Journal of Endodontics* **37**(1), 58–62. doi: 10.1016/j.joen.2010.09.004

International Organization for Standardization. (2001) *Dental root canal sealing materials ISO* 6786.

Islam, I., Chng, H. K., Yap, A. U. (2006). Comparison of the physical and mechanical properties of MTA and portland cement. *Journal of Endodontics* **32**(3), 193–7. doi: 10.1016/j.joen.2005.10.043

Kogan, P., He, J., Glickman, G. N., *et al.* (2006). The effects of various additives on setting properties of MTA. *Journal of Endodontics* **32**(6), 569–72. doi: 10.1016/j.joen.2005.08.006

Linsuwanont, P. (2003) MTA apexification combined with conventional root canal retreatment. *Australian Endodontics Journal* **29**(1), 45–9.

Loxley, E. C., Liewehr, F. R., Buxton, T. B., *et al.* 3rd (2003) The effect of various intracanal oxidizing agents on the push-out strength of various perforation repair materials. *Oral Surgery, Oral Medicine, Oral Pathology, Oral Radiology and Endodontics* **95**(4), 490–4. doi: 10.1067/moe.2003.32

Maroto, M., Barbería, E., Planells, P., *et al.* (2005) Dentin bridge formation after mineral trioxide aggregate (MTA) pulpotomies in primary teeth. *American Journal of Dentistry* **18**(3), 151–4.

Massi, S., Tanomaru-Filho, M., Silva, G. F., *et al.* (2011) pH, calcium ion release, and setting time of an experimental mineral trioxide aggregate-based root canal sealer. *Journal of Endodontics* **37**(6), 844–6. doi: 10.1016/j.joen.2011.02.033

Matt, G. D., Thorpe, J. R., Strother, J. M., *et al.* (2004) Comparative study of white and gray mineral trioxide aggregate (MTA) simulating a one- or two-step apical barrier technique. *Journal of Endodontics* **30**(12), 876–9.

Menezes, R., Bramante, C. M., Letra, A., *et al.* (2004) Histologic evaluation of pulpotomies in dog using two types of mineral trioxide aggregate and regular and white Portland cements as wound dressings. *Oral Surgery, Oral Medicine, Oral Pathology, Oral Radiology and Endodontics* **98**(3), 376–9. doi: 10.1016/s107921040400215x

Midy, V., Dard, M., Hollande, E. (2001). Evaluation of the effect of three calcium phosphate powders on osteoblast cells. *Journal of Materials Science: Materials in Medicine* **12**(3), 259–65.

Nagas, E., Uyanik, M. O., Eymirli, A., *et al.* (2012). Dentin moisture conditions affect the adhesion of root canal sealers. *Journal of Endodontics* **38**, 240–4.

Naik, S., Hegde, A. H. (2005) Mineral trioxide aggregate as a pulpotomy agent in primary molars: an in vivo study. *Journal of the Indian Society of Pedodontics and Preventive Dentistry* **23**(1), 13–16.

Namazikhah, M. S., Nekoofar, M. H., Sheykhrezae, M. S., *et al.* (2008) The effect of pH on surface hardness and microstructure of mineral trioxide aggregate. *International Endodics Journal* **41**(2), 108–16. doi: 10.1111/j.1365-2591.2007.01325.x

Oskoee, S. S., Kimyai, S., Bahari, M., *et al.* (2011) Comparison of shear bond strength of calcium-enriched mixture cement and mineral trioxide aggregate to composite resin. *Journal of Contemporary Dental Practice* **12**(6), 457–62.

Ozdemir, H. O. B., Ozçelik, Karabucak, B., Cehreli, Z. C. (2008) Calcium ion diffusion from mineral trioxide aggregate through simulated root resorption defects. *Dental Traumatology* **24**(1), 70–3. doi: 10.1111/j.1600-9657.2006.00512.x

Percinoto, C., de Castro, A. M., Pinto, L. M. (2006) Clinical and radiographic evaluation of pulpotomies employing calcium hydroxide and trioxide mineral aggregate. *General Dentistry* **54**(4), 258–61.

Poggio, C., Lombardini, M., Alessandro, C., *et al.* (2007) Solubility of root-end-filling materials: a comparative study. *Journal of Endodontics* **33**(9), 1094–7. doi: 10.1016/j.joen.2007.05.021

Porter, M. L., Bertó A, Primus, C. M., *et al.* (2010) Physical and chemical properties of new-generation endodontic materials. *Journal of Endodontics* **36**(3), 524–8. doi: 10.1016/j.joen.2009.11.012

Saghiri, M. A., Garcia-Godoy, F., Lotfi, M., *et al.* (2012) Effects of diode laser and MTAD on the push-out bond strength of mineral trioxide aggregate–dentin interface. *Photomedicine and Laser Surgery* **30**(10), 587–91. doi: 10.1089/pho.2012.3291

Saghiri, M. A., Lotfi, M., Saghiri, A. M., *et al.* (2009) Scanning electron micrograph and surface hardness of mineral trioxide aggregate in the presence of alkaline pH. *Journal of Endodontics* **35**(5), 706–10. doi: 10.1016/j.joen.2009.01.017

Santos, A. D., Moraes, J. C., Araujo, E. B., *et al.* (2005) Physico-chemical properties of MTA and a novel experimental cement. *International Endodontics Journal* **38**(7), 443–7. doi: 10.1111/j.1365-2591.2005.00963.x

Sarkar, N. K., Caicedo, R., Ritwik, P., *et al.* (2005) Physicochemical basis of the biologic properties of mineral trioxide aggregate. *Journal of Endodontics* **31**(2), 97–100.

Shahi, S., Rahimi, S., Yavari, H. R., *et al.* (2012) Effects of various mixing techniques on push-out bond strengths of white mineral trioxide aggregate. *Journal of Endodontics* **38**(4), 501–4. doi: 10.1016/j.joen.2012.01.001

Shie, M. Y., Huang, T. H., Kao, C. T., *et al.* (2009) The effect of a physiologic solution pH on properties of white mineral trioxide aggregate. *Journal of Endodontics* **35**(1), 98–101. doi: 10.1016/j.joen.2008.09.015

Shokouhinejad, N., Sabeti, M., Hasheminasab, M., *et al.* (2010) Push-out bond strength of resilon/epiphany self-etch to intraradicular dentin after retreatment: A preliminary. *Journal of Endodontics* **36** (3), 493–6 DOI: 10.1016/j.joen.2009.11.009

Silva, E. J. N. L., Rosa, T. P., Herrera, D. R., *et al.* (2013). Evaluation of cytotoxicity and physicochemical properties of calcium silicate-based endodontic sealer MTA Fillapex. *Journal of Endodontics* **39**, 274–7.

Storm, B., Eichmiller, F. C., Tordik, P. A., *et al.* (2008) Setting expansion of gray and white mineral trioxide aggregate and Portland cement. *Journal of Endodontics* **34**(1), 80–2. doi: 10.1016/j.joen.2007.10.006

Tanomaru-Filho, M., Morales, V., da Silva, G. F., *et al.* (2012) Compressive strength and setting time of MTA and Portland cement associated with different radiopacifying agents. *ISRN Dentistry* **1–4**, 898051. doi: 10.5402/2012/898051

Torabinejad, M., Chivian, N. (1999) Clinical applications of mineral trioxide aggregate. *Journal of Endodontics* **25**(3), 197–205. doi: 10.1016/s0099-2399(99)80142-3

Torabinejad, M., Hong, C. U., McDonald, F., *et al.* (1995) Physical and chemical properties of a new root-end filling material. *Journal of Endodontics* **21**(7), 349–53. doi: 10.1016/s0099-2399(06)80967-2

Tunç, E. S., Sönmez, I. S., Bayrak, S., *et al.* (2008) The evaluation of bond strength of a composite and a compomer to white mineral trioxide aggregate with two different bonding systems. *Journal of Endodontics* **34**(5), 603–5. doi: 10.1016/j.joen.2008.02.026

Viapiana, R., Guerreiro-Tanomaru, J.M., Tanomaru-Filho, M., *et al.* (2014) Investigation of the effect of sealer use on the heat generated at the external root surface during root canal obturation using warm vertical compaction technique with System B heat source. *Journal of Endodontics* in press.

Walker, M. P., Diliberto, A., Lee, C. (2006) Effect of setting conditions on mineral trioxide aggregate flexural strength. *Journal of Endodontics* **32**(4), 334–6. doi: 10.1016/j.joen.2005.09.012

Watts, J. D., Holt, D. M., Beeson, T. J., *et al.* (2007) Effects of pH and mixing agents on the temporal setting of tooth-colored and gray mineral trioxide aggregate. *Journal of Endodontics* **33**(8), 970–3. doi: 10.1016/j.joen.2007.01.024

Yan, P., Peng, B., Fan, B., *et al.* (2006) The effects of sodium hypochlorite (5.25%), chlorhexidine (2%), and Glyde File Prep on the bond strength of MTA-dentin. *Journal of Endodontics* **32**(1), 58–60. doi: 10.1016/j.joen.2005.10.016

4 MTA in Vital Pulp Therapy

Till Dammaschke,[1] Joe H. Camp,[2,3] and George Bogen[3]

[1] Department of Operative Dentistry,
Westphalian Wilhelms-University, Germany
[2] School of Dentistry, University of North Carolina, USA
[3] Private Practice, USA

Mineral Trioxide Aggregate: Properties and Clinical Applications, First Edition.
Edited by Mahmoud Torabinejad.
© 2014 John Wiley & Sons, Inc. Published 2014 by John Wiley & Sons, Inc.

Natural forces within us are the true healers of disease.

—Hippocrates

INTRODUCTION

Vital pulp therapy is a procedure designed to preserve the vitality of the dental pulp. Treatment selection is dependent on the extent of remaining healthy pulp tissue, and includes direct pulp capping and partial or complete pulpotomy. Exposure of the pulp can occur due to caries excavation, trauma, restorative procedures, or anatomical anomalies. The cellular mechanisms involved in pulp repair and bridge formation will be reviewed in order to describe the principles and strategy supporting vital pulp therapy.

When microorganisms challenge the dental pulp, the tissue has an innate capacity for protection and repair (Fig. 4.1). However, when bacteria are precluded from entering the pulp, the tissue exhibits a remarkable regenerative capacity. This phenomenon was demonstrated in a classic investigation where environmentally controlled conventional and germ-free laboratory rats were subjected to experimentally induced and untreated pulp exposures in molar teeth

(A) (B)

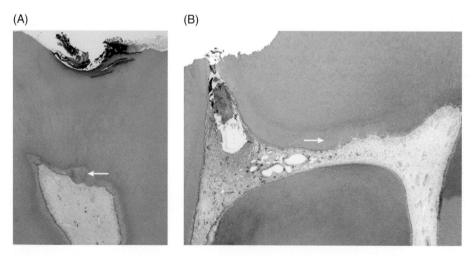

Fig. 4.1 (A) Photomicrograph of an asymptomatic human tooth with a carious lesion, bacterial invasion of dentinal tubules, tertiary dentin formation (arrow) and a vital pulp. (B) Photomicrograph of symptomatic human tooth with penetration of bacteria into distal pulp horn showing pulpal necrosis while mesial pulp tissue remains vital and is uninflamed with normal appearance of dentin, predentin and odontoblast layer. Note formation of tertiary dentin (arrow). Original magnification × 16, Taylor modified B & B Stain. Courtesy of Dr. Domenico Ricucci.

(Kakehashi *et al.* 1965). The conventional rats were exposed to the normal milieu of microflora while the gnotobiotic rats lived in a completely sterile environment and received sterile food. Both groups of test animals were sacrificed at intervals of 1 to 42 days and their teeth evaluated histologically. The conventional rats developed necrosis of the exposed pulps after 8 days, characterized by chronic inflammation and the formation of periapical lesions due to bacterial invasion. A completely different response was observed in the gnotobiotic rodents. Dentin bridging was evident at 14 days and all older specimens exhibited matrix formation and vital pulp tissue beneath completely sealed reparative dentin bridges. All specimens showed minimal pulpal inflammation histologically and more importantly, the germ-free rats did not develop periapical pathosis.

Histological examination of teeth from germ-free rats revealed an important feature of the healing process. Cells lining the newly-formed hard tissue (odontoblast-like cells) were organized into a single cell layer similar to primary odontoblasts; however, morphologically they were shorter than the original elongated cells. Odontoblasts are terminal, post-mitotic cells that, if damaged, do not have the capacity to divide and generate new odontoblasts. The hard tissue-forming cells observed in the germ-free rats were not conventional odontoblasts, but were specialized secretory cells differentiated from recruited mesenchymal cells (fibroblasts) found within the pulp stroma (Smith *et al.* 1995).

This study helps in understanding the basic concept and premise for vital pulp therapy. Bacterial contamination of the exposed pulp tissue must be abated by immune-component responses followed by cell recruitment from the dentin–pulp complex and hard tissue formation completed by differentiated progenitor cells rather than by survival or regeneration of the original cells. Minor indirect trauma to pulp tissue (without exposure of the tissue) stimulates existing primary odontoblasts to form reactionary dentin. This hard tissue is distinguished from the reparative dentin formed by differentiated mesenchymal cells after a pulp exposure. These two situations can describe certain instances of indirect and direct pulp capping where the original hard tissue-forming cells may either survive or be irreversibly damaged (American Association of Endodontists 2003).

Clearly, in clinical practice a sterile environment for an exposed pulp cannot be provided, so an artificial barrier between the vital pulp and external environment is placed to protect the pulp during the healing phase. These artificial barriers are pulp capping materials. The primary aim of pulp capping and pulpotomy has been to establish an environment that induces hard tissue formation by the remaining pulp cells and seals the exposure site, ultimately contributing to continued pulp vitality (Schröder 1985; Lim & Kirk 1987; Moghaddame-Jafari *et al.* 2005). The techniques and rationale for achieving this goal in vital pulp therapy will be described later in this chapter.

ADVANTAGES

Although the effectiveness of conventional root canal treatment is irrefutable, an important advantage of retaining pulp vitality appears to be the continued function of proprioceptive mechanisms and the protective avoidance of excessive occlusal forces during mastication. A root canal-treated tooth requires two and a half times greater occlusal loading to register a proprioceptive response than a tooth with a vital pulp (Randow & Glantz 1986; Stanley 1989). Therefore, greater pressure can be applied to a pulpless tooth before a reflexive response to relieve the force is activated. This diminished protective mechanism in root canal-treated teeth might produce a higher incidence of coronal and radicular tooth fractures (Fuss *et al.* 2001; Lertchirakarn *et al.* 2003; Mireku *et al.* 2010). Root filled teeth also exhibit an increased susceptibility to caries due to either substandard marginal integrity of restorations or a change in their biological environment (Merdad *et al.* 2011). Furthermore, vital pulp procedures are conservative, comparatively simple and inexpensive treatments that do not require more complex and costly restorative care (Hørsted-Bindslev & Bergenholtz 2003). The long-term retention of teeth with vital pulps and intact protective mechanisms provide superior survival rates compared with root filled teeth (Linn & Messer 1994, Caplan *et al.* 2005). Therefore, the overall objectives of vital pulp therapy include the elimination of bacteria from the dentin–pulp complex, protection, repair, and promotion of pulp healing in order to postpone more aggressive endodontic and restorative care (Weiger 2001).

PULP RESPONSES TO CAPPING MATERIALS

Many materials, medicaments, and methods have been used historically to treat and protect an exposed pulp. A short list of these agents includes formocresol, ferric sulfate, electrocautery, tricalcium phosphate, and calcium hydroxide (CH). However, all of these treatments and materials have shortcomings when the teeth are evaluated clinically and histologically. Consequently, vital pulp therapy and, specifically, direct pulp capping, have been considered controversial treatment options in permanent teeth due to the inability of traditional materials and treatment protocols to consistently provide a favorable outcome for the involved tooth (Tronstad & Mjör 1972; Langeland 1981; Ward 2002; Witherspoon 2008; Naito 2010).

In order to establish the reliability of materials used for vital pulp therapy, histological assessment of the pulp tissue response is required. Several months after direct pulp capping or pulpotomy, the following responses may be observed:

- regular pulp tissue without signs of inflammation and with a continuous layer of reparative dentin (hard tissue).

- chronically inflamed and infiltrated pulp tissue with the formation of a permeable layer of hard tissue interspersed with tunnel defects.
- highly inflamed pulp tissue with imperfect, incomplete or missing hard tissue formation or dense collagenous scar tissue in the area of pulp injury.

Only the first response can be considered as successful pulp healing because under this condition the pulp tissue will repair itself and survive after injury (Schroeder 1997). Calcium hydroxide is currently the most widely used pulp capping agent and its affect on pulpal tissue has been subjected to comprehensive investigations. Direct pulp capping with CH will be reviewed first to better understand the desirable properties and some disadvantages of this universally accepted pulp capping agent.

DIRECT PULP CAPPING WITH CALCIUM HYDROXIDE

The first published references to direct pulp capping using CH paste (aqueous suspension) were presented by Hermann (Hermann 1928, 1930) and, since the 1960s, hard setting CH salicylate ester cements have been the preferred material. Thus, for many decades, CH has been the standard material for maintaining pulp vitality. Currently, CH products are the best documented and most reliable materials for direct pulp capping, serving as the "gold standard" against which new materials have to be tested (Hørsted-Bindslev *et al.* 2003). However, more recently, innovative materials have been employed as pulp capping agents, including hydrophilic resins, resin-modified glass ionomer cements, ozone technology, lasers, resins combined with bioactive agents, and various calcium-silicate based cements including mineral trioxide aggregate (MTA; ProRoot MTA, Dentsply/Tulsa Dental Specialties, Tulsa, OK, USA).

Calcium hydroxide exhibits a high pH value and is initially bactericidal. Therefore, the material can neutralize the low pH of acid in carious lesions. It is well known that CH promotes the differentiation of odontoblasts or odontoblast-like cells, which form a hard tissue bridge in the region of the exposed pulp. CH contributes actively to the formation of new hard tissue by induction and up-regulation of the differentiation of odontoblast-like cells (Schröder 1972). Furthermore, low concentrations of CH induce the proliferation of pulp fibroblasts (Torneck *et al.* 1983).

In general, clinical studies show acceptable histological and clinical results for direct and indirect pulp capping procedures with CH (Dammaschke *et al.* 2010a). Basic research and clinical studies have reported success rates in excess of 80% for direct pulp capping procedures in humans (Baume & Holz 1981;

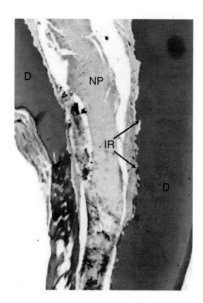

Fig. 4.2   Pulp tissue response to direct pulp capping with Dycal® after 5 months in primary tooth showing pulpal necrosis and internal resorption (D: dentin; NP: necrotic pulp; IR: internal resorption). Magnification×40. Source: Caicedo 2008. Reproduced with permission of John Wiley and Sons, Inc.

Hørsted *et al.* 1985; Duda & Dammaschke 2008; Duda & Dammaschke 2009). By contrast, Barthel *et al.* (2000) identified teeth with necrotic pulps, root canal fillings, or extractions after 10 years in approximately 75% of the cases examined after direct pulp capping with CH. Thus, pulp capping with CH is not without controversy, as it may not provide reliable bridge formation and pulpal protection for prolonged periods.

Calcium hydroxide has some major drawbacks to consider when selecting a material for pulp capping. The compound exhibits poor bonding to dentin, mechanical instability, and continued absorption after placement (Barnes & Kidd 1979; Cox *et al.* 1996; Goracci & Mori 1996) (Fig. 4.2). Moreover, the porosities in newly formed reparative dentin known as "tunnel defects" may act as portals of entry for microorganisms as the material absorbs. This can produce secondary inflammation of the pulp tissue and may be responsible for failed maintenance of tooth vitality and dystrophic calcification (Fig. 4.3). As a result, CH does not prevent microleakage over extended periods even when paired with a sealed restoration. Finally, the high pH (12.5) of calcium hydroxide suspensions also causes liquefaction necrosis at the pulp tissue interface (Barnes & Kidd 1979; Cox *et al.* 1996; Duda & Dammaschke 2008).

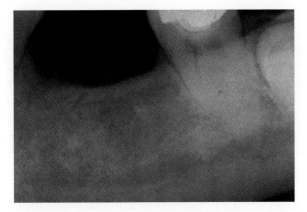

Fig. 4.3 Periapical radiograph of mandibular second molar in a 54-year-old patient. The molar received direct pulp capping approximately twelve years ago, using a hard setting calcium hydroxide (Dycal®). The pulp exhibits a delayed response to cold testing, pulpal calcification and diminished root canal lumen diameter.

MINERAL TRIOXIDE AGGREGATE

Physiochemical properties

The introduction of MTA as a pulp capping material in modern dentistry has transformed treatment outcomes in direct pulp capping from a procedure previously considered unpredictable and often avoided. MTA is a hydraulic calcium–silicate cement powder, which contains different oxide compounds (sodium and potassium oxides, calcium oxide, silicon oxide, ferric oxide, aluminum oxide and magnesium oxide). MTA's composition is similar to that of a refined Portland cement, which is available in most hardware stores (Camilleri *et al.* 2005; Dammaschke *et al.* 2005). Tricalcium silicate is a major component of both and the material is known to be biocompatible and bioactive (Laurent *et al.* 2009). Bioactivity denotes the positive effect of a medicament or a material on living tissue. A material is called bioactive if it can interact with cells of the human body or show a positive biological effect on cells (Hench & West 1996).

The introduction of MTA to dentistry was an historical milestone in the search and development of bioactive cements used for endodontic purposes. However, the first publications advocating the use of Portland cements in dentistry occurred before the end of the nineteenth century. In 1878 the German dentist D. Witte (Hanover, Germany) described the use of a commercial Portland cement to fill root canals and to treat vital pulp tissue (Witte 1878). Unfortunately, the use of this material was apparently not pursued after this period.

The first commercially available version of MTA (ProRoot MTA) was gray (GMTA) in color, and produced tooth discoloration if used within the clinical crown (Karabucak *et al.* 2005). The product was therefore reformulated in a yellow–white version as white MTA (WMTA) (Glickman & Koch 2000). GMTA contains chromomorphic ferrous compounds that include tetracalcium aluminum ferrite, which is absent in WMTA (Moghaddame-Jafari *et al.* 2005). Furthermore, the concentration of aluminum oxide, magnesium oxide, and ferric oxide in WMTA is significantly lower than in GMTA (Asgary *et al.* 2005). Despite component differences, direct pulp capping studies demonstrate that the histological reactions to GMTA and WMTA are similar (Faraco Júnior & Holland 2001, 2004; Parirokh *et al.* 2005).

Both GMTA and WMTA induce visible hard tissue formation with only mild signs of inflammation without substantial necrosis (Aeinehchi *et al.* 2003; Accorinte *et al.* 2008a, 2008b; Nair *et al.* 2008). The hard tissue formed is amorphous and without dentinal tubules (Faraco Júnior & Holland 2004; Parirokh *et al.* 2005) (Fig. 4.4). However, a recent study has shown tunnel defects in reparative dentin formed after MTA pulp capping in non-human primates. This feature of the dentin bridge may be of little consequence as set MTA is structurally stable and nonabsorbable (Al-Hezaimi *et al.* 2011). Unfortunately, tooth discoloration was also recently described after the use of WMTA in vital pulp therapy (Belobrov & Parashos 2011). This effect can be minimized by the use of dentin bonding agents inside the clinical crown in some MTA applications (Akbari *et al.* 2012).

In the clinical setting, MTA is mixed on a glass slab or in a Dappen dish with sterile water or anesthetic solution. After adding water to the MTA powder, it reacts to form a colloidal gel that sets within 4 hours (Torabinejad *et al.* 1995a). If set MTA comes in contact with tissue fluids, its calcium oxide converts into CH. The CH molecule dissociates into calcium and hydroxyl ions (Holland *et al.* 1999; Faraco Júnior & Holland 2001; Takita *et al.* 2006), increasing the pH to a value between 9.22 (Duarte *et al.* 2003) and 12.5 (Torabinejad *et al.* 1995a). Therefore, MTA and CH have similar features that include antimicrobial properties (Al-Hezaimi *et al.* 2005). Furthermore, MTA and CH may exhibit comparable mechanisms that induce new hard tissue formation when in contact with vital pulp tissue (Dominguez *et al.* 2003). However, MTA exhibits superior mechanical properties that discernibly differentiate the two materials.

The advantages of MTA in direct pulp capping, when compared with CH, include lower solubility, improved mechanical strength, and superior marginal adaptation to dentin (Sarkar *et al.* 2005). Furthermore, using MTA for direct pulp capping eliminates some of the disadvantages of CH, such as absorption of the capping material, mechanical instability, and subsequent inadequate long-term sealing ability due to leakage (Dammaschke *et al.* 2010c). MTA is a

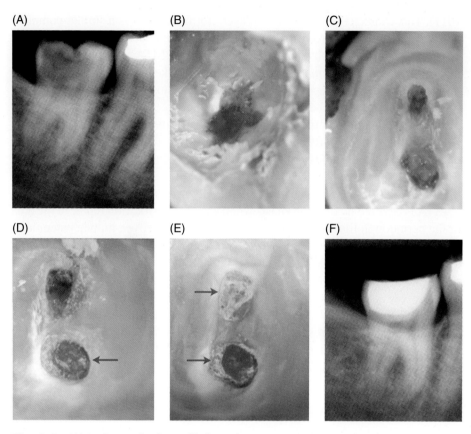

Fig. 4.4 (A) Radiograph of mandibular right asymptomatic second molar in 50-year old patient exhibiting deep caries proximal to pulp roof. (B) Photograph of initial pulp exposure during caries excavation. (C) Clinical photograph showing two large pulp exposures after hemostasis before direct MTA pulp capping. (D) Clinical photograph after re-entry and MTA removal at 3.5 months showing hard tissue formation at one exposure site (arrow). (E) Photograph of tertiary dentin formation after re-entry and MTA removal at 7 months (arrows). (F) Seven-month radiograph after permanent restoration placement. The patient was asymptomatic. Courtesy of Dr. Domenico Ricucci.

hydrophilic and hygroscopic cement that allows the material to set in the presence of blood and tissue fluids (Torabinejad *et al.* 1995a).

It is known that calcium silicate cements like MTA not only have the ability to release calcium and hydroxyl ions after contact with cell and tissue fluid (Borges *et al.* 2011), but also to form hydroxyapatite crystals on its surface (Sarkar *et al.* 2005; Bozeman *et al.* 2006; Gandolfi *et al.* 2010). The apatite formation contributes to leakage reduction not only by filling the gap along the interface but also via interactions with dentin during intrafibrillar apatite deposition (Han & Okiji

2011). This characteristic "interstitial layer" formation shows a similar composition and structure to hydroxyapatite when placed in contact with dentin and may be the most important physiochemical property of MTA in vital pulp therapy (Sarkar *et al*. 2005; Bozeman 2006). This feature makes it effective in preventing microleakage, thereby improving the treatment prognosis by providing a biologically active substrate for cell attachment (Sarkar *et al*. 2005). Furthermore, MTA is antibacterial (Torabinejad *et al*. 1995d; Ribeiro *et al*. 2006), not mutagenic (Kettering *et al*. 1995) and exhibits minor cytotoxicity (Keiser *et al*. 2000). It does not alter the cytomorphology of osteoblasts (Koh *et al*. 1998), promotes a biological cell reaction in these cells (Koh *et al*. 1997; Mitchell *et al*. 1999) and induces the formation of mineralized tissue (Abedi & Ingle 1995; Holland *et al*. 2001).

MTA is covered by cementoblasts when used for perforation repair in the area of the periodontal ligament (Holland *et al*. 2001). Moreover, human osteoblasts attach to MTA's surface, allowing cell survival (Zhu *et al*. 2000). Overall, all available studies show MTA to have excellent biocompatibility (Torabinejad *et al*. 1995b; Pitt Ford *et al*. 1996; Koh *et al*. 1997; Torabinejad & Chivian 1999; Keiser *et al*. 2000) with an exceptional sealing ability against microbial challenges (Torabinejad *et al*. 1993, 1995e; Torabinejad & Chivian 1999). It can be concluded that current research indicates MTA is the preferable material for direct pulp capping and the rational alternative to CH in vital pulp therapy (Holland *et al*. 2001; Cho *et al*. 2013) (Fig. 4.5).

Mode of action in pulp capping and pulpotomy

MTA has been shown to promote a variety of positive cellular responses *in vitro* when applied directly to the dental pulp (Bonson *et al*. 2004; Nakayama *et al*. 2005; Tani-Ishii *et al*. 2007). It also has a substantial effect on the mitosis index of progenitor cells and stimulates hard tissue formation after direct pulp capping (Dammaschke *et al*. 2010b). Progenitor cells are multipotent adult stem cells that have the potential to differentiate into odontoblast-like cells after injury or damage to the primary odontoblasts (Goldberg & Smith 2004, Goldberg *et al*. 2008). MTA most probably stimulates mineralization by up-regulation of bone morphogenic protein (Yasuda *et al*. 2008). *In vitro*, MTA promotes the production of mineralization matrix genes, mRNA, and a protein expression of cellular markers, which play a role in the mineralization process (Thomson *et al*. 2003).

When MTA is placed in direct contact with pulp cells, there is a significant increase in the induction and secretion of vascular endothelial growth factor (VEGF), a platelet-derived protein growth factor critical for angiogenesis and shown to be involved in dentinogenesis (Paranjpe *et al*. 2010, 2011). Moreover, in comparison with untreated control groups, MTA induces a significant increase of MDPC-23-cells in the S- and the G_2-phases and of OD-21-cells in the S-phase

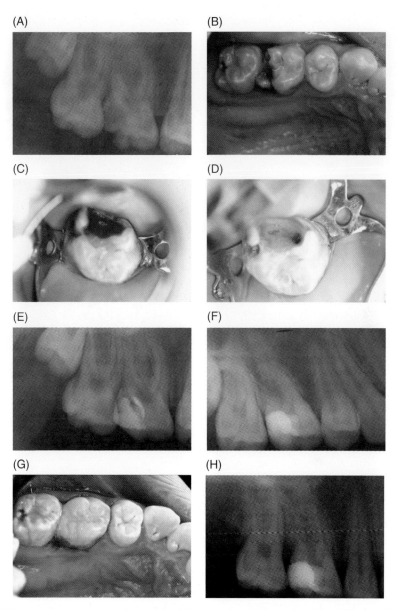

Fig. 4.5 (A) Preoperative radiograph of deep caries associated with maxillary right molar in symptomatic 15-year-old patient. (B) Clinical photograph of involved molar. (C) Caries removal using caries detector dye. (D) Clinical view of pulp exposures after 5.25% NaOCl hemostasis. (E) Radiograph of direct MTA pulp cap with wet cotton pellet and unbonded Photocore®. (F) Permanent bonded composite placed five days after MTA direct pulp cap. (G) Clinical photograph of final bonded composite restoration. (H) Fourteen-year recall radiograph without restorative intervention, patient responded normally to cold testing.

(A)

(B)

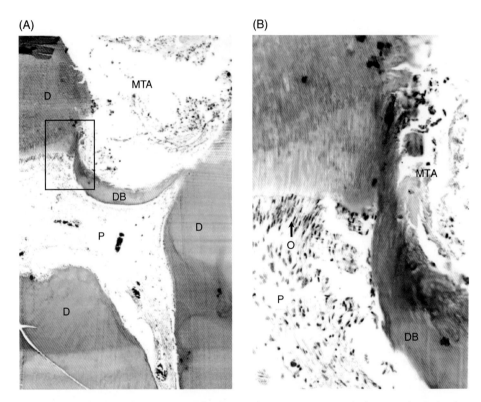

Fig. 4.6 (A) Direct pulp capping with MTA in a human primary tooth showing dentin bridge formation after five months (D: dentin; P: dental pulp; DB: dentin bridge). Magnification ×40. (B) Odontoblasts (O) proximal to MTA induced dentin (hard tissue) bridge. Magnification ×200. Source: Caicedo 2008. Reproduced with permission of John Wiley and Sons, Inc.

of the cell cycle *in vitro*. However, MTA does not influence the apoptosis of these cells. Therefore, it can be concluded that MTA promotes the proliferation, but not apoptosis of pulp cells. This may explain the regenerative processes observed after direct pulp capping with MTA *in vivo* (Moghaddame-Jafari *et al.* 2005; Caicedo *et al.* 2006) (Fig. 4.6).

Essential physiochemical properties attributed to MTA promote reparative dentinogenesis by uncoupling and activating growth factors nested in the proximal dentin (Koh *et al.* 1997; Tziafas *et al.* 2002; Okiji & Yoshiba 2009). Signaling molecules, including transforming growth factor-β (TGF-β), macrophage colony-stimulating factor (MCSF), and interleukins IL-1α and IL-β, are stimulated via the continued release of calcium ions during the setting process (Takita *et al.* 2006; An *et al.* 2012). MTA is able to improve the secretion of IL-1β significantly better compared with other capping materials like CH or hydrophilic bonding resins (Accorinte *et al.* 2008c; Reyes-Carmona *et al.* 2010; Cavalcanti *et al.* 2011; Galler *et al.* 2011). Interleukin-1 beta is a highly effective cytokine that controls the growth and differentiation of cells (Cavalcanti *et al.* 2011). It has been proposed that glycoproteins in the extracellular matrix can stimulate the formation of reparative or reactionary dentin (Smith *et al.* 1995; Goldberg & Smith 2004; Goldberg *et al.* 2008). In particular, tenascin and fibronectin have been identified as high molecular weight oligomeric proteins involved in odonto-blastic differentiation and odontogenesis in the presence of MTA (Thesleff *et al.* 1995; Leites *et al.* 2011; Zarrabi *et al.* 2011). Both glycoproteins are expressed during dentinogenesis and may be critical elements in pulp cell migration and differentiation (Zarrabi *et al.* 2011).

Proliferation and survival of human dental stromal cells is increased when cultured on set GMTA. Gene products such as osteocalcin, dental sialoprotein, and alkaline phosphatase are also up-regulated when in contact with set MTA and promote the differentiation of odontoblast-like cells essential for reparative dentin bridge formation. After MTA pulp capping, both sialoprotein and osteo-pontin have been identified during initial dentinogenesis at the exposure site (Kuratate *et al.* 2008). It is known that the presence of bone morphogenetic proteins BMP-2, BMP-4, BMP-7, signaling molecules such as TGF-β, and heme oxygenase-1 enzyme are required for differentiation of the odontoblastic cell line (Guven *et al.* 2011). The up-regulation of specific cytokines by MTA promotes mineralization by forming apatite-like clusters on collagen fibrils at the MTA-dentin interface (Ham *et al.* 2005; Yasuda *et al.* 2008; Reyes-Carmona *et al.* 2010). The up-regulated cytokines include cyclooxygenase-2, activating protein-1, myeloperoxidase, VEGF, nuclear factor-kappa B, and inducible nitric oxide synthase. MTA has been shown to improve the secretion of IL-1β and IL-8 and does not adversely affect the generation of reactive oxygen species and cell survival (Camargo *et al.* 2009). However, the release of aluminum ions by MTA may have a partial inhibitory effect on pulp stromal cells (Minamikawa *et al.* 2011).

Comparison with calcium hydroxide

The positive effect of MTA when in contact with vital pulp tissue has been experimentally evaluated in several species and compared with CH: in humans (Aeinehchi *et al.* 2003; Iwamoto *et al.* 2006; Caicedo *et al.* 2006; Accorinte *et al.* 2008a, b; Min *et al.* 2008; Nair *et al.* 2008; Sawicki *et al.* 2008; Mente *et al.* 2010; Parolia *et al.* 2010), monkeys (Pitt Ford *et al.* 1996), dogs (Faraco Júnior & Holland 2001; Dominguez *et al.* 2003, Queiroz *et al.* 2005; Asgary *et al.* 2008; Costa *et al.* 2008), pigs (Shayegan *et al.* 2009), and rodents (Dammaschke *et al.* 2010c). These investigations show that from a histological perspective, CH and MTA generate comparable reactions in vital pulp tissue.

Table 4.1 Histological results of direct pulp capping with MTA in comparison to CH (Literature review).

Authors	type of Ca(OH)$_2$	Species	Observation period	Result
Pitt Ford et al. 1996	Hard setting cement	Monkey	5 months	MTA significantly superior
Faraco Júnior and Holland 2001	Hard setting cement	Dog	2 months	MTA significantly superior
Aeinehchi et al. 2003	Hard setting cement	Human	1 week – 6 months	MTA significantly superior
Dominguez et al. 2003	Light curing	Dog	50 days + 150 days	MTA significantly superior
Accorinte et al. 2008	Hard setting cement	Human	30 days + 60 days	MTA significantly superior
Asgary et al. 2008	Hard setting cement	Dog	8 weeks	MTA significantly superior
Min et al. 2008	Hard setting cement	Human	2 months	MTA significantly superior
Nair et al. 2008	Hard setting cement	Human	1 week + 1 month + 3 months	MTA significantly superior
Mente et al. 2010	Aqueous paste	Human	12–80 months (median 27 months)	MTA significantly superior*
Hilton et al. 2013	Hard setting cement	Human	6–24 months (median 12.1 months)	MTA significantly superior
Queiroz et al. 2005	Aqueous paste	Dog	90 d	No significant difference
Iwamoto et al. 2006	Hard setting cement	Human	136 ± 24 days	No significant difference
Accorinte et al. 2008b	Powder	Human	30 days + 60 days	No significant difference
Costa et al. 2008	Aqueous paste	Dog	60 days	No significant difference
Sawicki et al. 2008	Hard setting cement	Human	47–609 days	No significant difference
Shayegan et al. 2009	Hard setting cement	Pigs	21 days	No significant difference
Dammaschke et al. 2010	Aqueous paste	Rat	1, 3, 7, 70 days	No significant difference
Parolia 2010	Hard setting cement	Human	15 days + 45 days	No significant difference

*The statistical results of Mente et al. (2010) were found by Naito (2010) to be inappropriate. Hence, these results should be regarded with care.

However, in direct contact with pulp tissue, MTA shows significantly less inflammation (Aeinehchi *et al.* 2003; Accorinte *et al.* 2008b; Nair *et al.* 2008; Parolia *et al.* 2010), a lower amount of hyperemia and necrosis (Aeinehchi *et al.* 2003; Dammaschke *et al.* 2010c), and a more homogeneous dentin bridge formation exhibiting fewer tunnel defects (Nair *et al.* 2008). The newly-formed reparative dentin is thicker and is characterized by a more uniform odontoblast-like cellular layer observed at the bridge interface (Aeinehchi *et al.* 2003; Min *et al.* 2008; Nair *et al.* 2008; Parolia *et al.* 2010). This may explain why MTA shows better results clinically when compared with CH in direct pulp capping (Mente *et al.* 2010; Hilton *et al.* 2013).

The majority of contemporary pulp capping studies show MTA to be superior to CH (Pitt Ford *et al.* 1996; Faraco Júnior & Holland 2001; Aeinehchi *et al.* 2003; Dominguez *et al.* 2003; Accorinte *et al.* 2008c; Asgary *et al.* 2008; Min *et al.* 2008; Nair *et al.* 2008; Mente *et al.* 2010; Leye Benoist *et al.* 2012; Hilton *et al.* 2013). However, some authors have found no significant differences in pulp healing between the two substances (Queiroz *et al.* 2005; Iwamoto *et al.* 2006; Accorinte *et al.* 2008b; Costa *et al.* 2008; Sawicki *et al.* 2008; Shayegan *et al.* 2009; Dammaschke *et al.* 2010c; Parolia *et al.* 2010) (Table 4.1). These investigations demonstrate that MTA is equal or superior to CH salicylate ester cement or CH powder when used for direct pulp capping (Accorinte el al. 2008a, b; Dammaschke *et al.* 2010c). Although it has been shown that CH paste generates a more favorable pulpal response than CH salicylate ester cements (Phaneuf *et al.* 1968; Retzlaff *et al.* & Castaldi 1969; Stanley & Lundy 1972; Liard-Dumtschin *et al.* 1984; Schröder 1985; Lim & Kirk 1987; Kirk *et al.* 1989; Staehle 1990), both materials are prone to absorption over time and therefore more vulnerable to microleakage. Furthermore, some additives necessary for the hard setting of CH may also be toxic to pulp tissue (Liard-Dumtschin *et al.* 1984). Therefore, MTA has advantages when compared to CH in pulp capping procedures due to better dimensional stability, sustained alkaline pH and equal or improved bioactive properties (Fridland & Rosado 2005; Sarkar *et al.* 2005; Dreger *et al.* 2012; Cho *et al.* 2013).

PULPOTOMY IN PRIMARY TEETH

Pulpotomy is defined as the amputation of the affected or infected coronal exposed pulp preserving the vitality and function of the remaining radicular pulp (American Academy of Pediatric Dentistry 2011). Pulpotomy on primary teeth is indicated for pulpal exposures in which the inflammation and/or infection has been judged to be confined to the coronal pulp. With more widespread inflammation into the radicular pulp the tooth is a candidate for pulpectomy and root canal filling or extraction. Hemorrhage control is the key diagnostic determinant in the assessment of irreversibly inflamed tissue and the decision for more aggressive treatment.

In the primary dentition with a mechanical or carious exposure, all the coronal pulp tissue is amputated. Following tissue removal, the pulp chamber should be thoroughly irrigated with a sodium hypochlorite (SH) soaked cotton pellet to remove debris and inspected for any remaining pulpal filaments. Hemostasis cannot be achieved with pulp filaments remaining in the chamber and is accomplished by applying pressure on the pulp stumps with a cotton pellet dampened with SH (1.25–6.0%). If hemostasis is not obtained in 2–3 minutes, this indicates the spread of inflammation into the radicular pulp and the pulpotomy is abandoned in favor of a pulpectomy or extraction. The pulp should never be capped with hemorrhage present as this will result in failure of the procedure (Matsuo *et al.* 1996). Once hemostasis is attained, the radicular pulp is covered with the medicament or pulp capping material of choice. The chamber is then sealed to prevent the ingress of microorganisms. In primary molars, the placement of a stainless steel crown is the preferred final restoration (Camp & Fuks 2006; Winters *et al.* 2008; McDonald *et al.* 2011).

Numerous pharmacotherapeutic agents have been utilized for pulpotomy in the primary dentition. These include CH, formocresol (FC), glutaraldehyde (GA), ferric sulfate (FS), MTA, and collagen. Formocresol continues to be the most widely used medicament for pulpotomy procedures today. However, major concerns about toxicity, allergicity, carcinogenicity, and mutagenicity have led to much criticism and decreased usage (Duggal 2009; Lewis 2010). Electrosurgery (Oringer 1975; Ruemping *et al.* 1983; Shaw *et al.* 1987, Shulman *et al.* 1987) and lasers (Elliot *et al.* 1999; Liu *et al.* 1999) also have been successfully implemented for tissue removal and hemostasis.

MTA PULPOTOMY

Primary teeth

Since its introduction, MTA has been used as a dressing in pulp capping and pulpotomy procedures in both primary and permanent teeth. Comparative studies have shown MTA to be equal to (Aeinehchi *et al.* 2007; Moretti *et al.* 2008; Subramaniam *et al.* 2009; Ansari *et al.* 2010; Erdem *et al.* 2011) or superior to (Salako *et al.* 2003; Agamy *et al.* 2004; Farsi *et al.* 2005; Holan *et al.* 2005; Fuks & Papagiannoulis 2006; Zealand *et al.* 2010) other medicaments and materials used for primary tooth pulpotomies. Most of the reports are comparative in nature, employing clinical signs and symptoms with radiographic interpretation to determine success or failure.

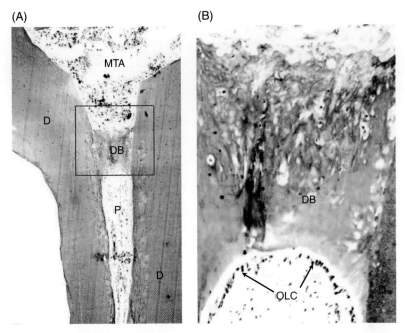

Fig. 4.7 (A) MTA pulpotomy in a human primary tooth showing dentin bridge (hard tissue) formation after five months. (D: dentin; P: dental pulp; DB: dentin bridge). Magnification×40. (B) Odontoblast-like cells (OLC) lining periphery of MTA induced dentin bridge. Magnification×200. Source: Caicedo 2008. Reproduced with permission of John Wiley and Sons, Inc.

Long-term clinical trials have also shown MTA to produce better results than FC when used for pulpotomy in primary teeth (Farsi *et al.* 2005; Holan *et al.* 2005; Zealand *et al.* 2010). Although radiopaque calcified tissue leading to canal obliteration can be seen in over half of the cases using both materials, MTA demonstrates dentin bridging absent with FC (Farsi *et al.* 2005; Caicedo *el al.* 2006; Zealand *et al.* 2010) (Fig. 4.7). Formocresol also has also been reported to show a greater amount of root resorption than MTA (Aeinehchi *et al.* 2007; Moretti *et al.* 2008; Subramaniam *et al.* 2009; Ansari *et al.* 2010; Erdem *et al.* 2011). A recent study comparing GMTA to WMTA revealed no statistical differences in the two materials over a study period of 84 months, although there was more bridging with GMTA (Cardosa-Silva *et al.* 2011). These outcomes suggest that MTA is a suitable replacement for FC in primary pulpotomies.

Another common medicament employed for primary pulpotomies is FS. Studies comparing MTA to FS have shown superior radiographic and clinical outcomes with MTA (Doyle *et al.* 2010, Erdem *et al.* 2011). The success rates were 96% and 88%, respectively, at two-years (Erdem *et al.* 2011). CH was abandoned as a

(A) (B)

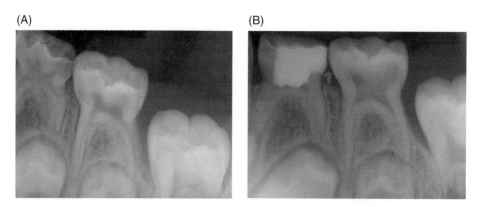

Fig. 4.8 (A) Radiograph of symptomatic primary left second mandibular molar with deep caries. (B) Post-operative 6-week radiograph after MTA pulpotomy, flowable compomer placement and bonded composite restoration. The patient was not symptomatic at recall.

pulpotomy agent many years ago because of the high incidence of root resorption and failure (Schröder & Granath 1971; Liu *et al.* 2011). A recent investigation (Moretti *et al.* 2011) compared MTA, FC, and CH in primary pulpotomies with a study period up to 24 months. Reported success with MTA and FC was 100%, while CH had a 64% failure rate. Because of the high success rates, dentinal bridge formation, preservation of healthy pulpal tissue, and a lack of root resorption, MTA has become the accepted standard for primary pulpotomies (Fig. 4.8).

Immature permanent teeth

Crown fractures or cariously exposed teeth with necrotic pulps and mature apices can be predictably treated with conventional root canal treatment. The overall prognosis for permanent retention of this group of teeth is excellent. However, loss of pulpal vitality in teeth with incomplete root development presents a more complicated treatment with a reduced prognosis. Conventional root canal procedures using inert materials such as gutta-percha will not induce root end maturation, and cannot be recommended for teeth with open apices. Moreover, the loss of pulpal vitality results in the cessation of root development, leaving the roots structurally weak and more prone to fracture than fully developed roots (Camp & Fuks 2006). Lack of complete root development may result in a poor crown/root ratio, leaving the teeth more susceptible to bone loss and periodontal involvement because of excessive mobility. Therefore, treatment should always be oriented toward preservation of pulpal tissue when possible in order to allow root maturation. (Video). These procedures include pulp capping, partial pulpotomy, full pulpotomy, and regenerative endodontic procedures (Iwaya *et al.* 2001; Bose *et al.* 2009; Jeeruphan *et al.* 2012).

(A)   (B)   (C)

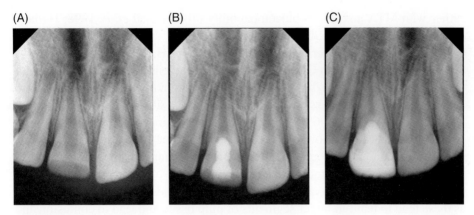

Fig. 4.9 MTA partial pulpotomy following traumatic injury. (A) Pre-op radiograph of a central incisor. Traumatic injury with large pulp exposure and hyperemic pulp. Inflammation in pulp required removal of tissue to cervical line before hemostasis was achieved with cotton pellets moistened with water and slight pressure after MTA placement. (B) Two month post-op radiograph shows MTA and composite placement. (C) Two year follow-up radiograph showing complete root formation and apical closure.

Pulp capping and pulpotomy procedures should be considered whenever possible in teeth with incompletely developed apices that have pulp exposures. The use of these conservative treatments does not preclude the use of more extensive procedures in the event of failure. With traumatic exposure, pulp capping is confined to small exposures treated within the first 24 hours after injury in which a restoration can be placed that assures a seal against bacterial invasion (Cvek 1993; Bakland & Andreasen 2012). Otherwise, a pulpotomy is indicated. Investigations have shown that pulp exposures from traumatic injuries usually exhibit a proliferative reaction with inflammation advancing only a few millimeters into the tissue (Cvek 1978; Cvek *et al.* 1982; Heide & Mjör 1983).

The AAPD guidelines (American Academy of Pediatric Dentistry 2011) define partial pulpotomy for carious exposures as the removal of pulpal tissue beneath the exposure to a depth of 1 to 3 mm in order to reach healthy tissue. For carious exposures with no evidence of radicular pathology, a partial pulpotomy or full pulpotomy (removal of all coronal pulp tissue) is indicated to assure root completion (Fig. 4.9).

Similar materials and drugs used for pulpotomy in primary teeth have been applied to permanent teeth. CH has been the traditional material employed to stimulate dentin bridge formation in permanent teeth. However, better results have been reported using MTA (Abedi *et al.* 1996; Myers *et al.* 1996; Pitt-Ford *et al.* 1996; Junn *et al.* 1998; Dominguez *et al.* 2003; Chacko & Kurikose 2006; El-Meligy & Avery 2006; Qudeimat *et al.* 2007; Nair *et al.* 2008). Dentin deposition also begins earlier with MTA and shows biocompatibility (Torabinejad *et al.* 1998; Holland *et al.* 1999; Brisco *et al.* 2006) and tissue cytoxicity (Torabinejad *et al.* 1995c; Osorio *et al.* 1998; Keiser *et al.* 2000) comparable to CH. MTA consistently shows better dentin bridging than CH, which is more homogeneous and continuous with the original dentin while exhibiting less pulpal inflammation in canine and human *in vivo* studies (Dominguez *et al.* 2003; Brisco *et al.* 2006; Chacko & Kurikose 2006; El-Meligy *et al.* 2006; Qudeimat *et al.* 2007; Nair *et al.* 2008).

During the partial pulpotomy procedure, only tissue judged to be inflamed is removed, which extends approximately 2 mm. A round diamond bur, used at high speed and with adequate water cooling removes the desired amount of pulpal tissue. Spoon excavators and slow-speed round burs are contraindicated as these tend to tear out larger segments of pulp tissue and lead to contusion and torsion (Sluka *et al.* 1981). The preparation is washed with sterile water or physiologic saline to remove debris and re-examined to assure a clean amputation. Hemostasis is achieved by placing cotton pellets dampened with SH and applying slight pressure with additional dry pellets. Hemostasis should occur in 30–60 s. If hemorrhage continues, the amputation is carried deeper. It is recommended not to blow excessive air on the exposed pulp as it may cause tissue damage by desiccation.

Once hemorrhage is controlled, the pulp is covered with a layer of MTA. After mixing, the MTA is loaded into a small amalgam carrier. For smaller amounts of MTA, the pellet is partially extruded from the amalgam carrier and all but 1–2 mm is removed with a plastic instrument. The MTA is gently placed over the remaining pulp tissue and teased into place with a moist cotton pellet using endodontic pliers. The MTA should be 1.5–3.0 mm in thickness. A thin layer of "flowable" glass ionomer or composite resin is gently placed over the MTA. This material should completely cover the MTA and contact a minimum amount of dentin around the periphery of the dressing. It is then light-cured if required. The tooth can then be restored with an acid-etched or self-etching primer and hydrophilic resin with a matched composite restoration without disturbing the MTA. The moisture necessary for setting of the MTA is derived from the pulp (Fig. 4.10).

Symptomatic permanent teeth

Conservative treatments applying vital therapy techniques, including pulp capping, partial pulpotomy, and full pulpotomy, in symptomatic permanent teeth have long been considered paradoxical. However, many recent pulpotomy studies have reported success in this area utilizing both CH (Mejare & Cvek 1993; Caliskan 1995) and MTA (Witherspoon *et al.* 2006; Eghbal *et al.* 2009). In a clinical case reported in 2001, Schmitt *et al.* submitted the first published case of the use of

(A)   (B)   (C)

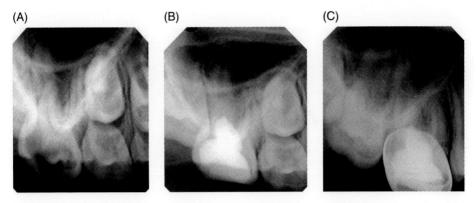

Fig. 4.10 MTA full pulpotomy. (A) Pre-op radiograph showing deep carious lesion and open apices in a maxillary first molar. The tooth was symptomatic but free of percussion sensitivity and no swelling. (B) Radiograph showing full pulpotomy to canal orifices. Hemostasis was achieved with 5.25% NaOCl and MTA placed and covered with composite. (C) Four year post-op radiograph. Complete root formation evident with stainless steel crown restoration. Note the eruption of the second molar and premolar.

MTA in a symptomatic permanent tooth diagnosed with reversible pulpitis and exhibiting open apices. Following partial pulpotomy, SH was used to achieve hemostasis and the pulp was capped directly with MTA. After 2 years, the apex had completed formation and the tooth was clinically and radiographically asymptomatic. Other studies included permanent teeth with lingering pain and carious pulpal exposure that demonstrated complete dentin bridge formation, with vital pulps free of inflammation when examined histologically after two months (Eghbal *et al.* 2009). These limited reports show the potential for MTA to reverse inflammatory changes in pulp tissue under ideal circumstances.

In order to better ensure favorable pulp capping and pulpotomy outcomes, SH is the preferred hemostatic agent when applied in both asymptomatic and symptomatic teeth with carious pulp exposures (Fig. 4.11). The solution is antibacterial and is neither toxic to pulpal cells nor inhibitory to healing when used for hemostasis in vital pulp therapy (Hafez *et al.* 2002; Demir & Cehreli 2007). Odontoblast-like cell formation with dentin bridging has consistently been shown when SH has been used to achieve hemostasis (Matsuo *et al.* 1996; Schmitt *et al.* 2001; Demir & Ceherli 2007; Bogen *et al.* 2008).

In the partial or complete pulpotomy procedure on symptomatic teeth, those with a fistula, swelling, or other obvious signs of pulpal necrosis are excluded. The pulp must be vital and free of suppuration. Following anesthetic injection, the tooth is isolated with a dental dam. A large carbide bur (#6 for molars and #4 for other teeth) is used with copious water spray to remove all caries. It is recommended that caries removal be augmented with the implementation of a

(A)   (B)

(C)   (D)

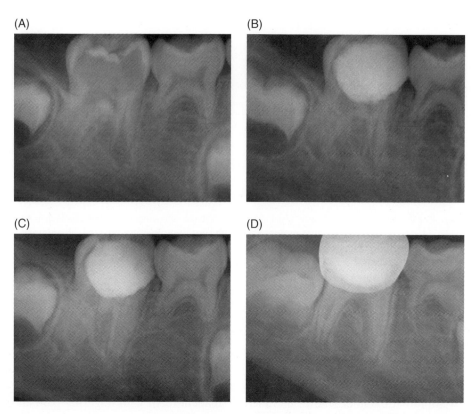

Fig. 4.11 MTA partial pulpotomy. (A) Pre-op radiograph of a mandibular right first permanent molar. The tooth was symptomatic. Note absence of the second premolar. (B) Radiograph showing partial pulpotomy, 5.25% NaOCl hemostasis and MTA placement after final composite. (C) Post-op radiograph at 1½ years. Note partial closure of apices. (D) Three year post-op radiograph. Closure of the apices and completed root formation is evident with stainless steel crown restoration.

caries detector dye and optical magnification (Fusayama *et al.* 1966; Fusayama & Terachima 1972).

Hemostasis of profuse hemorrhaging is achieved by lavaging the pulp with 1.25–6.0% SH. It is usually necessary to leave the solution in contact with the pulp stump for 10 to 15 minutes, with reapplication every 3 to 4 minutes to control bleeding. However, if hemostasis is not achieved after this time period while attempting a partial pulpotomy, then the procedure is abandoned in favor of a complete pulpotomy. Care must be exercised to avoid negative pressure over the remaining coronal or radicluar pulp tissue with the aspiration tip or bleeding will persist. If a full pulpotomy procedure is elected, MTA can be placed as one large aliquot and the mass compressed and shaped with a moist cotton pellet to create a uniform layer. Because of the large surface area of the MTA in a

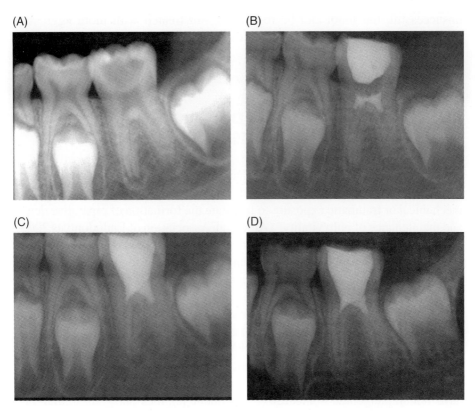

Fig. 4.12 Full MTA pulpotomy. (A) Mandibular right first molar exhibiting deep caries and open apices in seven year-old patient. (B) Radiograph after MTA pulpotomy with extrusion of MTA into the canal orifices. (C) Molar after placement of permanent bonded composite restoration. (D) One-year radiographic review showing maturation of roots and continued closure of apices. Courtesy of Dr. Laureen M. Roh, Los Angeles, California.

complete pulpotomy, permanent sealing of the lesion should be delayed until a subsequent appointment. Cotton wisps or customized and trimmed gauze moistened with sterile water are used to completely cover the MTA. Unlike the treatment of primary teeth, it is recommended that the tooth be provisionally sealed with Cavit™ (3M™ESPE™, St. Paul, MN, USA) or other temporary cement and the MTA be allowed to harden.

The treatment is completed at the following appointment at least 6 hours to several days later. The temporary seal and cotton or gauze is removed following isolation. Inspection of the MTA is performed to assure hardness and proper curing. If the MTA has failed to set, it is washed out and the pulp tissue is removed to the canal orifices and the procedure is repeated. After verifying set of the MTA, the tooth is sealed with an acid-etch and bonded composite restoration (Fig. 4.12). Should the conservative procedures described above be unsuccessful, the tooth can be re-entered and treated with more aggressive endodontic treatment such as apexification or regenerative therapy (Murray *et al*. 2007).

PULP CAPPING IN TEETH DIAGNOSED WITH REVERSIBLE PULPITIS

Direct pulp capping is specifically defined as the "treatment of an exposed vital pulp by sealing the pulpal wound with a dental material placed directly on a mechanical or traumatic exposure to facilitate the formation of reparative dentin and maintenance of pulp vitality" (American Association of Endodontists 2003). The first reported study examining direct pulp capping using MTA in humans showed that over a period of six months, histological examination of direct MTA pulp caps on maxillary third molars exhibited less hyperemia, less inflammation, and fewer areas of necrosis than CH. Moreover, the dentin bridge formation was thicker with a more consistent layer of odontoblasts (Aeinehchi *et al*. 2003). Recent human studies that examined carious exposures on reversibly inflamed permanent teeth using MTA as a direct pulp capping material have shown promising results when treatment protocols are standardized (Farsi *et al*. 2005; Bogen *et al*. 2008) . However, some prospective studies in humans that have not implemented standardized treatment regimes show dissimilar outcomes (Mente *et al*. 2010; Miles *et al*. 2010). These pulp capping investigations vary with respect to case selection, one versus two-step treatment strategies, caries removal protocols, hemostatic agents, MTA placement criteria and permanent restoration selection.

The modification in the treatment of cariously exposed permanent teeth requires procedural adjustments that include the use of a caries detector dye, SH hemostasis, broader and thicker MTA placement, time to allow proper MTA curing, and, more importantly, a sealed and bonded restoration. It appears that MTA direct pulp capping can be a valuable method for preserving pulp vitality in selected cases where the diagnosis is reversible pulpitis (Fig. 4.13). Moreover, the diagnosis can be confounded by the patient's subjective symptomatology, which may not accurately reflect the true histological condition of the involved tooth (Camp 2008). The diagnosis of reversible pulpitis is most reliably determined based on achieving hemostasis using SH after a 5 to 10 minute exposure period rather than cold testing (Matsuo *et al*. 1996; Bogen *et al*. 2008). SH can be a valuable diagnostic clinical tool in determining the extent and severity of pulpal inflammation and thus the treatment selection. For direct pulp capping in permanent teeth using MTA, the following

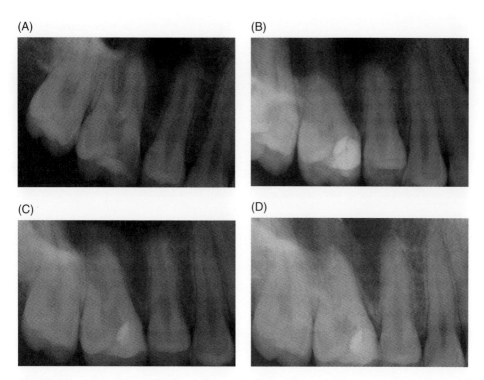

Fig. 4.13 (A) Radiograph of maxillary right first molar with deep caries in 16-year-old patient. Cold testing revealed a normal response to cold testing. (B) Post-treatment radiograph after MTA pulp capping, wet cotton pellet and unbonded Photocore® provisional restoration. (C) Radiograph after placement of bonded composite restoration. (D) Review radiograph at 5.5 years. Cold testing response was within normal limits.

treatment recommendations should be observed (adapted from Bogen & Chandler 2008):

1 Diagnosis must include radiographic and clinical evaluation, combined with vitality testing using cold stimulus.
2 Dental dam isolation and disinfection of the clinical crown with 6.0% SH or chlorhexidine.
3 Caries removal with slow speed round burs and spoon excavators using a caries detector dye with the aid of optical magnification.
4 Hemostasis using 1.25–6.0% SH soaked on a cotton pellet.
5 MTA placement over the exposure and surrounding dentin with a minimum thickness of 1.5 mm while leaving at least 1.0 mm of circumferential dentin for the final bonded restoration.
6 For one-step pulp capping, a flowable compomer is placed over the unset MTA and light-cured followed by a bonded composite restoration (Fig. 4.14).

(A)

(B)

(C)

(D)

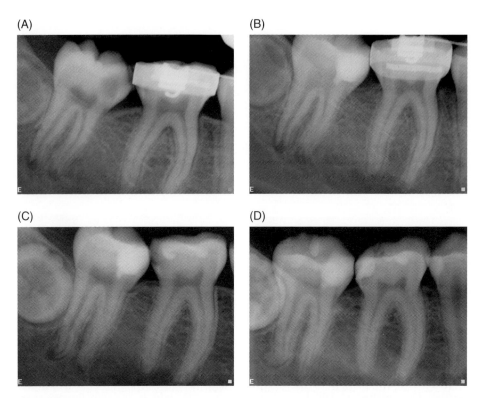

Fig. 4.14 One-visit pulp capping procedure. (A) Nine year-old patient exhibiting deep carious lesion in mandibular right second molar. (B) Radiograph showing final restoration placed over flowable composite after direct MTA pulp cap. (C) Six-month review. (D) Radiographic recall at 3.5 years. Pulp testing showed normal response to cold. Maturation and root closure evident. Courtesy of Dr. Adrian Silberman.

7   For two-step pulp capping, a wet cotton pellet or gauze is placed over the unset MTA and provisionalization is completed with unbonded Clearfil Photocore (Kuraray Co. LTD, Osaka, Japan) or similar product to allow for complete MTA curing before permanent restoration placement.

8   Placement of a bonded restoration on a return visit 5 to 10 days after reconfirming pulp vitality using a cold test.

TREATMENT CONSIDERATIONS

Several critical factors during treatment delivery can positively affect outcomes when MTA is employed as the pulp capping agent. Caries removal should be completed using a caries detector dye, optical magnification, and illumination

(Fusayama *et al*. 1966; Bogen *et al*. 2008). Fusayama and associates showed that two different carious layers are present during the carious process, and that the inner carious layer can remineralize when a sealed restoration is placed to prevent further bacterial ingress (Miyauchi *et al*. 1978; Tatsumi 1978; Tatsumi *et al*. 1992). Caries detectors allow for objective caries removal, thereby protecting the deep layer that contributes to pulp protection and continued pulp survival.

Investigations have shown that the control of hemorrhaging after pulp exposures is paramount to successful direct pulp capping (Matsuo *et al*. 1996; Bogen *et al*. 2008). SH has been shown to be an economical and clinically safe method to control bleeding. The solution is the medicament of choice in vital pulp therapy as it clears most dentinal chips, removes damaged cells from the exposure site, cleans the dentin interface, shows excellent hemostasis and exhibits efficacy against pathogenic microorganisms (Hafez *et al*. 2002; Demir & Ceherli 2007). The solution is highly recommended as an adjunct to successful pulp therapy, rather than sterile water or saline solution.

A primary and often overlooked aspect of direct pulp capping in a carious field is the presence of undetected microorganisms that can survive in the tubules of the surrounding dentin proximal to the exposure site after caries removal. These cariogenic pathogens can still be present after meticulous caries removal and SH disinfection. Pulp capping protocols historically have directed clinicians to place the pulp dressing conservatively over the pulp exposure but have failed to address the surrounding hard tissue that may remain contaminated with surviving bacteria. Therefore, the placement of MTA over the exposure site and the surrounding dentin may be critical if these bacteria are to be effectively neutralized. This strategy can improve successful outcomes, particularly in teeth that exhibit extensive caries with multiple exposures after caries removal (Bogen & Chandler 2008).

A thick layer of MTA over the exposure site and the surrounding dentin increases the probability that remaining microorganisms are entombed and incapable of challenging the pulp again. These residual pathogens can produce irreversible changes that can eventually lead to pulpal inflammation, necrosis, and possible endodontic therapy. This aspect of direct pulp capping is an important consideration in one-step protocols when flowable resin modified glass ionomer (RMGI) cements are used over unset MTA. Although RMGI materials exhibit acceptable bond strengths to dentin (Davidson 2006), the active chemical components are inflammatory and toxic when placed in direct contact with pulp tissue (do Nascimiento *et al*. 2000). However, RMGI cements have been shown to be mildly inflammatory to pulp tissue when in indirect contact on the remaining dentin and the materials appear to have substantial antibacterial properties (Herrera *et al*. 2000; Costa *et al*. 2011; Kotsanos & Arizos 2011).

RMGI cements are water-based bonding agents that are not affected by small amounts of water on the dentinal surface. The pH of unset RMGI cements is approximately 1.5 and the material acts as its own self-etching primer (Davidson 2006). There are no known characteristics of unset MTA that would affect the setting of RMGI cements. The material does not exhibit polymerization shrinkage stress and the bond strength to dentin and MTA should be approximately 10 MPa. Although RMGI cements provide the opportunity to provide one-step pulp capping using MTA, the effective killing of all remaining bacteria may be compromised when compared to a two-step protocol where a larger volume of MTA is placed over the exposure and surrounding dentin and RMGI cements are not utilized. Furthermore, the placement of RMGI cements over a large aliquot of unset MTA may be clinically challenging even for the most experienced operators.

DISADVANTAGES

Even though MTA appears to be the preferred material in vital pulp therapy with many positive features, the cement does have several drawbacks. The compressive and flexural strength as well as the microhardness of MTA are lower than that of dentin. The values for the compressive strength of MTA are between 45 and 98 MPa (Islam *et al.* 2006; Nekoofar *et al.* 2007, 2010c), the flexural strength is 11–15 MPa (Walker *et al.* 2006; Aggarwal *et al.* 2011), and the Vickers microhardness (HV) has been estimated between 40 and 60 HV (Danesh *et al.* 2006; Nekoofar *et al.* 2007; Namazikhah *et al.* 2008; Nekoofar *et al.* 2010a, b; Kang *et al.* 2012). In comparison, the values for dentin are about 200–350 MPa, 20 MPa, and 60–70 HV, respectively (Ryge *et al.* 1961; Motsch 1990; Fuentes *et al.* 2003) and thus considerably more than ProRoot MTA. Therefore, MTA seems to be unsuitable for long-term clinical use as a sole restorative base or to replace dentin after an indirect or direct pulp capping.

Another disadvantage of MTA is its extended setting time of more than 2.5 hours (Torabinejad *et al.* 1995a). This characteristic can compromise successful vital pulp procedures because of the added difficulty in delivering a sealed permanent restoration during the same visit (Duda & Dammaschke 2009; Dammaschke 2011). Due to the low mechanical properties and the long setting time of MTA, the material also requires coverage with a flowable RGMI cement, before a permanent restoration can be provided when one-visit treatment is elected. Moreover, mixed MTA exhibits a granular and sand-like consistency. Its handling, and application can be difficult and specialized devices are beneficial to attain best results (Stropko 2009; Gutmann & Lovedahl 2011). Gray

ProRoot MTA when originally introduced produced tooth discoloration (Karabucak *et al.* 2005) and this drawback has also been described after the use of WMTA for vital pulp therapy in the clinical crown due to the presence of metallic oxides (Belobrov & Parashos 2011). Finally, MTA is a relatively expensive material, especially in comparison to CH.

SUMMARY

Unfavorable outcomes in pulp capping are caused by infection, due to either remaining bacteria or exposure to new bacteria from defective restorations (Østravik & Pitt Ford 1998). The main advantage of MTA when used in vital pulp therapy is that it is a hard setting cement with low solubility with sustained antibacterial properties (Torabinejad *et al.* 1995a; Fridland & Rosado 2005). This hydraulic calcium-silicate cement used as a medication for pulp capping and pulpotomy may prevent the recontamination of pulp tissue (Pitt Ford *et al.* 1996).

MTA features pronounced biocompatibility, bioactivity, and the capacity to stimulate the formation of hard tissue. It appears to be the preferred material compared to CH as *in vivo* studies clearly demonstrate a superior or equal ability to stimulate reparative dentinogenesis in mechanically exposed, partially inflamed, and healthy pulps (Table 1.1). Other factors to consider that may contribute to successful outcomes in vital pulp therapy when using MTA:

- The pulp tissue should be cleared of bacteria and bacterial toxins.
- Complete hemostasis is required.
- Microbial contamination of the pulp tissue during treatment should be meticulously avoided.
- Sodium hypochlorite is the ideal solution for hemorrhage control.
- Provision of a bacteria-tight restoration should not be delayed.

By contrast, patient age, tooth location, subjective symptomatology, and the size or site of pulp exposure may play a secondary role when the final treatment outcome is considered.

ACKNOWLEDGMENT

The authors wish to thank Drs. Stephen Davis and Nicholas Chandler for their contributions to this chapter.

REFERENCES

Abedi, H.R., Ingle, J.I. (1995) Mineral trioxide aggregate: a review of a new cement. *Journal of the Californian Dental Association* **23**, 36–9.

Abedi, H.R., Torabinejad M., Pitt Ford T.R., *et al.* (1996) The use of mineral trioxide aggregate cement (MTA) as a direct pulp-capping agent. *Journal of Endodontics* **22**, 199 (abstract).

Accorinte, M.L., Holland, R., Reis, A., *et al.* (2008a) Evaluation of mineral trioxide aggregate and calcium hydroxide cement as pulp-capping agents in human teeth. *Journal of Endodontics* **34**, 1–6.

Accorinte, M.L., Loguercio, A.D., Reis, A., *et al.* (2008b) Response of human dental pulp capped with MTA and calcium hydroxide powder. *Operative Dentistry* **33**, 488–95.

Accorinte, M.L., Loguercio, A.D., Reis, A., *et al.* (2008c) Response of human pulps capped with different self-etch adhesive systems. *Clinical Oral Investigations* **12**, 119–27.

Aeinehchi, M., Dadvand, S., Fayazi, S., *et al.* (2007) Randomized controlled trial of mineral trioxide aggregate and formocresol for pulpotomy in primary molar teeth. *International Endodontic Journal* **40**, 261–7.

Aeinehchi, M., Eslami, B., Ghanbariha, M., *et al.* (2003) Mineral trioxide aggregate (MTA) and calcium hydroxide as pulp-capping agents in human teeth: a preliminary report. *International Endodontic Journal* **36**, 225–31.

Agamy, H.A., Bakry, N.S., Mounir, M.M., *et al.* (2004) Comparison of mineral trioxide aggregate and formocresol as pulp-capping agents in pulpotomized primary teeth. *Pediatric Dentistry* **26**, 302–9.

Aggarwal, V., Jain, A., Kabi, D. (2011) *In vitro* evaluation of effect of various endodontic solutions on selected physical properties of white mineral trioxide aggregate. *Australian Endodontic Journal* **37**, 61–4.

Akbari, M., Rouhani, A., Samiee, S., *et al.* (2012) Effect of dentin bonding agent on the prevention of tooth discoloration produced by mineral trioxide aggregate. *International Journal of Dentistry* **2012**:563203.

Al-Hezaimi, K., Al-Hamdan, K., Naghshbandi, J., *et al.* (2005) Effect of white-colored mineral trioxide aggregate in different concentrations on *Candida albicans* in vitro. *Journal of Endodontics* **3**, 684–6.

Al-Hezaimi, K., Salameh, Z., Al-Fouzan, K., *et al.* (2011) Histomorphometric and micro-computed tomography analysis of pulpal response to three different pulp capping materials. *Journal of Endodontics* **37**, 507–12.

American Academy of Pediatric Dentistry (2011) Reference manual: Guidelines on pulpal therapy for primary and immature permanent teeth. *Pediatric Dentistry* **33**, 214–15.

American Association of Endodontists (2003) *Glossary of Endodontic Terms*, 7th edn. American Association of Endodontists, Chicago.

An, S., Gao, Y., Ling, J., *et al.* (2012) Calcium ions promote osteogenic differentiation and mineralization of human dental pulp cells: implications for pulp capping materials. *Journal of Materials Science: Materials in Medicine* **23**, 789–95.

Ansari, G., Ranjpour, M. (2010) Mineral trioxide aggregate and formocresol pulpotomy in primary teeth: a 2 year follow-up. *International Endodontic Journal* **43**, 413–18.

Asgary, S., Parirokh, M., Eghbal, M.J., *et al.* (2005) Chemical differences between white and gray mineral trioxide aggregate. *Journal of Endodontics* **31**, 101–3.

Asgary, S., Eghbal, M.J., Parirokh, M., *et al.* (2008) A comparative study of histologic response to different pulp capping materials and a novel endodontic cement. *Oral Surgery Oral Medicine Oral Pathology Oral Radiology and Endodontics* **106**, 609–14.

Bakland, L.K., Andreasen, J.O. (2012) Will mineral trioxide aggregate replace calcium hydroxide in treating pulpal and periodontal healing complications subsequent to dental trauma? A review. *Dental Traumatology* **28**, 25–32.

Barnes, I.M., Kidd, E.A. (1979) Disappearing Dycal. *British Dental Journal* **147**, 111.

Barthel, C.R., Rosenkranz, B., Leuenberg, A., *et al.* (2000) Pulp capping of carious exposures: treatment outcome after 5 and 10 years: a retrospective study. *Journal of Endodontics* **26**, 525–8.

Baume, L.J., Holz, J. (1981) Long-term clinical assessment of direct pulp capping. *International Dental Journal* **31**, 251–60.

Belobrov, I., Parashos, P. (2011) Treatment of tooth discoloration after the use of white mineral trioxide aggregate. *Journal of Endodontics* **37**, 1017–20.

Bogen, G., Chandler, N.P. (2008) Vital pulp therapy. In: *Ingle's Endodontics* (J.I. Ingle, L.K. Bakand, J.C. Baumgartner, eds), 6th edn. BC Decker, Hamilton. pp. 1310–29.

Bogen, G., Kim, J.S., Bakland, L.K. (2008) Direct pulp capping with mineral trioxide aggregate: an observational study. *Journal of the American Dental Association* **139**, 305–15.

Bonson, S., Jeansonne, B.G., Laillier, T.E. (2004) Root-end filling materials alter fibroblast differentiation. *Journal of Dental Research* **83**, 408–13.

Borges, R.P., Sousa-Neto, M.D., Varsiani, M.A., *et al.* (2012) Changes in the surface of four calcium silicate-containing endodontic materials and an epoxy resin-based sealer after a solubility test. *International Endodontic Journal* **45**, 419–28.

Bose R., Nummikoski P., Hargreaves K (2009) A retrospective evaluation of radiographic outcomes in immature teeth with necrotic root canal systems treated with regenerative endodontic procedures. *Journal Endodontics* **35**, 1343–9.

Bozeman, T.B., Lemon, R.R., Eleazer, P.D. (2006) Elemental analysis of crystal precipitate from gray and white MTA. *Journal of Endodontics* **32**, 425–8.

Brisco, A.L., Rahal, V., Mestrener, S.R., *et al.* (2006) Biological response of pulps submitted to different capping materials. *Brazilian Oral Research* **20**, 219–25.

Caicedo R, Abbott PV, Alongi DJ, *et al.* (2006) Clinical, radiographic and histological analysis of the effects of mineral trioxide aggregate used in direct pulp capping and pulpotomies of primary teeth. *Australian Dental Journal* **51**, 297–305.

Caliskan, M.K. (1995) Pulpotomy of carious vital teeth with periapical involvement. *International Endodontic Journal* **28**, 172–7.

Camargo, S.E., Camargo, C.H., Hiller, K.A., *et al.* (2009) Cytotoxicity and genotoxicity of pulp capping materials in two cell lines. *International Endodontic Journal* **42**, 227–37.

Camilleri, J., Montesin, F.E., Brady, K., *et al.* (2005) The constitution of mineral trioxide aggregate. *Dental Materials* **21**, 297–303.

Camp, J.H., Fuks, A.B. (2006) Pediatric endodontics: endodontic treatment for the primary and young, permanent dentition. In: *Pathways of the Pulp* (S. Cohen & K. Hargreaves, eds), 9th edn. Mosby, St. Louis, pp. 822–82.

Camp, J.H. (2008) Diagnosis dilemmas in vital pulp therapy: treatment for the toothache is changing, especially in young, immature teeth. *Pediatric Dentistry* **30**, 197–205.

Caplan, D.J., Cai, J., Yin, G., *et al.* (2005) Root canal filled versus non-root canal filled teeth: a retrospective comparison of survival times. *Journal of Public Health Dentistry* **65**, 90–6.

Cardoso-Silva, C., Barberia, E., Maroto, M., *et al.* (2011) Clinical study of mineral trioxide aggregate in primary molars. Comparison between grey and white MTA – a long term follow-up (84 months). *Journal of Dentistry* **39**, 187–93.

Cavalcanti, B.N., de Mello Rode, S., França, C.M., *et al.* (2011) Pulp capping materials exert an effect of the secretion of IL-1β and IL-8 by migrating human neutrophils. *Brazilian Oral Research* **25**, 13–18.

Chacko, V., Kurikose, S. (2006) Human pulpal response to mineral trioxide aggregate (MTA): a histologic study. *Journal of Clinical Pediatric Dentistry* **30**, 203–9.

Cho, S.Y., Seo, D.G., Lee, S.J., *et al.* (2013) Prognostic factors for clinical outcomes according to time after direct pulp capping. *Journal of Endodontics* **39**, 327–31.

Costa, C.A.S., Duarte, P.T., de Souza, P.P., *et al.* (2008) Cytotoxic effects and pulpal response caused by a mineral trioxide aggregate formulation and calcium hydroxide. *American Journal of Dentistry* **21**, 255–61.

Costa, C.A.S., Ribeiro, A.P., Giro, E.M., *et al.* (2011) Pulp response after application of two resin modified glass ionomer cements (RMGICs) in deep cavities of prepared human teeth. *Dental Materials* **27**, e158–e170.

Cox, C.F., Sübay, R.K., Ostro, E., *et al.* (1996) Tunnel defects in dentinal bridges. Their formation following direct pulp capping. *Operative Dentistry* **21**, 4–11.

Cvek, M. (1978) A clinical report on partial pulpotomy and capping with calcium hydroxide in permanent incisors with complicated crown fractures. *Journal of Endodontics* **4**, 232–7.

Cvek, M. (1993) Endodontic management of traumatized teeth. In: *Textbook and Color Atlas of Traumatic Injuries to the Teeth* (J.O. Andreasen & F.M. Andreasen, eds), 3rd edn. Munksgaard, Copenhagen, pp. 517–86.

Cvek, M., Cleaton-Jones, P., Austin, J., *et al.* (1982) Pulp reactions to exposure after experimental crown fractures or grinding in adult monkeys. *Journal of Endodontics* **8**, 391–7.

Dammaschke, T. (2011) Direct pulp capping. *Dentist* **27**(8), 88–94.

Dammaschke, T., Gerth, H.U.V., Züchner, H., *et al.* (2005) Chemical and physical surface and bulk material characterization of white ProRoot MTA and two Portland cements. *Dental Materials* **21**, 731–8.

Dammaschke, T., Leidinger, J., Schäfer, E. (2010a) Long-term evaluation of direct pulp capping-treatment outcomes over an average period of 6.1 years. *Clinical Oral Investigations* **14**, 559–67.

Dammaschke, T., Stratmann, U., Wolff, P., *et al.* (2010b) Direct pulp capping with mineral trioxide aggregate: An immunohistological comparison with calcium hydroxide in rodents. *Journal of Endodontics* **36**, 814–19.

Dammaschke, T., Wolff, P., Sagheri, D., *et al.* (2010c) Mineral trioxide aggregate for direct pulp capping: a histologic comparison with calcium hydroxide in rat molars. *Quintessence International* **41**, e20–e30.

Danesh, G., Dammaschke, T., Gerth, H.U.V., *et al.* (2006) A comparative study of selected properties of ProRoot MTA and two Portland cements. *International Endodontic Journal* **39**, 213–19.

Davidson, C.L. (2006) Advances in glass-ionomer cements. *Journal of Applied Oral Science* **14** (Suppl.), 3–9.

Demir, T., Cehreli, Z.C. (2007) Clinical and radiographic evaluation of adhesive pulp capping in primary molars following hemostasis with 1.25 % sodium hypochlorite: 2-year results. *American Journal of Dentistry* **20**, 182–8.

do Nascimento, A.B., Fontana, U.F., Teixeira, H.M., *et al.* (2000) Biocompatibility of a resin-modified glass-ionomer cement applied as pulp capping in human teeth. *American Journal of Dentistry* **13**, 28–34.

Dominguez, M.S., Witherspoon, D.E., Gutmann, J.L., *et al.* (2003) Histological and scanning electron microscopy assessment of various vital pulp-therapy materials. *Journal of Endodontics* **29**, 324–33.

Doyle, T.L., Casas, M.J., Kenny, D.J., *et al.* (2010) Mineral trioxide aggregate produces superior outcomes in vital primary molar pulpotomy. *Pediatric Dentistry* **32**, 41–7.

Dreger L.A., Felippe W.T., Reyes-Carmona J.F., *et al.* (2010). Mineral trioxide aggregate and Portland cement promote biomineralization in vivo. *Journal Endodontics* **38**, 324–9.

Duarte, M.A.H., Demarchi, A.C.C.O., Yamashita, J.C., *et al.* (2003) pH and calcium ion release of 2 root-end filling materials. *Oral Surgery Oral Medicine Oral Pathology Oral Radiology and Endodontics* **95**, 345–7.

Duda, S., Dammaschke, T. (2008) Measures for maintain pulp vitality. Are there alternatives to calcium hydroxide in direct pulp capping? *Quintessenz* **59**, 1327–34, 1354 [in German].

Duda, S., Dammaschke, T. (2009) Direct pulp capping – prerequisites to clinical treatment success. *Endodontie* **18**, 21–31 [in German].

Duggal, M. (2009) Formocresol alternatives. *British Dental Journal* **206**, 3.

Eghbal, M.J., Asgary, S., Baglue, R.A., *et al.* (2009) MTA pulpotomy of human permanent molars with irreversible pulpitis. *Australian Endodontic Journal* **35**, 4–8.

Elliott, R.D., Roberts, M.W., Burkes, J., *et al.* (1999) Evaluation of the carbon dioxide laser on vital human primary pulp tissue. *Pediatric Dentistry* **21**, 327–31.

El-Meligy, O.A., Avery, D.R. (2006) Comparison of mineral trioxide aggregate and calcium hydroxide as pulpotomy agents in young permanent teeth (apexogenesis). *Pediatric Dentistry* **28**, 399–404.

Erdem, A.P., Guven, Y., Balli, B., *et al.* (2011) Success rates of mineral trioxide aggregate, ferric sulfate and formocresol pulpotomies: a 24 month study. *Pediatric Dentistry* **33**, 165–70.

Faraco Júnior, I.M., Holland, R. (2001) Response of the pulp of dogs to capping with mineral trioxide aggregate or a calcium hydroxide cement. *Dental Traumatology* **17**, 163–6.

Faraco Júnior, I.M., Holland, R. (2004) Histomorphological response of dogs'dental pulp capped with white Mineral Trioxide Aggregate. *Brazilian Dental Journal* **15**, 104–8.

Farsi, N., Alamoudi, N., Balto, K., *et al.* (2005) Success of mineral trioxide aggregate in pulpotomized primary molars. *Journal of Clinical Pediatric Dentistry* **29**, 307–11.

Fridland, M.,, Rosado, R. (2005) MTA solubility: a long term study. *Journal of Endodontics* **31**, 376–9.

Fuentes, V., Toledano, M., Osorio, R., *et al.* (2003) Microhardness of superficial and deep sound human dentin. *Journal of Biomedical Materials Research Part A* **66A**, 850–3.

Fuks, A.B., Papagiannoulis, L. (2006) Pulpotomy in primary teeth: review of the literature according to standardized criteria. *European Archives of Pediatric Dentistry* **7**, 64–72.

Fusayama, T., Okuse, K., Hosoda, H. (1966) Relationship between hardness, discoloration, and microbial invasion in carious dentin. *Journal of Dental Research* **45**, 1033–46.

Fusayama, T., Terachima, S. (1972) Differentiation of two layers of carious dentin by staining. *Journal of Dental Research* **51**, 866.

Fuss, Z., Lustig, J., Katz, A., *et al.* (2001) An evaluation of endodontically treated vertical root fractured teeth: impact of operative procedures. *Journal of Endodontics* **27**, 46–8.

Galler, K.M., Schweikl, H., Hiller, K.A., *et al.* (2011) TEGDMA reduces mineralization in dental pulp cells. *Journal of Dental Research* **90**, 257–62.

Gandolfi, M.G., van Lunduyt, K., Taddei, P., *et al.* (2010) Environmental scanning electron microscopy connected with energy dispersive X-ray analysis and Raman techniques to study ProRoot mineral trioxide aggregate and calcium silicate cements in wet conditions and in real time. *Journal of Endodontics* **36**, 851–7.

Glickman, G.N., Koch, K.A. (2000) 21st-century endodontics. *Journal of the American Dental Association* **131**(Suppl.), 39S–46S.

Goldberg, M., Smith, A.J. (2004) Cells and extracellular matrices of dentin and pulp: a biological basis for repair and tissue engineering. *Critical Reviews in Oral Biology and Medicine* **15**, 13–27.

Goldberg, M., Farges, J.-C., Lacerda-Pinheiro, S., *et al.* (2008) Inflammatory and immunological aspects of dental pulp repair. *Pharmacological Research* **58**, 137–47.

Goracci, G., Mori, G. (1996) Scanning electron microscopic evaluation of resin-dentin and calcium hydroxide-dentin interface with resin composite restorations. *Quintessence International* **27**, 129–35.

Gutmann, J.L., Lovedahl, P.E. (2011) Problem-solving challenges in periapical surgery. In: *Problem Solving in Endodontics* (J.L Gutmann, P.E. Lovedahl, eds), 5th edn. Elsevier Mosby, Maryland Heights, p 351.

Guven, E.P., Yalvac, M.E., Sahin, F., *et al.* (2011) Effect of dental materials calcium hydroxide-containing cement, mineral trioxide aggregate, and enamel matrix derivative on proliferation and differentiation of human tooth germ stem cells. *Journal of Endodontics* **37**, 650–6.

Hafez, A.A., Cox, C.F., Tarim, B., *et al.* (2002) An in vivo evaluation of hemorrhage control using sodium hypochlorite and direct pulp capping with a one- or two- component adhesive system in exposed nonhuman primate pulps. *Quintessence International* **33**, 261–72.

Ham, K.A., Witherspoon, D.E., Gutmann, J.L., *et al.* (2005) Preliminary evaluation of BMP-2 expression and histological characteristics during apexification with calcium hydroxide and Mineral Trioxide Aggregate. *Journal of Endodontics* **31**, 275–9.

Han, L., Okiji, T. (2011) Uptake of calcium and silicon released from calcium silicate-based endodontic materials into root canal dentine. *International Endodontic Journal* **44**, 1081–7.

Heide, S., Mjör, I.A. (1983) Pulp reactions to experimental exposures in young permanent monkey teeth. *International Endodontic Journal* **16**, 11–19.

Hench, L.L., West, J.K. (1996) Biological application of bioactive glasses. *Life Chemistry Reports* **13**, 187–241.

Hermann, B. (1928) Ein weiterer Beitrag zur Frage der Pulpenbehandlung. *Zahnärztliche Rundschau* **37**, 1327–76 [in German].

Hermann, B. (1930) Dentinobliteration der Wurzelkanäle nach Behandlung mit Calcium. *Zahnärztliche Rundschau* **39**, 888–99 [in German].

Herrera, M., Castillo, A., Bravo, M., *et al.* (2000) Antibacterial activity of resin adhesives, glass ionomer and resin-modified glass ionomer cements and a compomer in contact with dentin caries samples. *Operative Dentistry* **25**, 265–9.

Hilton TJ, Ferracane JL, Mancl L; for Northwest Practice-based Research Collaborative in Evidence-based Dentistry (NWP) (2013) Comparison of CaOH with MTA for Direct Pulp Capping: A PBRN Randomized Clinical Trial. *Journal of Dental Research* **92**, S16–22.

Holan, G., Eidelman, E., Fuks, A.B. (2005) Long-term evaluation of pulpotomy in primary molars using Mineral Trioxide Aggregate or formocresol. *Pediatric Dentistry* **27**, 129–36.

Holland, R., de Souza, V., Nery, M.J., *et al.* (1999) Reaction of dogs' teeth to root canal filling with Mineral Trioxide Aggregate or a glass ionomer sealer. *Journal of Endodontics* **25**, 728–30.

Holland, R., Otoboni-Filho, J.A., de Souza, V., *et al.* (2001) Mineral trioxide aggregate repair of lateral root perforations. *Journal of Endodontics* **27**, 281–4.

Hørsted, P., Sandergaard, B., Thylstrup, A., *et al.* (1985) A retrospective study of direct pulp capping with calcium hydroxide compounds. *Endodontics and Dental Traumatology* **1**, 29–34.

Hørsted-Bindslev, P., Bergenholtz, G. (2003) Vital pulp therapies. In: *Textbook of Endodontology* (eds G. Bergenholtz, P. Hørsted-Bindslev, C. Erik-Reit), Blackwell Munksgaard, Oxford, pp. 66–91.

Hørsted-Bindslev, P., Vilkinis, V., Sidlauskas, A. (2003) Direct pulp capping of human pulps with a dentin bonding system or with calcium hydroxide cement. *Oral Surgery Oral Medicine Oral Pathology Oral Radiology and Endodontics* **96**, 591–600.

Islam, I., Chng, H.K., Yap, A.U.J. (2006) Comparison of the physical and mechanical properties of MTA and Portland cement. *Journal of Endodontics* **32**, 193–7.

Iwamoto, C.E., Adachi, E., Pameijer, C.H., *et al.* (2006) Clinical and histological evaluation of white ProRoot MTA in direct pulp capping. *American Journal of Dentistry* **19**, 85–90.

Iwaya S.I., Ikawa M., Kubota M. (2001) Revascularization of an immature permanent tooth with apical periodontitis and sinus tract. *Dental Traumatology* **17**, 185–7.

Jeeruphan T., Jantarat J., Yanpiset K., *et al.* (2012) Mahidol study 1: comparison of radiographic and survival outcomes of immature teeth treated with either regenerative endodontic or apexification methods: a retrospective study. *Journal of Endodontics* **38**, 1330–6.

Junn, D.J., McMillan, P., Bakland, L.K., *et al.* (1998) Quantitative assessment of dentin bridge formation following pulp-capping with mineral trioxide aggregate (MTA). *Journal of Endodontics* **24**, 278 (abstract).

Kakehashi, S., Stanley, H.R., Fitzgerald, R.J. (1965) The effects of surgical exposure of dental pulps in germ-free and conventional laboratory rats. *Oral Surgery Oral Medicine Oral Pathology* **20**, 340–9.

Kang, J.S., Rhim, E.M., Huh, S.Y., *et al.* (2012) The effects of humidity and serum on the surface microhardness and morphology of five retrograde filling materials. *Scanning* **34**, 207–14.

Karabucak, B., Li, D., Lim, J., *et al.* (2005) Vital pulp therapy with mineral trioxide aggregate. *Dental Traumatology* **21**, 240–3.

Keiser, K., Johnson, C.C., Tipton, D.A. (2000) Cytotoxicity of mineral trioxide aggregate using human periodontal ligament fibroblasts. *Journal of Endodontics* **26**, 288–91.

Kettering, J.D., Torabinejad, M. (1995) Investigation of mutagenicity of mineral trioxide aggregate and other commonly used root-end filling materials. *Journal of Endodontics* **21**, 537–9.

Kirk, E.E.J., Lim, K.C., Khan, M.O.G. (1989) A comparison of dentinogenesis on pulp capping with calcium hydroxide in paste and cement form. *Oral Surgery Oral Medicine Oral Pathology* **68**, 210–19.

Koh, E.T., Torabinejad, M., Pitt Ford, T.R., *et al.* (1997) Mineral trioxide aggregate stimulates a biological response in human osteoblasts. *Journal of Biomedical Materials Research* **37**, 432–9.

Koh, E.T., McDonald, F., Pitt Ford, T.R., *et al.* (1998) Cellular response to mineral trioxide aggregate. *Journal of Endodontics* **24**, 543–7.

Kotsanos, N., Arizos, S. (2011) Evaluation of a resin modified glass ionomer serving both as indirect pulp therapy and as restorative material for primary molars. *European Archives of Pediatric Dentistry* **12**, 170–5.

Kuratate, M., Yoshiba, K., Shigetani, Y., *et al.* (2008) Immunohistochemical analysis of nestin, osteopontin, and proliferating cells in the reparative process of exposed dental pulp capped with mineral trioxide aggregate. *Journal of Endodontics* **34**, 970–4.

Langeland, K. (1981) Management of the inflamed pulp associated with deep carious lesion. *Journal of Endodontics* **7**, 169–81.

Laurent, P., Aubut, V., About, I. (2009) Development of a bioactive Ca_3SiO_5 based posterior restorative material (Biodentine™). In: *Biocompatibility or Cytotoxic Effects of Dental Composites* (M. Goldberg, ed.). Coxmoor, Oxford, pp. 195–200.

Leites, A.B., Baldissera, E.Z., Silva, A.F., *et al.* (2011) Histologic response and tenascin and fibronectin expression after pulp capping in pig primary teeth with mineral trioxide aggregate or calcium hydroxide. *Operative Dentistry* **36**, 448–56.

Lertchirakarn, V., Palamara, J.E., Messer, H.H. (2003) Patterns of vertical root fracture: Factors affecting stress distribution in the root canal. *Journal of Endodontics* **29**, 523–8.

Lewis, B. (2010) The obsolescence of formocresol. *Journal of the Californian Dental Association* **38**, 102–7.

Leye Benoist, F., Gaye Ndiaye, F., Kane, A.W., *et al.* (2012) Evaluation of mineral trioxide aggregate (MTA) versus calcium hydroxide cement (Dycal®) in the formation of a dentine bridge: a randomised controlled trial. *International Dental Journal* **62**, 33–9.

Liard-Dumtschin, D., Holz, J., Baume, L.J. (1984) Direct pulp capping - a biological trial of 8 products. *Schweizer Monatsschrift für Zahnmedizin* **94**, 4–22 [in French].

Lim, K.C., Kirk, E.E.J. (1987) Direct pulp capping: a review. *Endodontics and Dental Traumatology* **3**, 213–19.

Linn, J., Messer, H.H. (1994) Effect of restorative procedures on the strength of endodontically treated molars. *Journal of Endodontics* **20**, 479–85.

Liu, H., Zhou, Q., Qin, M. (2011) Mineral trioxide aggregate versus calcium hydroxide for pulpotomy in primary molars. *Chinese Journal of Dental Research* **14**, 121–5.

Liu, J., Chen, L.R., Chao, S.Y. (1999) Laser pulpotomy of primary teeth. *Pediatric Dentistry* **21**, 128–9.

Matsuo, T., Nakanishi, T., Shimizu, H., *et al.* (1996) A clinical study of direct pulp capping applied to carious-exposed pulps. *Journal of Endodontics* **22**, 551–6.

McDonald, R.E., Avery, D.R., Dean, J.A. (2011) Treatment of deep caries, vital pulp exposure, and pulpless teeth. In: *McDonald and Avery's Dentistry of the Child and Adolescent* (J.A. Dean, D.R. Avery, R.E. McDonald, eds), 9th edn. Mosby Elsevier, Maryland Heights, pp. 343–65.

Mejare, I., Cvek, M. (1993) Partial pulpotomy in young permanent teeth with deep carious lesions. *Endodontics and Dental Traumatology* **9**, 238–42.

Mente, J., Geletneky, B., Ohle, M., *et al.* (2010) Mineral trioxide aggregate or calcium hydroxide direct pulp capping: an analysis of the clinical treatment outcome. *Journal of Endodontics* **36**, 806–13.

Merdad, K., Sonbul, H., Bukhary, S. *et al.* (2011). Caries susceptibility of endodontically versus nonendodontically treated teeth. *Journal of Endodontics* **37**, 139–42.

Miles, J.P., Gluskin, A.H., Chambers, D., *et al.* (2010) Pulp capping with mineral trioxide aggregate (MTA): a retrospective analysis of carious pulp exposures treated by undergraduate dental students. *Operative Dentistry* **35**, 20–8.

Min, K.S., Park, H.J., Lee, S.K., *et al.* (2008) Effect of mineral trioxide aggregate on dentin bridge formation and expression of dentin sialoprotein and heme oxygenase-1 in human dental pulp. *Journal of Endodontics* **34**, 666–70.

Minamikawa, H., Yamada, M., Deyama, Y., *et al.* (2011) Effect of *N*-acetylcysteine on rat dental pulp cells cultured on mineral trioxide aggregate. *Journal of Endodontics* **37**, 637–41.

Mireku, A.S., Romberg, E., Fouad, A.F., *et al.* (2010) Vertical fracture of root filled teeth restored with posts: the effects of patient age and dentine thickness. *International Endodontic Journal* **43**, 218–25.

Mitchell, P.J.C., Pitt Ford, T.R., Torabinejad, M., *et al.* (1999) Osteoblast biocompatibility of mineral trioxide aggregate. *Biomaterials* **20**, 167–73.

Miyauchi, H., Iwaku, M., Fusayama, T. (1978) Physiological recalcification of carious dentin. *The Bulletin of Tokyo Medical and Dental University* **25**, 169–79.

Moghaddame-Jafari, S., Mantellini, M.G., Botero, T.M., *et al.* (2005) Effect of ProRoot MTA on pulp cell apoptosis and proliferation *in vitro*. *Journal of Endodontics* **31**, 387–91.

Moretti, A.B., Sakai, V.T., Oliveira, T.M., *et al.* (2008) The effectiveness of mineral trioxide aggregate, calcium hydroxide and formocresol for pulpotomies in primary teeth. *International Endodontic Journal* **41**, 547–55.

Motsch, A. (1990) Die Unterfüllung – eine kritische Diskussion der verschiedenen Zement und Präparate. In: Neue Füllungsmaterialien – *Indikation und Verarbeitung* (ed Akademie Praxis und Wissenschaft in der DGZMK), Carl Hanser, Munich, pp. 35–54 [in German].

Murray, P.E., Garcia-Godoy, F., Hargreaves, K.M. (2007) Regenerative endodontics: a review of current status and a call for action. *Journal of Endodontics* **33**, 377–90.

Myers, K., Kaminski, E., Lautenschlater, E. (1996) The effects of mineral trioxide aggregate on the dog pulp. *Journal of Endodontics* **22**, 198 (abstract).

Nair, P.N.R., Duncan, H.F., Pitt Ford, T.R., *et al.* (2008) Histological, ultrastructural and quantitative investigations on the response of healthy human pulps to experimental pulp capping with mineral trioxide aggregate: a randomized controlled trial. *International Endodontic Journal* **41**, 128–50.

Naito, T. (2010) Uncertainty remains regarding long-term success of mineral trioxide aggregate for direct pulp capping. *Journal of Evidence-Based Dental Practice* **10**, 250–1.

Nakayama, A., Ogiso, B., Tanabe, N., *et al.* (2005) Behavior of bone marrow osteoblast-like cells on mineral trioxide aggregate: morphology and expression of type I collagen and bone-related protein mRNAs. *International Endodontic Journal* **38**, 203–10.

Namazikhah, M.S., Nekoofar, M.H., Sheykhrezae, M.S., *et al.* (2008) The effect of pH on the surface hardness and microstructure of mineral trioxide aggregate. *International Endodontic Journal* **41**, 108–16.

Nekoofar, M.H., Adusei, G., Sheykhrezae, M.S., *et al.* (2007) The effect of condensation pressure on selected physical properties of mineral trioxide aggregate. *International Endodontic Journal* **40**, 453–61.

Nekoofar, M.H., Aseeley, Z., Dummer, P.M.H. (2010a) The effect of various mixing techniques on the surface microhardness of mineral trioxide aggregate. *International Endodontic Journal* **43**, 312–20.

Nekoofar, M.H., Oloomi, K., Sheykhrezae, M.S., *et al.* (2010b) An evaluation of the effect of blood and human serum on the surface microhardness and surface microstructure of mineral trioxide aggregate. *International Endodontic Journal* **43**, 849–58.

Nekoofar, M.H., Stone, D.F., Dummer, P.M.H. (2010c) The effect of blood contamination on the compressive strength and surface microstructure of mineral trioxide aggregate. *International Endodontic Journal* **43**, 782–91.

Okiji, T., Yoshiba, K. (2009) Reparative dentinogenesis induced by mineral trioxide aggregate: a review from the biological and physicochemical points of view. *International Journal of Dentistry* 2009:464280.

Oringer, M.J. (1975) *Electrosurgery in Dentistry*, 2nd edn. WB Saunders, Philadelphia.

Osorio, R.M., Hefti, A., Vertucci, F.J., *et al.* (1998) Cytotoxicity of endodontic materials. *Journal of Endodontics* **24**, 91–6.

Østravik, D., Pitt Ford, T.R. (1998) *Essential Endodontology: Prevention and Treatment of Apical Periodontitis*. Blackwell, Oxford, pp. 192–210.

Paranjpe, A., Zhang, H., Johnson, J.D. (2010) Effects of mineral trioxide aggregate on human pulp cells after pulp-capping procedures. *Journal of Endodontics* **36**, 1042–7.

Paranjpe, A., Smoot, T., Zhang, H., *et al.* (2011) Direct contact with mineral trioxide aggregate activates and differentiates human dental pulp cells. *Journal of Endodontics* **37**, 1691–5.

Parirokh, M., Asgary, S., Eghbal, M.J., *et al.* (2005) A comparative study of white and grey mineral trioxide aggregate as pulp capping agent in dog's teeth. *Dental Traumatology* **21**, 150–4.

Parolia, A., Kundabala, M., Rao, N.N., *et al.* (2010) A comparative histological analysis of human pulp following direct pulp capping with Propolis, mineral trioxide aggregate and Dycal. *Australian Dental Journal* **55**, 59–64.

Phaneuf, R.A., Frankl, S.N., Ruben, M.P. (1968) A comparative histological evaluation of three commercial calcium hydroxide preparations on the human primary dental pulp. *Journal of Dentistry for Children* **35**, 61–76.

Pitt Ford, T.R., Torabinejad, M., Abedi, H.R., *et al.* (1996) Using mineral trioxide aggregate as a pulp-capping material. *Journal of the American Dental Association* **127**, 1491–4.

Qudeimat, M.A., Barrieshi-Nusair, K.M., Owais, A.I. (2007) Calcium hydroxide vs. mineral trioxide aggregate for partial pulpotomy of permanent molars with deep caries. *European Archives of Pediatric Dentistry* **8**, 99–104.

Queiroz, A.M., Assed, S., Leonardo, M.R., *et al.* (2005) MTA and calcium hydroxide for pulp capping. *Journal of Applied Oral Science* **13**, 126–30.

Randow, K., Glantz, P.O. (1986) On cantilever loading of vital and non-vital teeth. An experimental clinical study. *Acta Odontologica Scandinavica* **44**, 271–7.

Retzlaff, A.E., Castaldi, C.R. (1969) Recent knowledge of the dental pulp and its application to clinical practice. *Journal of Prosthetic Dentistry* **22**, 449–57.

Reyes-Carmona, J.F., Santos, A.S., Figueiredo, C.P., *et al.* (2010) Host-mineral trioxide aggregate inflammatory molecular signaling and biomineralization ability. *Journal of Endodontics* **36**, 1347–53.

Ribeiro, C.S., Kuteken, F.A., Hirata Júnior, R., *et al.* (2006) Comparative evaluation of antimicrobial action of MTA, calcium hydroxide and Portland cement. *Journal of Applied Oral Science* **14**, 330–3.

Ruemping, D.R., Morton, T.H., Jr, Anderson, M.W. (1983) Electrosurgical pulpotomy in primates – a comparison with formocresol pulpotomy. *Pediatric Dentistry* **5**, 14–18.

Ryge, G., Foley, D.E., Fairhurst, C.W. (1961) Microindentation hardness. *Journal of Dental Research* **40**, 1116–26.

Salako, N., Joseph, B., Ritwik, P., *et al.* (2003) Comparison of bioactive glass, mineral trioxide aggregate, ferric sulfate and formocresol as pulpotomy agents in rat molar. *Dental Traumatology* **19**, 314–20.

Sarkar, N.K., Caicedo, R., Ritwik, P., *et al.* (2005) Physicochemical basis of the biological properties of Mineral Trioxide Aggregate. *Journal of Endodontics* **31**, 97–100.

Sawicki, L., Pameijer, C.H., Emerich, K., *et al.* (2008) Histological evaluation of mineral trioxide aggregate and calcium hydroxide in direct pulp capping of human immature permanent teeth. *American Journal of Dentistry* **21**, 262–6.

Schmitt, D., Lee, J., Bogen, G. (2001) Multifaceted use of ProRoot MTA root canal repair material. *Journal of Pediatric Dentistry* **23**, 326–30.

Schröder U. (1972) Evaluation of healing following experimental pulpotomy of intact human teeth and capping with calcium hydroxide. *Odontologisk Revy* **23**, 329–40.

Schröder U. (1985) Effects of calcium hydroxide-containing pulp-capping agents on pulp cell migration, proliferation, and differentiation. *Journal of Dental Research* **64** (Spec. Iss.), 541–8.

Schröder, U., Granath, L.E. (1971) On internal dentine resorption in deciduous molars treated by pulpotomy and capped with calcium hydroxide. *Odontologisk Revy* **22**, 179–88.

Schroeder, H.E. (1997) *Pathobiologie oraler Strukturen. Zähne, Pulpa, Parodont*, 3rd edn. Karger, Basel, p 136 [in German].

Shaw, D.W., Sheller, B., Barrus, B.D., *et al.* (1987) Electrosurgical pulpotomy – a 6-month study in primates. *Journal of Endodontics* **13**, 500–5.

Shayegan, A., Petein, M., Vanden Abbeele, A. (2009) The use of beta-tricalcium phosphate, white MTA, white Portland cement and calcium hydroxide for direct pulp capping of primary pig teeth. *Dental Traumatology* **25**, 413–19.

Shulman, E.R., Mulver, F.F., Burkes, E.J., Jr (1987) Comparison of electrosurgery and formocresol as pulpotomy techniques in monkey primary teeth. *Pediatric Dentistry* **9**, 189–94.

Sluka, H., Lehmann, H., Elgün, Z. (1981) Comparative experiments on treatment techniques in vital amputation in view of the preservation of the remaining pulp. *Quintessenz* **32**, 1571–7 [in German].

Smith, A.J., Cassidy, N., Perry, H., *et al.* (1995) Reactionary dentinogenesis. *International Journal of Developmental Biology* **39**, 273–80.

Staehle, H.J. (1990) *Calciumhydroxid in der Zahnheilkunde*. Hanser, Munich [in German].

Stanley, H.R., Lundy T. (1972) Dycal therapy for pulp exposure. *Oral Surgery Oral Medicine Oral Pathology* **34**, 818–25.

Stanley, H.R. (1989) Pulp capping: Conserving the dental pulp – Can it be done? Is it worth it? *Oral Surgery Oral Medicine Oral Pathology* **68**, 628–39.

Stropko, J.J. (2009) Micro-surgical endodontics. In: *Endodontics*. Vol. III (A. Castellucci, ed.). Edizioni Odontoiatriche Il Tridente, Florence, pp. 1118–25.

Subramaniam, P., Konde, S., Mathew, S., *et al.* (2009) Mineral trioxide aggregate as pulp capping agent for primary teeth pulpotomy: 2 year follow up study. *Journal of Clinical Pediatric Dentistry* **33**, 311–14.

Takita, T., Hayashi, M., Takeichi, O., *et al.* (2006) Effect of mineral trioxide aggregate on proliferation of cultured human dental pulp cells. *International Endodontic Journal* **39**, 415–22.

Tani-Ishii, N., Hamada, N., Watanabe, K., *et al.* (2007) Expression of bone extracellular matrix proteins on osteoblast cells in presence of mineral trioxide aggregate. *Journal of Endodontics* **33**, 836–9.

Tatsumi, T. (1989) Physiological remineralization of artificially decalcified monkey dentin under adhesive composite resin restoration. *Kokubyo Gakkai Zasshi* **56**, 47–74 [in Japanese].

Tatsumi, T., Inokoshi, S., Yamada, T., *et al.* (1992) Remineralization of etched dentin. *Journal of Prosthetic Dentistry* **67**, 617–20.

Thesleff, I., Vaahtokari, A., Partanen, A.M. (1995) Regulation of organogenesis: common molecular mechanisms regulating the development of teeth and other organs. *International Journal of Developmental Biology* **39**, 35–50.

Thomson, T.S., Berry, J.E., Somerman, M.J., *et al.* (2003) Cementoblasts maintain expression of osteocalcin in the presence of mineral trioxide aggregate. *Journal of Endodontics* **29**, 407–12.

Torabinejad, M., Chivian, N. (1999) Clinical applications of Mineral Trioxide Aggregate. *Journal of Endodontics* **25**, 197–205.

Torabinejad, M., Watson, T.F., Pitt Ford, T.R. (1993) Sealing ability of a mineral trioxide aggregate when used as a root end filling material. *Journal of Endodontics* **19**, 591–5.

Torabinejad, M., Hong, C.U., McDonald, F., *et al.* (1995a) Physical and chemical properties of a new root-end filling material. *Journal of Endodontics* **21**, 349–53.

Torabinejad, M., Hong, C.U., Pitt Ford, T.R., *et al.* (1995b) Tissue reaction to implanted super-EBA and mineral trioxide aggregate in the mandible of guinea pigs: a preliminary report. *Journal of Endodontics* **21**, 569–71.

Torabinejad, M., Hong, C.U., Pitt Ford, T.R., *et al.* (1995c) Cytotoxicity of four root end filling materials. *Journal of Endodontics* **21**, 489–92.

Torabinejad, M., Rastegar, A.F., Kettering, J.D., *et al.* (1995d) Bacterial leakage of mineral trioxide aggregate as a root-end filling material. *Journal of Endodontics* **21**, 109–12.

Torabinejad, M., Smith, P.W., Kettering, J.D., *et al.* (1995e) Comparative investigation of marginal adaptation of mineral trioxide aggregate and other commonly used root-end filling materials. *Journal of Endodontics* **21**, 295–99.

Torabinejad, M., Pitt Ford, T.R., Abedi, H.R., *et al.* (1998) Tissue reaction to implanted root-end filling materials in the tibia and mandible of guinea pigs. *Journal of Endodontics* **24**, 468–71.

Torneck, C.D., Moe, H., Howley, T.P. (1983) The effect of calcium hydroxide on porcine pulp fibroblasts *in vitro*. *Journal of Endodontics* **9**, 131–6.

Tronstad, L., Mjör, I.A. (1972) Capping of the inflamed pulp. *Oral Surgery Oral Medicine Oral Pathology* **34**, 477–85.

Tziafas, D., Pantelidou, O., Alvanou, A., *et al.* (2002) The dentinogenic effect of mineral trioxide aggregate (MTA) in short-term capping experiments. *International Endodontic Journal* **35**, 245–54.

Walker, M.P., Diliberto, A., Lee, C. (2006) Effect of setting conditions on mineral trioxide aggregate flexural strength. *Journal of Endodontics* **32**, 334–6.

Ward, J. (2002) Vital pulp therapy in cariously exposed permanent teeth and its limitations. *Australian Endodontic Journal* **28**, 29–37.

Weiger, R. (2001) Vitalerhaltende Therapie. In: *Endodontie* (D. Heidemann, ed.). Urban& Fischer, Munich, pp. 58–78 [in German].

Winters, J., Cameron, A.C., Widmer, R.P. (2008) Pulp therapy for primary and immature permanent teeth. In: *Handbook of Pediatric Dentistry* (A.C. Cameron, R.P. Widmer, eds), 3rd edn. Mosby Elsevier, Philadelphia, pp. 95–113.

Witherspoon, D.E. (2008) Vital pulp therapy with new materials: new directions and treatment perspectives - permanent teeth. *Journal of Endodontics* **34** (Suppl.), S25–S28.

Witherspoon, D.E., Small, J.C., Harris, G.Z. (2006) Mineral trioxide aggregate pulpotomies: a case series outcome assessment. *Journal of the American Dental Association* **137**, 610–18.

Witte, D. (1878) Das Füllen der Wurzelcanäle mit Portland-Cement. *Deutsche Vierteljahrsschrift für Zahnheilkunde* **18**, 153–4 [in German].

Yasuda, Y., Ogawa, M., Arakawa, T., *et al.* (2008) The effect of mineral trioxide aggregate on the mineralization ability of rat dental pulp cells: an *in vitro* study. *Journal of Endodontics* **34**, 1057–60.

Zarrabi, M.H., Javidi, M., Jafarian, A.H., *et al.* (2011) Immunohistochemical expression of fibronectin and tenascin in human tooth pulp capped with mineral trioxide aggregate and a novel endodontic cement. *Journal of Endodontics* **37**, 1613–18.

Zealand, C.M., Briskie, D.M., Botero, T.M., *et al.* (2010) Comparing gray mineral trioxide aggregate and diluted formocresol in pulpotomized human primary molars. *Pediatric Dentistry* **32**, 393–9.

Zhu, Q., Haglund, R., Safavi, K.E., *et al.* (2000) Adhesion of human osteoblasts on root-end filling materials. *Journal of Endodontics* **26**, 404–6.

5 Management of Teeth with Necrotic Pulps and Open Apices

Shahrokh Shabahang[1] and David E. Witherspoon[2]

[1] Department of Endodontics, Loma Linda University School of Dentistry, USA
[2] North Texas Endodontic Associates, USA

DIAGNOSIS IN IMMATURE TEETH

Development of the dental root structure requires a vital pulp. If the pulp is vital and the apex is not formed, it is imperative to take the necessary steps to maintain the vitality of the pulp. These measures promote the apex to complete its formation and calcification since it is only pulpal tissue that has the ability to form true dentin (Goldman 1974). Disruption of pulp vitality will interfere with continued root development. Ideally, where possible, pulp vitality must be

Mineral Trioxide Aggregate: Properties and Clinical Applications, First Edition.
Edited by Mahmoud Torabinejad.
© 2014 John Wiley & Sons, Inc. Published 2014 by John Wiley & Sons, Inc.

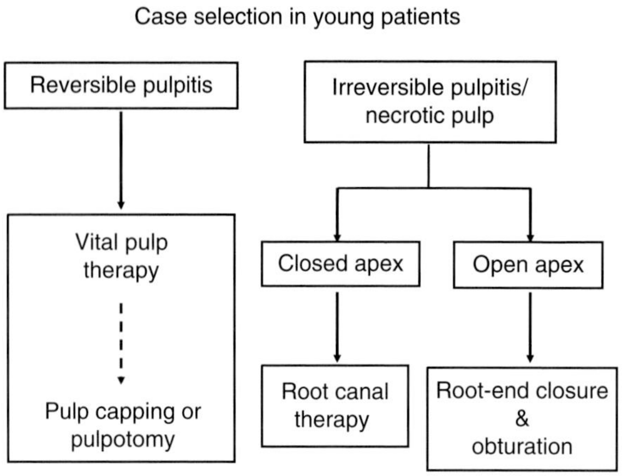

Case selection in young patients

```
┌─────────────────────┐        ┌─────────────────────┐
│ Reversible pulpitis  │        │ Irreversible pulpitis/│
│                      │        │    necrotic pulp     │
└─────────────────────┘        └─────────────────────┘
          │                        │            │
          ▼                        ▼            ▼
┌─────────────────────┐   ┌──────────────┐  ┌──────────────┐
│    Vital pulp       │   │ Closed apex  │  │  Open apex   │
│    therapy          │   └──────────────┘  └──────────────┘
│      ┊              │          │                │
│      ┊              │          ▼                ▼
│      ▼              │   ┌──────────────┐  ┌──────────────┐
│ Pulp capping or     │   │ Root canal   │  │Root-end closure│
│   pulpotomy         │   │  therapy     │  │     &        │
└─────────────────────┘   └──────────────┘  │  obturation  │
                                            └──────────────┘
```

Fig. 5.1   Case selection for treatment of permanent teeth with incomplete root development.

maintained in immature permanent teeth to allow completion of root development. The pulp tissues should be removed only when irreversibly inflamed or
necrotic. Typically, the dental pulp tissue in young patients has been exposed
to less irritation, is more cellular and therefore better able to recover from injury.
Cvek and coworkers (Cvek *et al.* 1982) demonstrated that complex crown
fractured teeth show vital pulp tissue after being exposed for up to seven days
post injury, with only 2 mm of the pulp beneath the exposure level exhibiting
inflammation.

Clearly, proper assessment of the pulpal status to allow an accurate diagnosis
is critical prior to determining the treatment plan for teeth with underdeveloped
roots. Before determination of the best treatment option, pulp vitality must be
assessed. If vital, every effort must be made to maintain its vitality to allow
continued root development. Figure 5.1 presents a flow chart to facilitate the
decision-making process when treating permanent teeth with incompletely
developed roots.

Assessment of the tooth in question is made using radiographic evaluation
to determine the maturity of the developing root and clinical evaluation based
on history and clinical testing. Immature teeth are usually encountered in children. Pulp testing in children is a complex procedure and subjective in nature.
It is impacted by their linguistic development and expectations (Pinkham
1997; Toole *et al.* 2000; Harman *et al.* 2005). The less linguistically developed
and the higher their expectations of a negative experience, the less discriminat-
ing their response might be (Toole *et al.* 2000; Harman *et al.* 2005). Diagnosis
can be confused by the patient's subjective symptomatology, which may not
correctly echo the real histological status of the pulp (Camp 2008). The

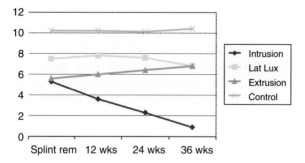

Fig. 5.2 Pulpal blood flow measurement using laser Doppler shows negative impact of intrusive injuries.

response to pulp testing is also less predictable than in adults, leading to a greater possibility of false negatives. Generally, the response to cold stimulus produces the most reliable result (Fulling & Andreasen 1976; Fuss *et al.* 1986). Electric pulp testing in teeth with open immature apices can produce a high percentage of false negatives (Klein 1978). The history is also important not only to determine any predisposing conditions, which may impact pulpal healing, but also symptoms and presence of certain complicating factors such as traumatic injuries to the tooth. For instance, hyperglycemia may significantly impact pulpal healing (Garber *et al.* 2009). Using laser doppler measurement of pulpal blood flow (PBF), Strobl and coworkers (2004) were able to show that lateral and extrusive subluxation injuries do not significantly impact PBF. On the other hand, intrusive injuries lead to diminished PBF and pulp necrosis (Fig. 5.2). Additionally, determination of pulp status may be accomplished by direct viewing of the pulpal tissues if it is exposed. Diagnosing reversible pulpitis can be most reliably established by assessing the clinical ability to achieve hemostasis using NaOCl for 5 to 10 min after the pulp has been clinically exposed (Matsuo *et al.* 1996; Bogen *et al.* 2008).

A comprehensive understanding of the radiographic appearance of normal root formation is indispensable in correctly diagnosing periradicular pathosis associated with immature teeth. In developing stages, the buccal–lingual dimension of the root canal of incisors is typically greater than the mesial–distal dimension. A root canal with parallel walls mesiodistally is inclined to have divergent walls and greater width labio-lingually; a canal with tapering walls mesiodistally tends to have parallel walls and greater width labio-lingually. The lag in root development usually exists for more than three years after eruption of the tooth (Duell 1973). This developmental pattern can be misleading with respect to convergence and divergence. Since the buccal–lingual aspect of the root canal is the last to become convergent as the root develops, it is possible to have a radiograph showing an apically convergent root canal, which in the buccal-lingual plane is divergent (Camp 1980). There are factors aside from the apical anatomy that can be misleading. The tissue forming apically may appear radiographically complete, but is often porous as the developing root diaphragm in the labio-lingual plane lags behind that in the mesio-distal plane of the immature root (Gutmann & Heaton 1981). However, with the advent of cone beam computerized tomography, the difficulty in assessing apical formation is minimized (Patel 2010).

As Fig. 5.1 shows, if the pulp is deemed necrotic, root canal therapy is indicated; however, because of the presence of an open apex, root end closure must be achieved prior to completion of root canal therapy.

HISTORY OF TREATING IMMATURE TEETH

Traditionally, the treatment of immature teeth has been challenging. Typically, these teeth inherently have several treatment challenges that are not encountered when teeth in adult patients. The apical diameter of the canal is often larger than the coronal diameter (Friend 1969), rendering mechanical root canal debridement difficult. The lack of an apical constriction makes canal obturation in all dimensions difficult. The thin walls of the root canal are prone to fracture, rendering surgical intervention and non-surgical root canal therapy techniques that require significant compaction during obturation as undesirable options. Historically, techniques for the management of non-vital immature teeth have included custom fitting gutta-percha cones as the filling material without a prior apexification procedure (Stewart 1963; Friend 1966), paste fills (Friend 1967), apical surgery (Ingle 1965), and often extraction (Rule & Winter 1966).

In 1940, Rohner (1940) described the use of a Calxyl paste to be placed over the pulp remnant after vital pulpectomy. The result was formation of an apical barrier. The first description of the use of calcium hydroxide (CH) as an agent to induce apical closure was in 1953 (Marmasse 1953). This was followed by Granath in 1959 (Granath 1959); subsequently in 1962 Matsumiya (Matsumiya *et al.* 1962) and in 1964 Kaiser (Kaiser 1964) also reported on the use of CH in apical closure procedures. At this time several other materials were also being utilized for this procedure; these included Tricresol and formalin (Cooke & Rowbotham 1960) and antibiotic pastes (Herbert 1959; Ball 1964). The term apexification was used to describe the procedure for inducing apical closure to facilitate obturation of the root canal system and was popularized in the 1960s (Frank 1966; Steiner *et al.* 1968). It thus became the treatment protocol of choice for immature necrotic teeth. In addition to the use of CH, various other procedures and medicaments have been recommended for inducing apexification with varying degrees of success. These include inducing a blood clot (Ham *et al.* 1972), and placement of materials such as Tricresol and formalin (Cooke & Rowbotham 1960), antibiotic pastes (Ball 1964), tricalcium phosphate (Koenigs *et al.* 1975; Roberts & Brilliant 1975), collagen–calcium phosphate gel (Nevins *et al.* 1977, 1978; Citrome *et al.* 1979), CH in different mixes such as camphorated parachlorophenol (CMCP) (Frank 1966; Dylewski 1971; Steiner & Van Hassel 1971; Ham *et al.* 1972; Torneck *et al.* 1973), iodoform (Holland *et al.* 1973), water (Binnie & Rowe 1973; Wechsler *et al.* 1978), local anesthetic solution, isotonic saline solution, glycerol, and others (Heithersay 1970; Vojinovic & Srnie 1975; Camp 1980; Webber *et al.* 1981). Several case reports have also demonstrated continued apical development in non-vital teeth after removal of the non-vital tissue and control of infection alone (Das 1980; Cameron 1986). Additionally, Lieberman and Trowbridge (1983) reported a case in which apical closures of non-vital permanent incisors were observed without any treatment at all.

Regardless of the many approaches to apexification, CH has become the material of choice for this procedure since the 1960s. This is mainly due to Frank's (1966) landmark paper where he proposed the use of a thick paste of CH and CMCP. After placement of the paste, the tooth would require evaluations every 3–6 months until closure of the apex as determined radiographically or clinically (manifested by a hard barrier at the root-end detected with an endodontic instrument). He further proposed that, with this procedure, the clinical results might vary and present as follows: (1) an apex that closes with a definite, though minimal, recession of the root canal (the apical aspect continues to develop with a seemingly obliterated apex); (2) the obliterated apex may develop without any change in the root canal space; (3) there may be no radiographic evidence of any development in the periapex or root canal, however, an instrument inserted into the canal encounters a definite stop that would allow for the filling procedure; or (4) a calcific bridge may form just coronal to the apex, which can be determined radiographically. Feiglin (1985), similarly classified various categories of apex formation following apexification procedures with CH and listed them as follows: (1) The apex bridged over with hard tissue that would presumably be osteocementum or osteodentin; (2) a perfectly normal apex formed from the point of trauma to the apex of the tooth; (3–4) variable amounts of vital tissue remained above the point of trauma, which allowed the root canal to heal or bridge over and the apex to continue forming and to calcify; and (5) apex lifted off during tooth movement.

INFECTION CONTROL IN IMMATURE TEETH

Immature permanent teeth pose special challenges during endodontic procedures not only because of the wide-open root apex, but also because of the thin dentin walls (Fig. 5.3). As such, debridement is completed primarily by chemical means to remove any remaining pulp tissues and to disinfect the canal system. Furthermore, an accurate determination of root length is required to ensure complete canal debridement and to confine treatment materials to the canal space. This would prevent damaging of the very valuable remnants of the Hertwig's epithelial root sheath (HERS) (Fig. 5.4).

Generally, electronic apex locators are not accurate in teeth with wide open apices (Hulsmann and Pieper 1989). Radiographic root determination is the best means to obtain accurate root length measurement (Fig. 5.5).

Sodium hypochlorite (NaOCl) and CH have good tissue dissolving properties as well as antimicrobial activity (The 1979; Cunningham & Balekjian 1980; Cunningham & Joseph 1980; Morgan *et al.* 1991; Baumgartner & Cuenin 1992; Yang *et al.* 1995; Turkun & Cengiz 1997; Wadachi *et al.* 1998; Gomes *et al.* 2001). While NaOCl exerts its effect during the course of the procedure, CH requires additional exposure time. A 1-week obturation of the canal space with CH will allow disinfection along with dissolution and removal of pulpal remnants (Sjogren *et al.* 1991; Turkun & Cengiz 1997). Despite its convenient availability, several investigators have reported shortcomings with respect to NaOCl's ability to completely disinfect the root canal space (Shabahang *et al.* 2003; Waltimo *et al.* 2005; Siqueira & Rocas 2008). Inconsistencies in reports may be due to differences in methodologies or the actual usage protocols. In fact,

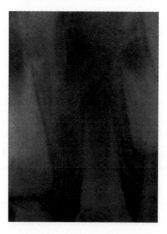

Fig. 5.3 Radiographic view of an immature permanent incisor with open apex and thin dentin walls.

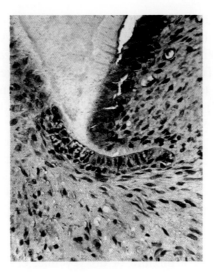

Fig. 5.4 Hertwig's epithelial root sheath with BMP-2 immunoreactivity stain.

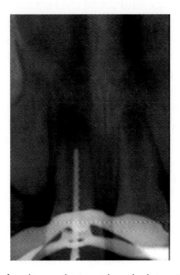

Fig. 5.5 Demonstration of radiographic root length determination in an incisor with a wide-open apical foramen.

NaOCl is most effective when mixed into solution just before use (Johnson & Remeikis 1993). Heat, light and exposure to oxygen may readily inactivate NaOCl (Gerhardt & Williams 1991; Clarkson *et al.* 2001).

Long-term exposure to CH may also have detrimental effects on dentin. Studies have shown that long-term CH therapy that would expose root dentin to

CH for periods exceeding one month results in structural changes in dentin that yield significantly higher susceptibility to root fracture (Andreasen *et al.* 2002, 2006; White *et al.* 2002; Doyon *et al.* 2005; Rosenberg *et al.* 2007; Hatibovic-Kofman *et al.* 2008; Tuna *et al.* 2011; Bakland and Andreasen 2012). Previous reports of failures of teeth with a history of apexification due to cervical root fractures (Cvek 1992) may be attributed, not only to the thin dentin walls, but also to excessive exposure of the dentin to CH.

In recent years, several investigative groups have revisited antibiotic agents for root canal disinfection. Use of antibiotics is not a new approach to root canal disinfection. In 1980, Das (1980) reported successful apexification of a tooth after root canal debridement and intracanal antibiotic therapy with an oxytetracycline HCl ointment. During the past decade, addition of antibiotic products to debridement protocols has regained popularity.

In 2003, Torabinejad and his group published a series of reports to demonstrate the advantages of a mixture of doxycycline, citric acid, and detergent (BioPure MTAD) over NaOCl and other commonly used root canal irrigants (Beltz *et al.* 2003; Shabahang *et al.* 2003; Shabahang & Torabinejad 2003; Torabinejad *et al.* 2003a, b, c). BioPure MTAD is effective as a final rinse prior to obturation to disinfect the root canal system and to remove the smear layer.

In 2001, Iwaya and associates (2001) published a case that demonstrated the effectiveness of a double antibiotic paste to disinfect a premolar with a necrotic pulp and a large periradicular radiolucent lesion; subsequently Banchs and Trope (2004) published a similar case. In this case report and subsequent studies, Trope's group recommended a mixture of metronidazole, ciprofloxacin, and minocycline. In *in-vitro* studies, this antibiotic combination has shown potential to disinfect the root canal system (Hoshino *et al.* 1996; Sato *et al.* 1996). In an animal experiment, significantly better disinfection was achieved after dressing with the triple antibiotic paste compared with biomechanical debridement using 1.25% NaOCl (Windley *et al.* 2005). Due to potential staining caused by longer exposures to minocycline (Kim *et al.* 2010; Nosrat *et al.* 2012), some investigators have opted to omit the minocycline and use a double antibiotic mix.

APEXIFICATION

If pulpal necrosis occurs in immature teeth, an alternative treatment approach to conventional root canal therapy must be employed due to the presence of an open apex. The young pulpless tooth, frequently, has thin, fragile walls making it difficult to adequately clean and to obtain the necessary apical seal (Frank 1966).

Traditionally, the approach has been to utilize CH to induce apexification following disinfection of the root canals in the conventional manner (Seltzer 1988). Completion of endodontic therapy has been typically delayed until root-end closure has been completed through apexification. Apexification is defined as "a method of inducing a calcified barrier in a root with an open apex or the continued apical development of an incompletely formed root in teeth with a necrotic pulp" (Anonymous 2003). Apexification employing CH in one form or another has a long history in the treatment of non-vital immature teeth.

CALCIUM HYDROXIDE APEXIFICATION THERAPY: OUTCOMES

A number of studies have examined apexification outcomes both in terms of success and length of time it takes to achieve apical closure using CH. In 1970, Heithersay (1970) reported on 21 clinical cases, which were treated with CH in a methylcellulose carrier (Pulpdent) over an observation period of 14–75 months. The results showed that in teeth with continued apical development, a definite fine apical canal could be seen radiographically, but there was no definite apical barrier clinically. In their 1987 report, Ghose and associates (1987) used Calasept in traumatized, partially developed permanent central incisors of 43 patients between the ages of 8 and 12 years. All of the teeth had crown fractures with pulp exposures. The pulps had been exposed to the oral environment for one month to three years and all were necrotic. Forty-nine of 51 teeth developed an apical barrier that could be confirmed clinically and radiographically. The time needed to form an apical barrier of hard tissue ranged from 3–10 months. Morfis and Siskos (1991) reported on the outcomes of 34 cases in which apexification was performed using CH. In all cases, chemically pure CH powder was mixed with anesthetic solution. Twelve patients were aged 27–40 years and the other 22 were aged 8–20 years. Continuation of root development was achieved in 6 cases, continuation and bridge formation occurred in 3 cases, bridge formation alone was seen in 21 cases and in 4 cases no root-end closure was observed. Hard tissue bridge formation was the most common form of root-end closure (Morfis & Siskos, 1991). In a similar study of 32 trauma-induced necrotic immature permanent incisors in 7–10-year-olds with or without a periradicular lesion, the mean duration for apical closure was 10 to 14 weeks (Lee *et al.* 2010). In a retrospective analysis of apical closure using CH in 15 non-vital immature incisor teeth, a success rate of 100% was reported within 1 year (Walia *et al.* 2000). Several variables were identified that influenced the time required for complete apexification. Older children with a narrow open

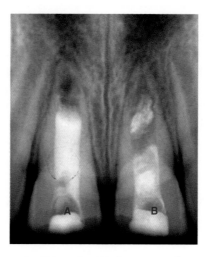

Fig. 5.6 Apexification with CH tooth: (A) has incomplete apical barrier formation; (B) has complete apical barrier formation.

apex had a shorter treatment time than younger children; teeth without periradicular infection showed some amount of root growth and apical closure that was faster than those with periradicular infection. Additionally, the investigators reported that the calcified bridge formed following apexification was a porous structure (Walia *et al.* 2000). Dominguez Reyes *et al.* (2005) examined the time taken to obtain apical closure in a sample comprised of 26 young permanent incisors with necrotic pulps and open apices. Apical closure was obtained in 100% of the cases studied. Of these, 88.4% needed three to four sessions of CH treatment (an average of 3.23 sessions) in order to obtain apical closure; the average time employed was 12.19 months. Preoperative symptoms and periradicular pathosis did not affect outcome (Dominguez Reyes *et al.* 2005). In a study of 28 necrotic incisors in children with an age range of 6 and 13 years, apical closure was achieved in all cases. The mean duration to achieve apical closure was 8.6 months with a range of 3.24 to 13.96 months. The type of tissue in the apical region was categorized as cementoid tissue (85.72%) or osseous tissue (14.28%). The teeth were monitored over a 2-year period following completion of the non-surgical endodontic treatment. In 7.1 % of the cases re-infection occurred (Mendoza *et al.* 2010).

Unfortunately, the Frank technique is sometimes unpredictable (Fig. 5.6). In addition to the various types of apical barriers formed, other inconsistencies relating to the use of CH for apexification include: the time for root apices to close, the number of dressings necessary to complete closure, and the role of infection. Depending on the study, the speed of barrier formation varies from 3 to 24 months (Frank 1966; Finucane & Kinirons 1999; Kinirons *et al.* 2001).

There is also variation in the recommended number of reapplications of CH (Webber 1984; Yates 1988; Morse *et al.* 1990; Sheehy & Roberts 1997; Abbott 1998; Mackie 1998; Mackie & Hill 1999). There is no consensus on the impact of changing the dressing material on the rate and quality of apical barrier formation. Recommendations regarding the proper timing to change the CH have varied from monthly, once every 3 months, once every 6–8 months, to no change at all (Chosack *et al.* 1997; Sheehy & Roberts 1997; Abbott 1998; Kinirons *et al.* 2001; Felippe *et al.* 2005). Finally, there appears to be no consensus on the role of infection. Some studies report an increase in the time for apexification when infection is present (Cvek 1972; Kleier & Barr 1991) and others have demonstrated no statistically significant differences (Ghose *et al.* 1987; Yates 1988; Mackie 1998; Finucane & Kinirons 1999). Additionally, Torneck and Smith (1970) have indicated that there may be incomplete bridging of the apex even though a two-dimensional radiograph may give the appearance of complete bridging. Periradicular inflammation may persist around the apices of many teeth due to the presence of necrotic tissue in the crevices of the apical bridge. Therefore, the presence of a radiographically and clinically closed apex is not necessarily indicative of a normal periodontium (Koenigs *et al.* 1975).

Another major drawback of the apexification protocol using CH is the effect that a long-term application of CH has on the structural integrity of the root dentin. As previously stated, several studies have demonstrated that with longer exposures of dentin to CH, the dentin's ability to with stand fracture is significantly decreased (Andreasen *et al.* 2002, 2006; White *et al.* 2002; Doyon *et al.* 2005; Rosenberg *et al.* 2007; Hatibovic-Kofman *et al.* 2008; Tuna *et al.* 2011; Bakland & Andreasen 2012).

NON-VITAL PULP THERAPY

Root-end closure via the use of apical barriers

Any treatment requiring several visits over a long period of time risks patient attrition caused by diminished tolerance to treatment and geographic relocation. If a child moves away during the course of treatment, it is difficult to ensure the dressing changes are made as needed until a barrier is formed. Likewise, patient compliance can be a problem when multiple visits are involved. Repeated visits to the dentist can be disruptive and difficult in a busy schedule so that the parent and child become wary of the routine and discontinue required visits (Heling *et al.* 1999). Also, appointments are easily forgotten because the patient usually has no discomfort and the tooth appears normal clinically. Another problem, which is avoided by one-visit apexification, is subjecting an unwilling child through treatments that may be very unpleasant to a young patient. Many children who fear trips to the dentist are even more traumatized by repeated visits. This response is even further heightened in younger children who present with wide open apices that require more treatment appointments. Given the complexity of apexification using CH, clinicians have frequently sought an alternative treatment protocol. Thus, the need for a reliable one-visit apexification treatment is clear.

Several investigators have demonstrated the use of dentin apical plugs in non-surgical root canal therapy of mature teeth (Tronstad 1978; Holland *et al.* 1980, 1983; Holland 1984; Brady *et al.* 1985). In 1967, Michanowicz & Michanowicz described a technique of using CH for an apical plug before gutta-percha filling in non-vital teeth with an open apex. Teeth with apical plugs of CH have also demonstrated mean leakage values that are significantly less than those obturated without plugs (Weisenseel *et al.* 1987). Pitts and associates (1984) histologically compared CH and dentin plugs in 36 overinstrumented canine teeth of nine mature cats. Their findings demonstrated that both plugs were effective in controlling the filling materials within the confines of the canals; however, a significant number of CH plugs washed out by 1 month. In contrast, the dentin plugs remained fully intact. Calcified tissue matrix formation was evident in the majority of the specimens containing dentin plugs after 1 month of placing them, whereas no foraminal calcification was seen until 3 months in samples treated with CH plugs. Tricalcium phosphate has also been proposed as an apical barrier in a single-appointment technique (Coviello & Brilliant 1979; Harbert 1991, 1996). When compared to multi-appointment CH–CMCP paste treatment of open apices, tricalcium phosphate resulted in no overfills in the apices of permanent human teeth. In contrast, CH treatment resulted in several cases that were associated with overextension of the root canal filling material. Because of its larger particle size, the experimental material offered improved resistance against compaction, and therefore, less material was extruded compared to the CH plugs (Coviello & Brilliant 1979). Brandell and associates (1986) evaluated the apical closures produced by demineralized dentin, hydroxyapatite, and dentin chips in monkeys. At the 6-month observation period, none of the demineralized dentin plugs showed complete apical closure. In contrast, 66% of the roots filled with hydroxyapatite exhibited complete apical closure, and 50% of roots with dentin chip plugs had complete apical closure. The authors concluded that the organic component of dentin might not be effective in inducing apical hard tissue formation.

Mineral trioxide aggregate apical plug

Mineral trioxide aggregate (MTA), whose principal components include tricalcium silicate, tricalcium aluminate, tricalcium oxide, and silicate oxide, has been commercially available for approximately 20 years. MTA was introduced to dentistry in 1993, primarily as a root-end filling material. While the majority of the studies involving MTA have noted its obvious benefits with its use in root-end fillings, these same attributes make MTA an attractive material for use in the treatment of immature non-vital teeth. The physical, chemical and structural aspects of this material are discussed in depth elsewhere within this text. MTA is a powder consisting of fine hydrophilic particles, which set in the presence of moisture, and result in a colloidal gel that solidifies to a hard structure (Torabinejad *et al.* 1995b). Numerous leakage studies (Torabinejad *et al.* 1993) have demonstrated that MTA leaks significantly less than many restorative materials, including amalgam, Intermediate Restorative Material (IRM), Super EBA, and traditional root canal filling material of gutta-percha and sealer. Additionally, MTA offers the added advantage of setting even in the presence of blood. Furthermore, the high pH of MTA (reported to be 10.2, rising to 12.5 at 3 hours and thereafter) (Torabinejad *et al.* 1995b), which is similar to CH, may be one of the factors that promotes hard tissue formation. One of the most significant aspects of MTA in relation to its use as an apical plug in immature non-vital teeth is its ability to induce a cemental tissue in the periradicular region of the tooth (Torabinejad *et al.* 1995a). Thus, the use of MTA as apical plug in the treatment of immature non-vital teeth has enormous potential to simplify a complex procedure. Finally, MTA's ability to promote formation of hard tissue presents the potential of a biological seal of cementum over the material (Shabahang *et al.* 1999). The majority of the biological perimeters for the role that MTA plays in healing of the periradicular tissues following treatment of non-vital immature teeth have been inferred from its role in healing when placed as a root-end filling in surgical endodontics. An exception to this is the study carried out by Shabahang and coworkers (1999). They focused on evaluating MTA's role in periradicular healing when placed as an apical plug in open apex teeth. They histomorphometrically examined hard tissue formation and inflammation after treating teeth with open apices in dogs with osteogenic protein-1, MTA, and CH. While the amount of hard tissue formation and degree of inflammation in each tooth was not statistically different among the three materials, MTA induced hard tissue formation most consistently. In another study that compared the healing of immature non-vital teeth in monkeys treated with MTA or traditional CH apexification, MTA displayed less inflammation and a greater amount of hard tissue formation (Ham *et al.* 2005). A study conducted in dogs, examined the requirement of using CH paste before placing an MTA apical plug. Their findings showed that MTA used after root canal preparation favored apical root formation and periradicular healing. The initial use of CH paste was not necessary for apical root formation to occur. Furthermore the use of CH was strongly correlated with extrusion of MTA and formation of barriers beyond the limits of the root canal walls (Felippe *et al.* 2006). Hachmeister *et al.* examined the bacterial leakage patterns in a simulated model of immature non-vital teeth. The authors suggest that it was the technique of placing the MTA rather than the MTA itself that had the greatest impact on treatment outcome (Hachmeister *et al.* 2002). Intracanal application of CH for 1 week may improve the marginal adaptation of an apical plug of MTA (Bidar *et al.* 2010). This finding may be related to CH's ability to remove tissue remnants, thereby allowing better adaptation of MTA to the dentin walls.

Technical placement

Once cleaning of the root canal system is complete, a series of pluggers that are customarily used for warm vertical compaction of gutta percha are loosely fitted sequentially in the root canal system (Fig. 5.7A–D). The smallest plugger should fit loosely ~0.5 mm from the working length. MTA is then placed in the middle to apical third of the root canal system using one of several commercially available delivery systems. It is then compacted with a series of pluggers previously fitted to the root canal system. The pluggers can be vibrated ultrasonically to help advance MTA towards the apex of the tooth. Additionally the ultrasonic activity will compact the MTA apically (Matt *et al.* 2004; Yeung *et al.* 2006; Holden *et al.* 2008; Kim *et al.* 2009). Typically an additional apical matrix to limit the movement of MTA into the periradicular tissues is not warranted. Once an adequate apical plug of MTA is compacted to the working length and confirmed with a radiograph, the excess can be removed from the coronal and middle third of the canal system by irrigating with sterile water. The remaining fluid is removed with sterile paper points. The apical plug of MTA should be approximately 3–5 mm thick to allow minimal leakage (de Leimburg *et al.* 2004; Lawley *et al.* 2004; Matt *et al.* 2004; Al-Kahtani *et al.* 2005; Martin *et al.* 2007; Holden *et al.* 2008; Kim *et al.* 2009; Lolayekar *et al.* 2009). The remainder of the canal system can be restored with a core material adjacent to the MTA. The core layer can extend into the coronal third of the canal to enhance fracture resistance of the tooth (Lawley *et al.* 2004). Lastly, composite is layered against the core material, extending coronally to fill the access opening (Fig. 5.7E–F). (Video).

Outcomes

Several case reports have detailed the successful use of MTA in the management of non-vital immature teeth (Torabinejad & Chivian, 1999; Shabahang & Torabinejad, 2000; Witherspoon & Ham, 2001; Bishop & Woollard, 2002; Giuliani *et al.* 2002; Levenstein, 2002; Lynn & Einbender, 2003; Maroto *et al.* 2003; Steinig, *et al.* 2003; Hayashi *et al.* 2004). One of the case reports is of particular interest in that the tooth was initially treated with the traditional CH apexification

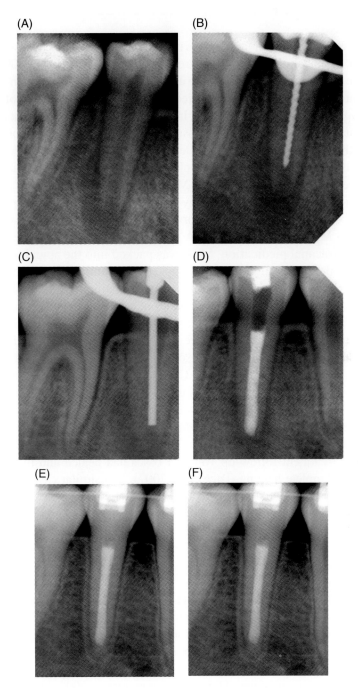

Fig. 5.7 (A) Preoperative radiograph of an immature 2nd premolar tooth with pulpal necrosis in a 12-year-old male patient; (B) working length radiograph; (C) plugger fit radiograph; (D) immediate postoperative radiograph. (E) 15-month recall radiograph; (F) 33-month recall radiograph.

approach; when the initial treatment was unsuccessful, the authors then successfully employed an apical plug of MTA to treat the tooth (Maroto *et al.* 2003). Since then several studies have examined the use of MTA as an apical plug in immature permanent teeth. Two studies have directly compared the outcomes of an MTA apical plug to traditional apexification. In 15 children, each with at least 2 necrotic permanent teeth requiring root-end closure, El-Meligy and Avery reported that at a 12 month follow-up period, two of the CH teeth had become re-infected whislt all the teeth treated with MTA apical plug remained clinically and radiographically successful. They concluded that MTA is a suitable replacement for CH for the apexification procedure (El-Meligy & Avery, 2006). In a similar study of 20 non-vital permanent maxillary incisors with immature apices, the teeth were treated with MTA or CH. In the MTA group, after 7 days of disinfection with CH as an intracanal medication, MTA was packed into the apical one third of the root canal and the remaining canal space was obturated with gutta-percha and sealer. In the apexification group, CH was maintained in the tooth until there was clinical and radiographic evidence of an apical stop. The canals where then obturated with gutta-percha and sealer in the same manner as the MTA group. In the CH group, apical closure was observed in 7 ± 2.5 months on average. Periradicular radiolucencies resolved in 4.6 ± 1.5 months for the MTA group and in 4.4 ± 1.3 months for the CH group. The total treatment was completed in 0.75 ± 0.5 months for the MTA group and 7 ± 2.5 months for the CH group (Pradhan *et al.* 2006).

In a case series, 11 teeth with immature root apices were treated with intracanal CH for 1–2 weeks followed by an apical plug of 3–5 mm of MTA. At the 2-year post-treatment follow-up 10 of 11 cases had healed and the remaining exhibited incomplete healing (Pace *et al.* 2007). In a similar case series report, five immature teeth with necrotic pulps were medicated with CH paste for 1–6 weeks and subsequently received an apical plug of MTA. Four of the five teeth were considered clinically and radiographically healed at a 2-year follow-up. One case in which the MTA was extruded beyond the apex did not heal (Erdem & Sepet, 2008).

Sarris and coworkers (2008) evaluated 17 non-vital permanent immature incisors in 15 children with a mean age of 11.7 years. The teeth were medicated with CH for at least 1 week before receiving a 3–4 mm plug of MTA. MTA placement was considered adequate in 13 of the 17 teeth. The mean follow-up time was 12.5 months ranging from 6–16 months. Overall, a clinical success rate of 94.1% and a radiographic success rate of 76.5% were reported.

In a retrospective analysis, Holden and coworkers (2008) studied 20 open apex teeth in 19 patients. All teeth were medicated with CH for at least a week and then obturated with a 4 mm plug of MTA. Overall, 85% of the cases were considered healed at the final recall. This included several retreatment cases of mature teeth. Excluding these cases from the data and focusing on immature teeth resulted in 16 cases, with follow-ups ranging from 12–44 months with an average of 26.7 months. For these cases, the healing rate was 93.75% based on periradicular index scores of 1 or 2 and no clinical signs or symptoms at follow-up examinations (Holden *et al.* 2008).

Nayar and Bishop reported on the outcomes of 38 cases of immature permanent teeth treated with an apical plug of MTA. All teeth were clinically and radiographically successful at the last follow-up period 12 months post treatment. They concluded that placement of an apical plug of MTA in these cases results in predictably successful outcomes. Furthermore, the number of visits and the total time required to achieve an apical barrier was markedly less than conventional techniques using CH. Interestingly, the presence of a preoperative periradicular radiolucency had no effect on the outcome (Nayar *et al.* 2009).

Annamalai and Mungara (2010) published a report on 30 non vital young permanent, single rooted teeth treated with apical plugs of 4–5 mm of MTA. In this study, they showed a 100% success rate based on clinical and radiographic findings at the 12-month follow-up. Total root-end closure was seen in 86.6% of cases and root growth in 30% of cases. Moore and coworkers reported on the outcomes of 22 non-vital immature permanent incisors in 21 children. The mean age for the cohort was 10 years. They placed a white MTA apical barrier in the teeth following an initial dressing with CH. The mean follow-up time was 23.4 months. They reported a clinical and radiographic success rate of 95.5% (Moore *et al.* 2011). Coronal discoloration was observed in 22.7% of the teeth.

Two larger studies have examined the outcomes of MTA in non-vital immature teeth. A prospective study that examined the outcomes of 57 teeth with open apices in 50 patients that were treated with a MTA apical plug placed in one appointment. No interim medication of CH was used in this study. Forty-three cases had a minimum of 12-month follow-up. Using the periapical index (PAI) score (Orstavik, *et al.* 1986; Orstavik, 1988) and the decrease in size of the apical lesion, healing was reported in 81% of the cases. The authors concluded that "apexification" in one step using an apical plug of MTA can be considered a predictable treatment, and may be an alternative to the use of CH (Simon *et al.* 2007). The other study was a retrospective analysis of 144 teeth in 116 patients treated in a single private endodontic office between 1999 and 2006. Ninety-two of the treatments were completed in one visit with the remaining 52 teeth treated in two visits with an intra-canal CH medication, typically placed for 3 weeks. Fifty-four percent (78/144) of the teeth were available for follow-up evaluation (60.3% one visit and 39.7%

(A) (B) (C)

(D) (E) (F)

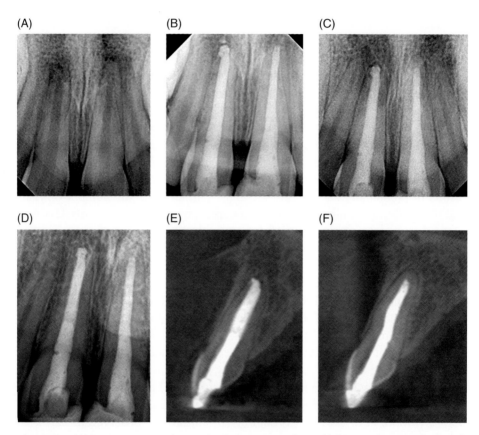

Fig. 5.8 (A) Preoperative radiograph of immature right and left central incisor teeth with pulpal necrosis as a result of a traumatic injury. (11-year-old male patient). (B) Immediate postoperative radiograph; (C) 36-month recall radiograph; (D) 85-month recall radiograph; (E) sagittal view from a CBCT taken at the 85-month recall of the left central incisor; (F) sagittal view from a CBCT taken at the 85-month recall of the left central incisor.

two visits). The maximum time of follow-up was 4.87 years. The mean time of follow-up was 19.4 months. For the cases followed for periods of 1 year or longer, 93.5% of teeth treated in 1 visit healed, and 90.5% of teeth treated in 2 visits healed (Witherspoon *et al.* 2008). This study contained several teeth that would not be classified as immature even though they had an open apex. If these cases are excluded from the results, then the results are as follows: The data consist of 119 immature non-vital teeth. Seventy-four of the treatments were completed in one visit with the remaining 45 teeth treated in two visits with an intracanal CH medication, typically placed for 3 weeks. Fifty-seven percent (68/119) of the teeth were available for follow-up evaluation (60.3% one visit and 39.7% two visits). For the cases followed for periods of 1 year or longer, 96.5% of teeth treated in 1 visit healed (Fig. 5.8),

Table 5.1 Summary of MTA apical plug: outcome studies.

Reference	No. cases	No recalled	Success	Failure	Median recall (months)	No. visits
Moore et al. Dent Trauma. 27:166–73, 2011	22	22	21	1	23.4	2
Annamalai & Mungara J Clin Ped Dent. 35:149–55, 2010	30	30	30	0	12	?
Nayar et al. Eur J Prosth & Rest Dent. 17:150–6, 2009	38	38	38	0	?	?
Mente et al. J Endod. 35:1354–8, 2009	78	56	47	8	30.9	2
Erdem & Sepet Dent Trauma. 24:e38–41, 2008	5	5	5	0	24	2
Witherspoon et al. J Endod. 34:1171–6, 2008	92	47	46	1	19.4	1
Witherspoon et al. J Endod. 34:1171–6, 2008	52	31	26	1	19.4	2
Holden et al. J Endod. 34:812–7, 2008	43	20	17	2	24.45	2
Sarris et al. Dent Trauma. 24:79–85, 2008	17	17	13	1	12.5	3
Pace et al. Int Endod J 40:478–84, 2007	11	11	10	0	24	2
Simon et al. Int Endod J. 40:186–97, 2007	57	43	35	6	15.8	1
El-Meligy & Avery Ped Dent. 28:248–53, 2006	15	15	15	0	12	?
Pradhan et al. J Dent Child 73:79–85, 2006	10	10	10	0	12	?
Totals	470	345	313	20	19.45	
Cumulative percentages		73%	91%	6%		

(A) (B) (C)

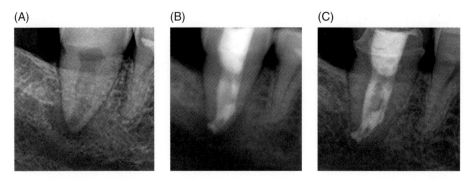

Fig. 5.9 (A) Preoperative radiograph of an open apex 2nd molar tooth with pulpal necrosis; (B) immediate postoperative radiograph; (C) 36-month recall radiograph.

and 89% of teeth treated in two visits healed. Only one case in each treatment category was unsuccessful. However, four cases that were initially treated with CH failed to return to complete treatment in a timely manner; when they did return, in one case up to 6 years later, the teeth were no longer restorable (Witherspoon *et al.* 2008). A large retrospective study on mature teeth with a MTA apical plug obturation has also been published. Overall 84% of cases healed (Mente *et al.* 2009). This topic is address in greater detail elsewhere in the text.

In a systematic review and meta-analysis comparing the outcomes of CH apexification and MTA apical plug, the authors concluded that clinical success rates for both procedures was similar (Chala *et al.* 2011). Two studies comparing the two materials reported on a total of 50 teeth: one by El Meligy and Avery (2006) and the other by Pradhan *et al.* (Pradhan *et al.* 2006) – both are discussed above. Based on the combined data of the two studies, the difference in initial clinical success between the two treatment regimens was not statistically significant. Nevertheless, 100% of the MTA cases where successful at the final follow-up visit compared to 92% of the CH cases (Chala *et al.* 2011).

Overall, these results indicate that the MTA apical barrier technique is a predictable method (Table 5.1) for obturating teeth with immature apices (Fig. 5.9). Nevertheless, there are several questions regarding the use of MTA as an apical plug in immature non-vital teeth that require clarification. One is whether measuring apical barrier formation represents a valid measure in assessing outcomes of this treatment protocol. Perhaps more importantly, the role of CH as an interim intracanal medication prior to the placement of the apical plug requires further study. Most importantly, the long-term outcomes of this procedure must be further evaluated.

REFERENCES

Abbott, P. V. (1998) Apexification with calcium hydroxide – when should the dressing be changed? The case for regular dressing changes. *Australian Endodontic Journal: the Journal of the Australian Society of Endodontology* **24**(1), 27–32.

Al-Kahtani, A., Shostad, S., Schifferle R, *et al.* (2005) In-vitro evaluation of microleakage of an orthograde apical plug of mineral trioxide aggregate in permanent teeth with simulated immature apices. *Journal of Endodontics* **31**(2), 117–19.

Andreasen, J. O., Farik, B., Munksgaard, E. C., *et al.* (2002) Long-term calcium hydroxide as a root canal dressing may increase risk of root fracture. *Dental Traumatology* **18**(3), 134–7.

Andreasen, J. O., Munksgaard, E. C., Bakland, L. K., *et al.* (2006) Comparison of fracture resistance in root canals of immature sheep teeth after filling with calcium hydroxide or MTA. *Dental Traumatology* **22**(3), 154–6.

Annamalai, S., Mungara, J. (2010) Efficacy of mineral trioxide aggregate as an apical plug in non-vital young permanent teeth: preliminary results. *Journal of Clinical Pediatric Dentistry* **35**(2), 149–55.

Anonymous (2003) *Glossary of Endodontic Terms*. Chicago, American Association of Endodontists.

Bakland, L. K., Andreasen, J. O. (2012) Will mineral trioxide aggregate replace calcium hydroxide in treating pulpal and periodontal healing complications subsequent to dental trauma? A review. *Dental Traumatology* **28**(1), 25–32.

Ball, J. (1964) Apical root formation in a non-vital immature permanent incisor. *British Dental Journal* **116**: 166–7.

Banchs, F., Trope, M. (2004) Revascularization of immature permanent teeth with apical periodontitis: new treatment protocol? *Journal of Endodontics* **30**(4), 196–200.

Baumgartner, J. C., Cuenin, P. R. (1992) Efficacy of several concentrations of sodium hypochlorite for root canal irrigation. *Journal of Endodontics* **18**(12), 605–12.

Beltz, R. E., Torabinejad, M., Pouresmail, M. (2003) Quantitative analysis of the solubilizing action of MTAD, sodium hypochlorite, and EDTA on bovine pulp and dentin. *Journal of Endodontics* **29**(5), 334–7.

Bidar, M., Disfani, R., Gharagozloo, S., *et al.* (2010) Medication with calcium hydroxide improved marginal adaptation of mineral trioxide aggregate apical barrier. *Journal of Endodontics* **36**(10), 1679–82.

Binnie, W. H., Rowe, A. H. (1973) A histological study of the periapical tissues of incompletely formed pulpless teeth filled with calcium hydroxide. *Journal of Dental Research* **52**(5), 1110–16.

Bishop, B. G., Woollard, G. W. (2002) Modern endodontic therapy for an incompletely developed tooth. *General Dentistry* **50**(3), 252–6; quiz 257–8.

Bogen, G., Kim, J. S., Bakland, L. K. (2008). Direct pulp capping with mineral trioxide aggregate: an observational study. [Erratum appears in J Am Dent Assoc. 2008 May;139(5), 541]. *Journal of the American Dental Association* **139**(3), 305–15; quiz 305–15.

Brady, J. E., Himel, V. T., Weir, J. C. (1985) Periapical response to an apical plug of dentin filings intentionally placed after root canal overinstrumentation. *Journal of Endodontics* **11**(8), 323–9.

Brandell, D. W., Torabinejad, M., Bakland, L. K., *et al.* (1986) Demineralized dentin, hydroxylapatite and dentin chips as apical plugs. *Endodontics & Dental Traumatology* **2**(5), 210–14.

Cameron, J. A. (1986) The use of sodium hypochlorite activated by ultrasound for the debridement of infected, immature root canals. *Journal of Endodontics* **12**(11), 550–4.

Camp, J. H. (1980) Pedodontic endodontic treatment. In: *Pathways of the Pulp* (S. Cohen and R. C. Burns, eds), Mosby, St Louis, pp 622–56.

Camp, J. H. (2008) Diagnosis dilemmas in vital pulp therapy: treatment for the toothache is changing, especially in young, immature teeth. *Journal of Endodontics* **34**(7 Suppl), S6–12.

Chala, S., Abouqal, R., Rida, S. (2011) Apexification of immature teeth with calcium hydroxide or mineral trioxide aggregate: systematic review and meta-analysis. *Oral Surgery Oral Medicine Oral Pathology Oral Radiology & Endodontics* **112**(4), e36–42.

Chosack, A., Sela, J., Cleaton-Jones, P. (1997) A histological and quantitative histomorphometric study of apexification of nonvital permanent incisors of vervet monkeys after repeated root filling with a calcium hydroxide paste. *Endodontics & Dental Traumatology* **13**(5), 211–17.

Citrome, G. P., Kaminski, E. J., Heuer, M. A. (1979) A comparative study of tooth apexification in the dog. *Journal of Endodontics* **5**(10), 290–7.

Clarkson, R. M., Moule, A. J., Podlich, H. M. (2001) The shelf-life of sodium hypochlorite irrigating solutions. *Australian Dental Journal* **46**(4), 269–76.

Cooke, C., Rowbotham, T. C. (1960) The closure of open apices in non-vital immature incisor teeth. *British Dental Journal* **108**, 147.

Coviello, J., Brilliant, J. D. (1979) A preliminary clinical study on the use of tricalcium phosphate as an apical barrier. *Journal of Endodontics* **5**(1), 6–13.

Cunningham, W. T., Balekjian, A. Y. (1980) Effect of temperature on collagen-dissolving ability of sodium hypochlorite endodontic irrigant. *Oral Surgery, Oral Medicine, Oral Pathology* **49**(2), 175–7.

Cunningham, W. T., Joseph, S. W. (1980) Effect of temperature on the bactericidal action of sodium hypochlorite endodontic irrigant. *Oral Surgery, Oral Medicine, Oral Pathology* **50**(6), 569–71.

Cvek, M. (1972) Treatment of non-vital permanent incisors with calcium hydroxide. *I. Follow-up of periapical repair and apical closure of immature roots. Odontologisk Revy* **23**(1), 27–44.

Cvek, M. (1992) Prognosis of luxated non-vital maxillary incisors treated with calcium hydroxide and filled with gutta-percha. A retrospective clinical study. *Endodontics & Dental Traumatology* **8**(2), 45–55.

Cvek, M., Cleaton-Jones, P. E., Austin, J.C., *et al.* (1982). Pulp reactions to exposure after experimental crown fractures or grinding in adult monkeys. *Journal of Endodontics* **8**(9), 391–7.

Das, S. (1980) Apexification in a nonvital tooth by control of infection. *Journal of the American Dental Association* **100**(6), 880–1.

de Leimburg, M. L., Angeretti, A., Ceruti, P., *et al.* (2004) MTA obturation of pulpless teeth with open apices: bacterial leakage as detected by polymerase chain reaction assay. *Journal of Endodontics* **30**(12), 883–6.

Dominguez Reyes, A., Munoz Munoz, L., Aznar Martín, T. (2005) Study of calcium hydroxide apexification in 26 young permanent incisors. *Dental Traumatology* **21**(3), 141–5.

Doyon, G. E., Dumsha, T., von Fraunhofer, J.A. (2005) Fracture resistance of human root dentin exposed to intracanal calcium hydroxide. *Journal of Endodontics* **31**(12), 895–7.

Duell, R. C. (1973) Conservative endodontic treatment of the open apex in three dimensions. *Dental Clinics of North America* **17**(1), 125–34.

Dylewski, J. J. (1971) Apical closure of nonvital teeth. *Oral Surgery, Oral Medicine, Oral Pathology* **32**(1), 82–9.

El-Meligy, O. A. S., Avery, D. R. (2006) Comparison of apexification with mineral trioxide aggregate and calcium hydroxide. *Pediatric Dentistry* **28**(3), 248–53.

Erdem, A. P., Sepet, E. (2008) Mineral trioxide aggregate for obturation of maxillary central incisors with necrotic pulp and open apices. *Dental Traumatology* **24**(5), e38–41.

Feiglin, B. (1985) Differences in apex formation during apexification with calcium hydroxide paste. *Endodontics & Dental Traumatology* **1**(5), 195–9.

Felippe, M. C. S., Felippe, W. T., Marques, M. M., *et al.* (2005) The effect of the renewal of calcium hydroxide paste on the apexification and periapical healing of teeth with incomplete root formation. *International Endodontic Journal* **38**(7), 436–42.

Felippe, W. T., Felippe, M. C. S., Rocha, M. J. (2006) The effect of mineral trioxide aggregate on the apexification and periapical healing of teeth with incomplete root formation. *International Endodontic Journal* **39**(1), 2–9.

Finucane, D., Kinirons, M. J. (1999) Non-vital immature permanent incisors: factors that may influence treatment outcome. *Endodontics & Dental Traumatology* **15**(6), 273–7.

Frank, A. L. (1966) Therapy for the divergent pulpless tooth by continued apical formation. *Journal of the American Dental Association* **72**(1), 87–93.

Friend, L. A. (1966) The root treatment of teeth with open apices. *Proceedings of the Royal Society of Medicine* **59**(10), 1035–6.

Friend, L. A. (1967) The treatment of immature teeth with non-vital pulps. *Journal of the British Endodontic Society* **1**(2), 28–33.

Friend, L. A. (1969) Root canal morphology in incisor teeth in the 6–15 year old child. *Journal of the British Endodontic Society* **3**(3), 35–42.

Fulling, H. J., Andreasen, J. O. (1976) Influence of maturation status and tooth type of permanent teeth upon electrometric and thermal pulp testing. *Scandinavian Journal of Dental Research* **84**(5), 286–90.

Fuss, Z., Trowbridge, H., Bender, I. B., *et al.* (1986) Assessment of reliability of electrical and thermal pulp testing agents. *Journal of Endodontics.* **12**(7), 301–5.

Garber, S. E., Shabahang, S., Escher, A.P., *et al.* (2009) The effect of hyperglycemia on pulpal healing in rats. *Journal of Endodontics* **35**(1), 60–2.

Gerhardt, D. E., Williams, H. N. (1991) Factors affecting the stability of sodium hypochlorite solutions used to disinfect dental impressions. *Quintessence International* **22**(7), 587–91.

Ghose, L. J., Baghdady, V. S., Hikmat, Y. M. (1987) Apexification of immature apices of pulpless permanent anterior teeth with calcium hydroxide. *Journal of Endodontics* **13**(6), 285–90.

Giuliani, V., Baccetti, T., Pace, R., *et al.* (2002) The use of MTA in teeth with necrotic pulps and open apices. *Dental Traumatology* **18**(4), 217–21.

Goldman, M. (1974) Root-end closure techniques including apexification. *Dental Clinics of North America* **18**(2), 297–308.

Gomes, B. P., Ferraz, C. C., Vianna, M. E., *et al.* (2001) In vitro antimicrobial activity of several concentrations of sodium hypochlorite and chlorhexidine gluconate in the elimination of *Enterococcus faecalis*. *International Endodontic Journal* **34**(6), 424–8.

Granath, L. E. (1959) Some notes on the treatment of traumatized incisors in children. *Odontology Reviews* **10**: 272.

Gutmann, J. L., Heaton, J. F. (1981) Management of the open (immature) apex. 2. Non-vital teeth. *International Endodontic Journal* **14**(3), 173–8.

Hachmeister, D. R., Schindler, W. G., Walker, W. A. 3rd, *et al.* (2002) The sealing ability and retention characteristics of mineral trioxide aggregate in a model of apexification. *Journal of Endodontics* **28**(5), 386–90.

Ham, J. W., Patterson, S. S., Mitchell, D. F. (1972) Induced apical closure of immature pulpless teeth in monkeys. *Oral Surgery, Oral Medicine, Oral Pathology* **33**(3), 438–49.

Ham, K. A., Witherspoon, D. E., Gutmann, J. L., (2005). Preliminary evaluation of BMP-2 expression and histological characteristics during apexification with calcium hydroxide and mineral trioxide aggregate. *Journal of Endodontics* **31**(4), 275–9.

Harbert, H. (1991) Generic tricalcium phosphate plugs: an adjunct in endodontics. *Journal of Endodontics* **17**(3), 131–4.

Harbert, H. (1996) One-step apexification without calcium hydroxide. *Journal of Endodontics* **22**(12), 690–2.

Harman, K., Lindsay, S., Adewami, A., *et al.* (2005) An investigation of language used by children to describe discomfort expected and experienced during dental treatment. *International Journal of Paediatric Dentistry* **15**(5), 319–26.

Hatibovic-Kofman, S., Raimundo, L., Zheng, L, (2008) Fracture resistance and histological findings of immature teeth treated with mineral trioxide aggregate. *Dental Traumatology* **24**(3), 272–6.

Hayashi, M., Shimizu, A., Ebisu, S. (2004) MTA for obturation of mandibular central incisors with open apices: case report. *Journal of Endodontics* **30**(2), 120–2.

Heithersay, G. S. (1970) Stimulation of root formation in incompletely developed pulpless teeth. *Oral Surgery, Oral Medicine, Oral Pathology* **29**(4), 620–30.

Heling, I., Lustmann, J., . Hover, R., *et al.* (1999) Complications of apexification resulting from poor patient compliance: report of case. *Journal of Dentistry for Children* **66**(6), 415–18.

Herbert, W. E. (1959) Three cases of disturbance of calcification of a tooth and infection of the dental pulp following trauma. *Dental Practice* **9**, 176–80.

Holden, D. T., Schwartz, S. A., Kirkpatrick, T. C., *et al.* (2008) Clinical outcomes of artificial root-end barriers with mineral trioxide aggregate in teeth with immature apices. *Journal of Endodontics* **34**(7), 812–17.

Holland, G. R. (1984) Periapical response to apical plugs of dentin and calcium hydroxide in ferret canines. *Journal of Endodontics* **10**(2), 71–4.

Holland, R., de Souza, V., Russo, M. de C. (1973) Healing process after root canal therapy in immature human teeth. *Revista Da Faculdade de Odontologia de Aracatuba* **2**(2), 269–79.

Holland, R., De Souza, V., Nery, M.J. *et al.* (1980) Tissue reactions following apical plugging of the root canal with infected dentin chips. A histologic study in dogs' teeth. *Oral Surgery, Oral Medicine, Oral Pathology* **49**(4), 366–9.

Holland, R., Nery, M. J., Souza, V, (1983) The effect of the filling material in the tissue reactions following apical plugging of the root canal with dentin chips. A histologic study in monkeys' teeth. *Oral Surgery, Oral Medicine, Oral Pathology* **55**(4), 398–401.

Hoshino, E., Kurihara-Ando, N., Sato, I, (1996). In-vitro antibacterial susceptibility of bacteria taken from infected root dentine to a mixture of ciprofloxacin, metronidazole and minocycline. *International Endodontic Journal* **29**(2), 125–30.

Hulsmann, M., Pieper, K. (1989) Use of an electronic apex locator in the treatment of teeth with incomplete root formation. *Endodontics & Dental Traumatology* **5**(5), 238–41.

Ingle, J. I. (1965) *Endodontics*. Lea & Febiger, Philadelphia.

Iwaya, S. I., Ikawa, M., Kubota, M. (2001) Revascularization of an immature permanent tooth with apical periodontitis and sinus tract. *Dental Traumatology* **17**(4), 185–7.

Johnson, B. R., Remeikis, N. A. (1993) Effective shelf-life of prepared sodium hypochlorite solution. *Journal of Endodontics* **19**(1), 40–3.

Kaiser, H. J. (1964) Management of wide open apex canals with calcium hydroxide. *21st Annual Meeting of the American Association of Endodontists*. Washington DC.

Kim, J.-H., Kim, Y., Shin, S. J., *et al.* (2010) Tooth discoloration of immature permanent incisor associated with triple antibiotic therapy: a case report. *Journal of Endodontics* **36**(6), 1086–91.

Kim, U.-S., Shin, S.-J., Chang, S. W, (2009) In vitro evaluation of bacterial leakage resistance of an ultrasonically placed mineral trioxide aggregate orthograde apical plug in teeth with wide open apexes: a preliminary study. *Oral Surgery Oral Medicine Oral Pathology Oral Radiology & Endodontics* **107**(4), e52–6.

Kinirons, M. J., Srinivasan, V., Welbury, R.R., *et al.* (2001) A study in two centres of variations in the time of apical barrier detection and barrier position in nonvital immature permanent incisors. *International Journal of Paediatric Dentistry* **11**(6), 447–51.

Kleier, D. J., Barr, E. S. (1991) A study of endodontically apexified teeth. *Endodontics & Dental Traumatology* **7**(3), 112–17.

Klein, H. (1978) Pulp responses to an electric pulp stimulator in the developing permanent anterior dentition. *Journal of Dentistry for Children* **45**(3), 199–202.

Koenigs, J. F., Heller, A. L., Brilliant, J. D., *et al.* (1975) Induced apical closure of permanent teeth in adult primates using a resorbable form of tricalcium phosphate ceramic. *Journal of Endodontics* **1**(3), 102–6.

Lawley, G. R., Schindler, W. G., Walker, W. A. 3rd, *et al.* (2004) Evaluation of ultrasonically placed MTA and fracture resistance with intracanal composite resin in a model of apexification. *Journal of Endodontics* **30**(3), 167–72.

Lee, L.-W., Hsiao, S.-H., Chang, C. C., *et al.* (2010) Duration for apical barrier formation in necrotic immature permanent incisors treated with calcium hydroxide apexification using ultrasonic or hand filing. *Journal of the Formosan Medical Association* **109**(8), 596–602.

Levenstein, H. (2002) Obturating teeth with wide open apices using mineral trioxide aggregate: a case report. *South African Dental Journal* **57**(7), 270–3.

Lieberman, J,. Trowbridge, H. (1983) Apical closure of nonvital permanent incisor teeth where no treatment was performed: case report. *Journal of Endodontics* **9**(6), 257–60.

Lolayekar, N., Bhat, S. S., Hegde, S. (2009). Sealing ability of ProRoot MTA and MTA-Angelus simulating a one-step apical barrier technique – an in vitro study. *Journal of Clinical Pediatric Dentistry* **33**(4), 305–310.

Lynn, E. A., Einbender, S. (2003) The use of mineral trioxide aggregate to create an apical stop in previously traumatized adult tooth with blunderbuss canal. Case report. *New York State Dental Journal* **69**(2), 30–2.

Mackie, I. C. (1998) UK National Clinical Guidelines in Paediatric Dentistry. Management and root canal treatment of non-vital immature permanent incisor teeth. Faculty of Dental Surgery, Royal College of Surgeons. *International Journal of Paediatric Dentistry* **8**(4), 289–93.

Mackie, I. C., Hill, F. J. (1999) A clinical guide to the endodontic treatment of non-vital immature permanent teeth. *British Dental Journal* **186**(2), 54–8.

Marmasse, A. (1953) *Dentisterie Operatoire*. JB Bailliére, Paris.

Maroto, M., Barberia, E., Planells, P., *et al.* (2003) Treatment of a non-vital immature incisor with mineral trioxide aggregate (MTA). *Dental Traumatology* **19**(3), 165–9.

Martin, R. L., Monticelli, F., Brackett, W. W, (2007) Sealing properties of mineral trioxide aggregate orthograde apical plugs and root fillings in an in vitro apexification model. *Journal of Endodontics* **33**(3), 272–5.

Matsumiya, S., Susuki, A., Takuma, S. (1962) Atlas of clinical pathology. *The Tokyo Dental College Press* **1**.

Matsuo, T., Nakanishi, T., Shimizu, H., *et al.* (1996) A clinical study of direct pulp capping applied to carious-exposed pulps. *Journal of Endodontics* **22**(10), 551–6.

Matt, G. D., Thorpe, J. R., Strother, J. M., *et al.* (2004) Comparative study of white and gray mineral trioxide aggregate (MTA) simulating a one- or two-step apical barrier technique. *Journal of Endodontics* **30**(12), 876–9.

Mendoza, A. M., Reina, E. S., García-Godoy, F. (2010) Evolution of apical formation on immature necrotic permanent teeth. *American Journal of Dentistry* **23**(5), 269–74.

Mente, J., Hage, N., Pfefferle, T, (2009) Mineral trioxide aggregate apical plugs in teeth with open apical foramina: a retrospective analysis of treatment outcome. *Journal of Endodontics* **35**(10), 1354–8.

Michanowicz, J. P., Michanowicz, A. E. (1967) A conservative approach and procedure to fill an incompletely formed root using calcium hydroxide as an adjunct. *Journal of Dentistry for Children* **34**(1), 42–7.

Moore, A., Howley, M. F., O'Connell, A. C. (2011) Treatment of open apex teeth using two types of white mineral trioxide aggregate after initial dressing with calcium hydroxide in children. *Dental Traumatology* **27**(3), 166–73.

Morfis, A. S., Siskos, G. (1991) Apexification with the use of calcium hydroxide: a clinical study. *Journal of Clinical Pediatric Dentistry* **16**(1), 13–19.

Morgan, R. W., Carnes, Jr., D. L., Montgomery, S. (1991) The solvent effects of calcium hydroxide irrigating solution on bovine pulp tissue. *Journal of Endodontics* **17**(4), 165–8.

Morse, D. R., O'Larnic, J., Yesilsoy, C. (1990) Apexification: review of the literature. *Quintessence International* **21**(7), 589–98.

Nayar, S., Bishop, K., Alani, A. (2009) A report on the clinical and radiographic outcomes of 38 cases of apexification with mineral trioxide aggregate.[Erratum appears in Eur J Prosthodont Restor Dent. 2010 Mar;18(1),42]. *European Journal of Prosthodontics & Restorative Dentistry* **17**(4), 150–6.

Nevins, A., Wrobel, W., Valachovic, R., *et al.* (1977) Hard tissue induction into pulpless open-apex teeth using collagen-calcium phosphate gel. *Journal of Endodontics* **3**(11), 431–3.

Nevins, A., Finkelstein, F. *et al.* (1978) Induction of hard tissue into pulpless open-apex teeth using collagen-calcium phosphate gel. *Journal of Endodontics* **4**(3), 76–81.

Nosrat, A., Homayounfar, N., Laporta, R., *et al.* (2012) Drawbacks and unfavorable outcomes of regenerative endodontic treatments of necrotic immature teeth: a literature review and report of a case. *Journal of Endodontics* **38**(10), 1428–34.

Orstavik, D. (1988) Reliability of the periapical index scoring system. *Scandinavian Journal of Dental Research* **96**(2), 108–11.

Orstavik, D., Kerekes, K., Eriksen, H. M. (1986) The periapical index: a scoring system for radiographic assessment of apical periodontitis. *Endodontics & Dental Traumatology* **2**(1), 20–34.

Pace, R., Giuliani, V., Pini Prato, L. (2007) Apical plug technique using mineral trioxide aggregate: results from a case series. *International Endodontic Journal* **40**(6), 478–84.

Patel, S. (2010) The use of cone beam computed tomography in the conservative management of dens invaginatus: a case report. *International Endodontic Journal* **43**(8), 707–13.

Pinkham, J. R. (1997) Linguistic maturity as a determinant of child patient behavior in the dental office. *Journal of Dentistry for Children* **64**(5), 322–6.

Pitts, D. L., Jones, J. E., Oswald, R. J. (1984) A histological comparison of calcium hydroxide plugs and dentin plugs used for the control of Gutta-percha root canal filling material. *Journal of Endodontics* **10**(7), 283–93.

Pradhan, D. P., Chawla, H. S., Gauba, K., *et al.* (2006) Comparative evaluation of endodontic management of teeth with unformed apices with mineral trioxide aggregate and calcium hydroxide. *Journal of Dentistry for Children (Chicago, Ill)* **73**(2), 79–85.

Roberts, S. C., Jr., Brilliant, J. D. (1975) Tricalcium phosphate as an adjunct to apical closure in pulpless permanent teeth. *Journal of Endodontics* **1**(8), 263–9.

Rohner, W. (1940) Calxyl als wurzelfullings material nach pulpa extirpation. *Schweizer Monatsschrift fur Zahnmedicin* **50**, 903–48.

Rosenberg, B., Murray, P. E., Namerow, K. (2007) The effect of calcium hydroxide root filling on dentin fracture strength. *Dental Traumatology* **23**(1), 26–9.

Rule, D. C., Winter, G. B. (1966) Root growth and apical repair subsequent to pulpal necrosis in children. *British Dental Journal* **120**(12), 586–90.

Sarris, S., Tahmassebi, J. F., Duggal, M. S., *et al.* (2008) A clinical evaluation of mineral trioxide aggregate for root-end closure of non-vital immature permanent incisors in children- a pilot study. *Dental Traumatology* **24**(1), 79–85.

Sato, I., Ando-Kurihara, N., Kota, K., *et al.* (1996) Sterilization of infected root-canal dentine by topical application of a mixture of ciprofloxacin, metronidazole and minocycline in situ. *International Endodontic Journal* **29**(2), 118–24.

Seltzer, S. (1988) The root apex. In: *Endodontology: Biologic Considerations in Endodontic Procedures* (S. Seltzer & P. Krasner, eds) Lea & Febiger, Philadelphia, pp 1–30.

Shabahang, S., Torabinejad, M. (2000) Treatment of teeth with open apices using mineral trioxide aggregate. *Practical Periodontics & Aesthetic Dentistry* **12**(3), 315–20; quiz 322.

Shabahang, S., Torabinejad, M. (2003) Effect of MTAD on *Enterococcus faecalis*-contaminated root canals of extracted human teeth. [Miscellaneous Article]. *Journal of Endodontics September* **29**(9), 576–9.

Shabahang, S., Pouresmail, M., Torabinejad, M. (2003) In vitro antimicrobial efficacy of MTAD and sodium hypochlorite. *Journal of Endodontics* **29**(7), 450–2.

Shabahang, S., Torabinejad, M., Boyne, P.P., *et al.* (1999) A comparative study of root-end induction using osteogenic protein-1, calcium hydroxide, and mineral trioxide aggregate in dogs. *Journal of Endodontics* **25**(1), 1–5.

Sheehy, E. C., Roberts, G. J. (1997) Use of calcium hydroxide for apical barrier formation and healing in non-vital immature permanent teeth: a review. *British Dental Journal* **183**(7), 241–6.

Simon, S., Rilliard, F., Berdal, A., *et al.* (2007) The use of mineral trioxide aggregate in one-visit apexification treatment: a prospective study. *International Endodontic Journal* **40**(3), 186–97.

Siqueira, J. F., Jr., Rocas, I. N. (2008) Clinical implications and microbiology of bacterial persistence after treatment procedures. *Journal of Endodontics* **34**(11), 1291–301.e1293.

Sjogren, U., Figdor, D., Spångberg, L., *et al.* (1991) The antimicrobial effect of calcium hydroxide as a short-term intracanal dressing. *International Endodontic Journal* **24**(3), 119–25.

Steiner, J. C., Dow, P. R., Cathey, G. M. (1968) Inducing root end closure of nonvital permanent teeth. *Journal of Dentistry for Children* **35**(1), 47–54.

Steiner, J. C., Van Hassel, H. J. (1971) Experimental root apexification in primates. *Oral Surgery, Oral Medicine, Oral Pathology* **31**(3), 409–15.

Steinig, T. H., Regan, J. D., Gutmann, J. L. (2003) The use and predictable placement of Mineral Trioxide Aggregate in one-visit apexification cases. *Australian Endodontic Journal: the Journal of the Australian Society of Endodontology* **29**(1), 34–42.

Stewart, D. J. (1963) Root canal therapy in incisor teeth with open apices. *British Dental Journal* **114**: 249–54.

Strobl, H., Haas, M., Norer, B., *et al.* (2004) Evaluation of pulpal blood flow after tooth splinting of luxated permanent maxillary incisors. *Dental Traumatology* **20**(1), 36–41.

The, S. D. (1979) The solvent action of sodium hypochlorite on fixed and unfixed necrotic tissue. *Oral Surgery, Oral Medicine, Oral Pathology* **47**(6), 558–61.

Toole, R. J., Lindsay, S. J., Johnstone, S., *et al.* (2000) An investigation of language used by children to describe discomfort during dental pulp-testing. *International Journal of Paediatric Dentistry* **10**(3), 221–8.

Torabinejad, M., Chivian, N. (1999) Clinical applications of mineral trioxide aggregate. *Journal of Endodontics* **25**(3), 197–205.

Torabinejad, M., Watson, T. F., Pitt Ford, T. R. (1993) Sealing ability of a mineral trioxide aggregate when used as a root end filling material. *Journal of Endodontics* **19**(12), 591–5.

Torabinejad, M., Hong, C. U., Lee, S. J., *et al.* (1995a) Investigation of mineral trioxide aggregate for root-end filling in dogs. *Journal of Endodontics* **21**(12), 603–8.

Torabinejad, M., Hong, C. U., McDonald, F., *et al.* (1995b) Physical and chemical properties of a new root-end filling material. *Journal of Endodontics* **21**(7), 349–53.

Torabinejad, M., Cho, Y., Khademi, A.A., *et al.* (2003a) The effect of various concentrations of sodium hypochlorite on the ability of MTAD to remove the smear layer. *Journal of Endodontics* **29**(4), 233–9.

Torabinejad, M., Khademi, A. A., Babagoli, J, (2003b) A new solution for the removal of the smear layer. *Journal of Endodontics* **29**(3), 170–5.

Torabinejad, M., Shabahang, S., Aprecio, R. M., *et al.* (2003c) The antimicrobial effect of MTAD: an in vitro investigation. *Journal of Endodontics* **29**(6), 400–3.

Torneck, C. D., Smith, J. (1970) Biologic effects of endodontic procedures on developing incisor teeth. I. Effect of partial and total pulp removal. *Oral Surgery, Oral Medicine, Oral Pathology* **30**(2), 258–66.

Torneck, C. D., Smith, J. S., Grindall, P. (1973) Biologic effects of endodontic procedures on developing incisor teeth. IV. Effect of debridement procedures and calcium hydroxide-camphorated parachlorophenol paste in the treatment of experimentally induced pulp and periapical disease. *Oral Surgery, Oral Medicine, Oral Pathology* **35**(4), 541–54.

Tronstad, L. (1978) Tissue reactions following apical plugging of the root canal with dentin chips in monkey teeth subjected to pulpectomy. *Oral Surgery, Oral Medicine, Oral Pathology* **45**(2), 297–304.

Tuna, E. B., Dincol, M. E., Gençay, K., *et al.* (2011) Fracture resistance of immature teeth filled with BioAggregate, mineral trioxide aggregate and calcium hydroxide. *Dental Traumatology* **27**(3), 174–178.

Turkun, M., Cengiz, T. (1997) The effects of sodium hypochlorite and calcium hydroxide on tissue dissolution and root canal cleanliness. *International Endodontic Journal* **30**(5), 335–42.

Vojinovic, O., Srnie, E. (1975) Introduction of apical formation by the use of calcium hydroxide and Iodoform-Chlumsky paste in the endodontic treatment of immature teeth. *Journal of the British Endodontic Society* **8**(1), 16–22.

Wadachi, R., Araki, K., Suda, H. (1998) Effect of calcium hydroxide on the dissolution of soft tissue on the root canal wall. *Journal of Endodontics* **24**(5), 326–30.

Walia, T., Chawla, H. S., Gauba, K. (2000) Management of wide open apices in non-vital permanent teeth with Ca(OH)$_2$ paste. *Journal of Clinical Pediatric Dentistry* **25**(1), 51–6.

Waltimo, T., Trope, M., Haapasalo, M., *et al.* (2005) Clinical efficacy of treatment procedures in endodontic infection control and one year follow-up of periapical healing. *Journal of Endodontics* **31**(12), 863–6.

Webber, R. T. (1984) Apexogenesis versus apexification. *Dental Clinics of North America* **28**(4), 669–97.

Webber, R. T., Schwiebert, K. A., Cathey, G. M. (1981) A technique for placement of calcium hydroxide in the root canal system. *Journal of the American Dental Association* **103**(3), 417–21.

Wechsler, S. M., Fishelberg, G., Opderbeck, W. R. (1978). Apexification: a valuable and effective clinical procedure. *General Dentistry* **26**(5), 40–43.

Weisenseel, J. A., Jr., Hicks, M. L., Pelleu, G. B. Jr (1987). Calcium hydroxide as an apical barrier. *Journal of Endodontics* **13**(1), 1–5.

White, J. D., Lacefield, W. R., Chavers, L. S., *et al.* (2002) The effect of three commonly used endodontic materials on the strength and hardness of root dentin. *Journal of Endodontics* **28**(12), 828–30.

Windley III, W., Teixeira, F., Levin, L., *et al.* (2005) Disinfection of immature teeth with a triple antibiotic paste. *Journal of Endodontics* **31**(6), 439–43.

Witherspoon, D. E., Ham, K. (2001) One-visit apexification: technique for inducing root-end barrier formation in apical closures. *Practical Procedures & Aesthetic Dentistry: Ppad* **13**(6), 455–60; quiz 462.

Witherspoon, D. E., Small, J. C., Regan, J. D., *et al.* (2008) Retrospective analysis of open apex teeth obturated with mineral trioxide aggregate. *Journal of Endodontics* **34**(10), 1171–6.

Yang, S. F., Rivera, E. M., Baumgardner, K. R., *et al.* (1995) Anaerobic tissue-dissolving abilities of calcium hydroxide and sodium hypochlorite. *Journal of Endodontics* **21**(12), 613–16.

Yates, J. A. (1988) Barrier formation time in non-vital teeth with open apices. *International Endodontic Journal* **21**(5), 313–19.

Yeung, P., Liewehr, F. R., Moon, P. C. (2006) A quantitative comparison of the fill density of MTA produced by two placement techniques. *Journal of Endodontics* **32**(5), 456–9.

6 Regenerative Endodontics (Revitalization/Revascularization)

Mahmoud Torabinejad,[1] Robert P. Corr,[2] and George T.-J. Huang[3]

[1] Department of Endodontics, Loma Linda University School of Dentistry, USA
[2] Private Practice, USA
[3] Department of Bioscience Research, University of Tennessee Health Science Center, USA

Mineral Trioxide Aggregate: Properties and Clinical Applications, First Edition.
Edited by Mahmoud Torabinejad.
© 2014 John Wiley & Sons, Inc. Published 2014 by John Wiley & Sons, Inc.

INTRODUCTION

Pulpal necrosis generally occurs as a result of bacterial infection from caries, infractions, or frank exposure of the pulp to contamination of the oral cavity (Kakehashi *et al.* 1965). Traumatic luxation or avulsion injuries associated with severance of the blood supply result in pulpal ischemia, which also leads to necrosis and often a secondary infection with bacteria (Tsukamoto-Tanaka *et al.* 2006). Teeth with necrotic and infected pulps are routinely treated with endodontic procedures involving cleaning, shaping, and obturation of the root canal systems with a high rate of long-term success (Torabinejad *et al.* 2007). The consequence of pulpal necrosis in immature teeth, however, is the cessation of root development, making endodontic treatment with conventional techniques and materials difficult or impossible. Immature teeth have open and often divergent apices that are not suitable for complete cleaning and obturation with traditional materials. In addition, because of their thin walls, these teeth are susceptible to fracture after treatment (Kerekes *et al.* 1980).

Obtaining an adequate apical seal is widely accepted as a tenet of endodontic therapy (Schilder 1967). Teeth with necrotic pulps and immature apices present special challenges to clinicians during obturation. Apexification procedures that involve the production of an induced or artificial apical stop can allow for condensation of obturation materials. However, apexification procedures do not promote continuation of root development, nor do they increase fracture resistance of the root walls.

The ideal outcome for a necrotic immature tooth would be the regeneration of pulp tissue into a canal which is capable of promoting the continuation of normal root development. The advantages of pulp regeneration lie in the potential for reinforcement of dentinal walls by deposition of hard tissue and the potential for the development of an apical morphology more appropriate for conventional endodontic therapy if future treatment becomes necessary.

The potential for revascularization and continued development of replanted teeth has been well-documented in the dental literature. However, the presence of infection has been shown to interfere with this process (Ham *et al.* 1972; Kling *et al.* 1986; Cvek *et al.* 1990b). It has therefore traditionally been thought that successful revascularization cannot be an expected outcome after a tooth has become infected. However, there is a growing body of evidence to suggest that revitalization of the pulp space, along with continued growth of the root, may in fact be possible after pulpal necrosis and apical pathosis in teeth with immature apices. Nineteen case reports and 14 case series have been published demonstrating apparent continuation of root development of immature teeth with acute apical abscesses, as evidenced by deposition of hard tissue along the canal walls (Rule & Winter 1966; Nevins *et al.* 1977; Iwaya *et al.* 2001;

Banchs & Trope 2004; Chueh & Huang 2006; Cotti *et al.* 2008; Jung *et al.* 2008; Shah *et al.* 2008; Chueh *et al.* 2009; Ding *et al.* 2009; Bose *et al.* 2009; Reynolds *et al.* 2009; Shin *et al.* 2009; Mendoza *et al.* 2010; Petrino *et al.* 2010; Thomson & Kahler 2010; Nosrat *et al.* 2011; Cehreli *et al.* 2011, 2012; Chen *et al.* 2011; Jung *et al.* 2011; Aggarwal *et al.* 2012; Jadhav *et al.* 2012; Jeeruphan *et al.* 2012; Kim *et al.* 2012; Lenzi & Trope 2012; Miller *et al.* 2012; Chen *et al.* 2013; Keswani & Pandey 2013; Soares Ade *et al.* 2013; Yang *et al.* 2013). A majority of these cases have predominantly used a blood clot as a scaffold. Platelet-rich plasma (PRP) (Alsousou *et al.* 2009) has been suggested to be an ideal scaffold for revitalization and regenerative endodontic procedures (Hargreaves *et al.* 2008; Ding *et al.* 2009). Platelet-rich plasma has been shown to contain growth factors, stimulate collagen production, recruit other cells to the site of injury, produce anti-inflammatory agents, initiate vascular in-growth, induce cell differentiation, control the local inflammatory response, and improve soft and hard tissue wound healing (Hiremath *et al.* 2008). Torabinejad and Turman used PRP instead of whole blood as a scaffold for a revitalization procedure in a maxillary premolar with necrotic pulp and open apex (Torabinejad & Turman 2011). After 5.5months, there was radiographic evidence of resolution of periapical lesion, continual root development, and dentinal thickening. Clinically, the tooth responded to vitality tests. The authors suggested that PRP can be an ideal scaffold for regenerative/revitalization procedures.

REVASCULARIZATION AFTER REPLANTATION AND AUTOTRANSPLANTATION

Dental trauma resulting in the severance of blood supply to the pulp has been shown to cause necrosis of the tissue from ischemia (Tsukamoto-Tanaka *et al.* 2006). The potential for revascularization of the pulp space with functional tissue capable of hard tissue deposition after such dental trauma has been well-documented in the literature. A number of case reports present evidence of revascularization of replanted immature teeth, with reports of continued root thickening and apical closure, sensitivity to thermal stimulus and electrical pulp testing, and normal laser Doppler flowmetry readings (Fuss 1985; Johnson *et al.* 1985; Mesaros & Trope 1997). Andreasen *et al.* reported a successful revascularization rate of 34 percent in a prospective study that included 94 replanted immature teeth (Andreasen *et al.* 1995). Similar results have been found by other investigators (Sheppard & Burich 1980; Kling *et al.* 1986; Cvek *et al.* 1990a; Yanpiset & Trope 2000). Although these revascularization rates appear relatively low, *in vivo* animal studies suggest that pretreatment with topical antibiotics may increase the success of revascularization to 90 percent (Yanpiset & Trope 2000; Ritter *et al.* 2004).

A number of animal studies in rats, cats, dogs, and monkeys have been published, which provide the histological picture of revascularization after experimental replantation (Kvinnsland & Heyeraas 1989; Yanpiset & Trope 2000; Ritter *et al.* 2004; Tsukamoto-Tanaka *et al.* 2006). Replanted teeth in animal models generally show a pattern of slow pulpal degeneration, followed by replacement of the degenerated tissue by in-growth of new tissue through the apical foramen. Soft tissue has been observed to advance coronally to eliminate all the necrotic pulp tissue and fill the pulp chamber in 30 days (Monsour 1971; Skoglund & Tronstad 1981; Kvinnsland & Heyeraas 1989; Tsukamoto-Tanaka *et al.* 2006). However, few teeth in these studies showed normal pulp tissue with a normal odontoblastic layer and tubular dentin. Instead, the majority of specimens were reported to show an absence of odontoblasts and large areas of the original pulpal cavity filled with hard tissue resembling bone or cementum, which has been described as osteodentin by many investigators (Kvinnsland & Heyeraas 1989; Yanpiset & Trope 2000; Ritter *et al.* 2004). Soft tissue with morphological characteristics of normal pulp is a rare finding in experimentally replanted immature teeth. Osteodentin formation represents the typical healing pattern reported after revascularization of the pulp space.

Autotransplantation is a clinical situation that is very similar to that of the traumatically avulsed tooth, although performed under controlled surgical and aseptic conditions with minimal extraoral time. Under optimal conditions, success has been reported at 94% (Bauss *et al.* 2002). Zhao *et al.* transplanted teeth from green fluorescent protein (GFP) transgenic rats into extraction sockets of wild-type recipient rats (Zhao *et al.* 2007). The use of the GFP-transgenic rats allowed for later differentiation of donor versus host cells. Using immunohistochemical markers, they confirmed the presence of both bone matrix and dentin matrix in the revascularized pulp tissue. All of the cells associated with the dentin matrix were immunopositive for GFP indicating that the donor pulp tissue formed the matrix. The absence of GFP-negative cells (host cells) implies that the periapical mesenchymal tissues in the socket were not responsible for differentiation into odontoblasts. These findings suggest that some of the original pulp tissue may need to persist in order for odontoblasts to be present after healing.

Despite the large body of literature regarding the revascularization process in transplanted and replanted teeth, the findings cannot be directly applied to non-traumatized teeth with necrotic pulps. The pulp of an avulsed tooth is generally uncontaminated, unless exposed to bacterial insult from exposure during extraoral storage (Love 1996). Furthermore, the replanted tooth contains the amputated pulp tissue graft within the pulp space that likely influences the revascularization process. Although this amputated pulp has been shown to degenerate after extraction (Skoglund 1981), some of the tissue may survive the trauma due to diffusion of nutrients at the apical extent. It has also been suggested that the blood vessels of tissue grafts may re-anastamose with, or provide a nonvital conduit for, the new vasculature during angiogenesis (Barrett & Reade 1981; Goncalves *et al.* 2007).

REVITALIZATION OF NONVITAL-INFECTED TEETH IN ANIMALS

In 1972, Ham and colleagues experimentally exposed 17 immature teeth in three monkeys to induce development of apical periodontitis (Ham *et al.* 1972). The canals were then cleaned using broaches and hypochlorite. A paper point saturated in camphorated parachlorophenol was sealed in each canal for 3 days. The walls were subsequently filed with large diameter hedstrom files and beechwood creosote was sealed in the canals for a number of days. Some teeth were filled with calcium hydroxide and Cavit. After producing a blood clot in the remaining teeth, a coronal restoration was placed. The animals were euthanized at varying intervals of up to 165 days. More than half of the controls that remained open to the oral cavity had some degree of vital pulp tissue from one-third to one-half of the canal. Some apical bridging was observed in the calcium hydroxide-treated teeth. However, none of the teeth in the blood clot group showed apical bridging. Bone extended into the canals of some teeth, with some calcified tissue deposited along the walls. Cellular cementum extended into the canal as far as connective tissue migrated. None of the teeth with positive cultures developed any degree of apical closure, and no tissue identifiable as dentin was observed in any of the experimental teeth. Failure to observe consistent revitalization in the experimental groups may be the result of positive bacterial cultures before filling the canals, the use of inadequate coronal restorative materials, or the use of caustic medications in the canal.

Torneck *et al.* also examined the effects of debridement and disinfection in infected teeth (Torneck *et al.* 1973). Eight immature teeth in monkeys were exposed to the oral environment to induce pulp and periapical disease. The canal walls were filed and irrigated with saline. Camphorated parachlorophenol was then placed and sealed in the canal with amalgam for intervals of up to two months before obtaining histological samples. The presence of residual pulp and inflamed tissue was noted at the apical end. There was deposition of hard tissue in and about the apical part of the root canal despite severe inflammation (Fig. 6.1). The authors concluded that either the mechanical instrumentation reduced the cell populations that offer potential for regeneration, or the irritating medicament impeded the cellular activity of the pulp. They did not report on how inadequate disinfection may have impacted their results.

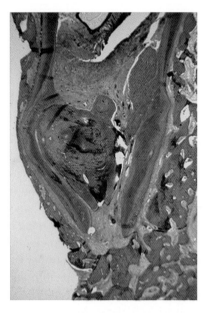

Fig. 6.1 Histological section of a tooth in which the pulp was removed and the root canal was contaminated and then sealed. Despite the presence of an abscess at a lower level, some of Hertwig's epithelial root sheath survived and produced a dentin-like tissue at the end of the root canal. Courtesy of Dr Calvin Torneck.

Myers and Founatin, in 1974, also infected the pulps of teeth in monkeys. The root canals were then biomechanically cleaned by instrumenting 2 mm beyond the apex and irrigated using 5.25% sodium hypochlorite irrigation (Myers & Fountain 1974). They filled the pulp space with blood only, blood and gelfoam, or nothing, and sealed the coronal access only with Cavit. Histological specimens were examined at intervals up to six months. Very limited in-growth of tissue was observed at the apical extent. The authors reported that the majority of cases demonstrated periapical inflammation, and colonies of microorganisms could be found in the canals. Some of the teeth developed fulminate infections that were reopened to drain. The authors suggested that the lack of successful revitalization might have been due to coronal leakage.

In 1976, Nevins *et al.* exposed the root canals of rhesus monkeys to oral contamination for one week after removing their dental pulps in order to induce endodontic infections (Nevins *et al.* 1976). The teeth were then instrumented and initially sealed with a cotton pellet and IRM only. Despite obtaining positive bacterial cultures in all teeth, an experimental collagen phosphate gel was introduced into all of the canals 3 days later. Histology was observed after 12 weeks. The teeth treated with calcium hydroxide showed apexification as anticipated. Fifteen of the 21 teeth filled with the collagen-calcium phosphate

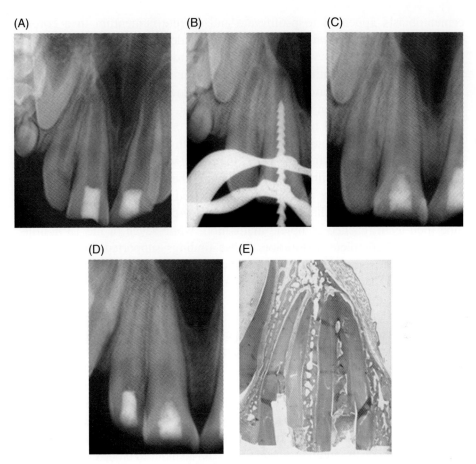

Fig. 6.2 (A), After removing dental pulps in monkeys and contamination of their root canals for a few days (B), they were then biomechanically instrumented (C), filled with an experimental collagen-phosphate gel or calcium hydroxide and then sealed with IRM (D). Radiographic examination of these teeth 6 months later shows closure of the apecies and thickening of the root canal walls (E). Histological examinations of these samples show apexification teeth treated with calcium hydroxide (right incisor) and formation of cementum, bone and reparative dentin lining the wall of the root canal of the left central incisor filled with experimental collagen-phosphate gel. Courtesy of Dr. Alan Nevins

gel were considered successfully revitalized with apposition of cementum-like tissue onto the canal walls narrowing the lumen and apical foramen. Teeth that were revitalized successfully showed tissues characteristic for cementum, bone, and reparative dentin lining the wall of the root canal for most of its length (Fig. 6.2). Lacerated remnants of pulpal tissue appeared to be actively producing reparative dentin. The authors concluded from their findings that cementoblasts appeared to proliferate and secrete cementum in a coronal direction in close proximity to the root canal dentin. They also postulated that mesenchymal cells within the apical periodontal ligament might have proliferated and differentiated to form hard tissue within the root canal space.

Das and colleagues removed the pulps from 22 teeth in baboons and allowed the canals to remain open to the oral cavity for 60 days (Das *et al.* 1997). The teeth were then cleaned by conventional filing or with broaches only. After cleaning, half of each group was treated either with formocresol or tetracycline-saturated paper points. After one week, the points were removed, and the coronal portion was sealed with IRM and amalgam. The animals were euthanized at six months. Seven of the nine tetracycline-treated teeth reached root completion, compared to only three of the 10 treated with formocresol. Three of the nine filed teeth reached complete maturation, while seven of the 13 nonfiled teeth reached complete maturation. These findings supported the hypothesis that some tissue remnants may persist that contribute to organizing the in-growth of tissue, and that mechanical shaping or the use of caustic chemicals might remove these important cells.

Thibodeau *et al.* conducted a study involving immature dog teeth with preexisting necrotic pulps and apical periodontitis (Thibodeau *et al.* 2007). They sealed oral plaque into their pulp chambers until there was radiographic evidence of apical periodontitis in 48 contaminated canine teeth. The teeth were re-accessed, irrigated with 1.25% sodium hypochlorite without any mechanical instrumentation, and a triple antibiotic paste was placed into the canal. One group of teeth was sealed coronally with MTA and amalgam and received no further treatment. Teeth in the other groups were re-accessed and irrigated to remove the antibiotics, and filled with an induced blood clot, a collagen solution, or a combination of the collagen solution and a blood clot before being sealed coronally. Radiographic and histological evaluation was performed up to three months post-operatively to assess for apical closure, root wall thickening, and the presence of vital tissue in the canals. Overall, the authors found thickened walls and apical closure in 49% and 55% of teeth respectively. Vital tissue was observed in 29% of the teeth. Although no statistical differences between treatment groups were reported, the authors reported that the inclusion of a blood clot in the canal favored revitalization.

Wang *et al.* later histologically assessed the type of tissues that had grown into the canal space in the study by Thibodeau (Wang *et al.* 2010). Similar to previous animal studies, cementum-like and bone-like tissue were noted to be present inside the canal spaces. It was found that the cementum-like and bone-like tissues were responsible for the thickening of the canal walls. The cementum deposition at the apex was responsible for the increase of the root length (Fig. 6.3). They concluded that the tissues found were not of pulpal origin, and

(A)   (B)

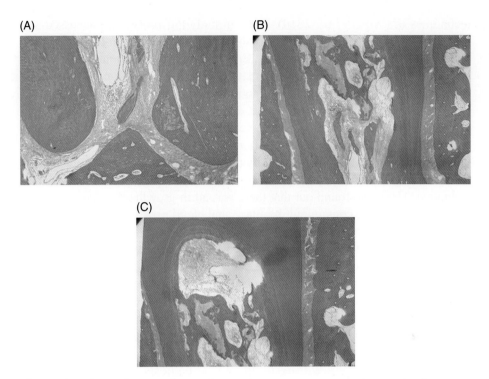

(C)

Fig. 6.3 After induction of apical periodontitis in immature dog teeth, they were disinfected using triple antibiotics. After removing the antibiotics, blood clot, a collagen solution, or a combination of the collagen solution and a blood clot were used as scaffolds. The teeth were then sealed coronally with MTA and amalgam. Histological examinations of the specimens three months later show an in-growth of bone into the (A) apical, (B) middle and (C), coronal sections of the root canal space. Courtesy of Dr B Thibodeau.

that the outcome of the revitalization process may not be tissue regeneration, but instead be tissue repair.

Zuong and associates compared root development and periapical healing between revitalization and apexification of immature dog teeth after inducing periapical periodontitis (Zuong *et al.* 2010). Revitalization and apexification were done in three teeth each, and radiographic examination was done at 1, 4, and 8 weeks postoperatively. After 8 weeks, the animals were euthanized. The revitalization group showed more consistent periapical healing. Apical closure was apparent with no significant change in dentin thickness in comparison to the apexification group. Histologically, the revitalized roots contained granulation tissue with large amounts of calcification on the canal walls.

da Silva and colleagues investigated the amount of inflammation and degree of repair of periapical tissues in infected immature dog teeth using two different techniques (da Silva *et al.* 2010). In their study, 56 roots were accessed and irrigated with hydrogen peroxide and sodium hypochlorite. In 28 roots, apical negative pressure irrigation using the EndoVac system was done with sodium hypochlorite. In 28 other roots, positive pressure irrigation with sodium hypochlorite followed by triple antibiotic dressing for 2 weeks was done. All canals were irrigated with sterile saline, dried with paper points, and the coronal accesses were restored with a double seal of MTA and amalgam. Histological assessment was carried out after 3 months and the authors reported that the negative pressure group showed significantly less inflammatory infiltrate at the periapical region compared to those samples treated with the positive irrigation technique. They also found out that there was an in-growth of connective tissue of periodontal origin containing fibroblasts and blood vessels inside the canals of both groups. They suggested that the EndoVac system may be an alternative to triple antibiotic paste for the revitalization process in necrotic immature teeth with apical periodontitis.

Yamauchi *et al.* treated 64 teeth in six dogs with apical periodontitis using a revitalization procedure (Yamauchi *et al.* 2011). Four different materials were left in the canals: blood clot, blood clot and collagen scaffold, blood clot with exposure of dentin matrix from ethylenediaminetetra-acetic acid (EDTA) treatment, and blood clot with collagen matrix and EDTA. All teeth showed increased wall thickness with resolving apical pathosis after 3.5 months. In the groups containing the collagen scaffold, more apical closure and a statistically significant amount of mineralized tissue was observed in comparison to groups not containing a collagen scaffold. When EDTA was used, histological evidence of hair-like projections from the dentin-associated mineralized tissue appeared to embed into the dentin wall. This illustrates the effects of EDTA, which promotes adherence of the mineralized tissue to the root canal walls.

Scarparo and colleagues compared the root development between teeth with vital pulp tissue, teeth with necrotic pulps, and teeth with necrotic pulps that subsequently underwent revitalization treatment procedures in immature rat molars (Scarparo *et al.* 2011). Initially, 36 teeth were accessed, their pulps were removed and left open to the oral cavity for 3 weeks to produce apical lesions. Eighteen teeth were left open for the remainder of the experiment. The remaining 18 teeth were then instrumented only in the cervical third of the canals, irrigated with sodium hypochlorite, dressed with a triple antibiotic paste, and sealed with a cotton pellet and an amalgam restoration. Histological samples were harvested after 3, 6, and 9 weeks. The results show that the control teeth with vital pulp showed no inflammation and normal signs of root development as expected. The control teeth with necrotic pulp showed periapical lesions and reduced root length and wall thickness. The teeth that were treated using revitalization procedures showed reduced periapical lesions with increased root

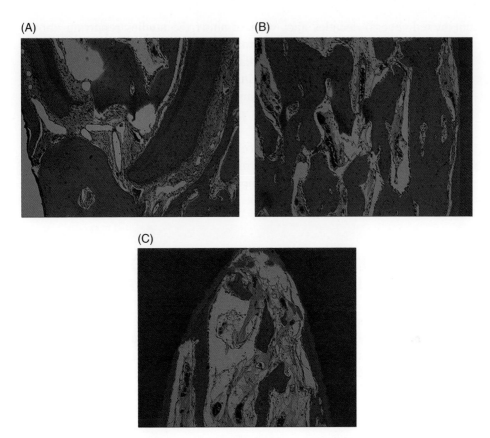

Fig. 6.4 After pulp extirpation in immature ferret cuspid teeth, blood clots were formed and covered with MTA and permanent filling material. Histological samples after 3 months illustrated an in-growth of bone into the (A), apical, (B), middle and (C), coronal sections of the root canal space.

length and wall thickness. About half of the revitalized group showed formation of cementum-like tissue in the apical portion of the roots while other samples in the same group showed an ingrowth of connective tissue into the root canal.

In 2011, Buhrley *et al.* evaluated the healing response in noninfected immature ferret cuspid teeth after extirpation of the pulp tissues followed by induction of a blood clot (Buhrley *et al.* 2011). Histological samples obtained three months after the procedures illustrated an ingrowth of bone that was contiguous with surrounding periapical bone (Fig. 6.4).

Based on the available literature, there appears to be compelling evidence that revitalization is possible despite pulpal necrosis and apical periodontitis. From previous studies, the evidence regarding the phenotypes of tissues has been found to consist of tissues similar to bone, cementum, and connective tissue. Much of the histological evidence available is from studies that were conducted several decades ago, with some of the studies reporting known bacterial contamination or the use of materials that are inadequate to provide an effective resistance to coronal leakage. Other limitations in the previous studies include the use of standard instrumentation to debride the canals, and the use of caustic medicaments and disinfectants, both of which could be detrimental to the tissues that potentially provide the genesis for revitalization.

Although the radiographic appearance of apical closure and canal wall thickening can give the impression that a normal, functional pulp has regenerated, the present histological evidence does not support this assumption, and more research is needed to incorporate current protocols.

CLINICAL EVIDENCE FOR REVITALIZATION IN NONVITAL-INFECTED TEETH IN HUMANS

Several case reports and series have demonstrated the potential for a nonvital, necrotic and infected immature tooth to revitalize, as evidenced by radiographic root thickening, apical closure, or a return of sensibility to thermal and electric pulp testing. In 1966, Rule and Winter presented a case report of continued maturation of a nonvital, immature mandibular premolar with a sinus tract stoma (Rule & Winter 1966). The tooth was accessed without anesthesia and cleaned to the level of bleeding tissue, then dressed with a polyantibiotic paste. Two weeks later, the canal was re-accessed, the antibiotics removed, and resorbable iodoform was introduced before double sealing with zinc oxide–eugenol (ZOE) and amalgam. The root showed continued thickening and apical closure 3 years post-operatively.

Nevins and colleagues reported on a child with a traumatically intruded maxillary lateral incisor that had developed symptoms of irreversible pulpitis and apical periodontitis (Nevins *et al.* 1977). Endodontic access was made, purulence was observed in the pulp space, and the canal was mechanically debrided while using saline irrigation, removing all but the apical stump of pulp tissue. Collagen-calcium phosphate gel was introduced into the pulp space and the canal was sealed. The child remained asymptomatic; apexogenesis was observed to continue at 7 weeks, and was more pronounced at longer follow up periods (Fig. 6.5).

Iwaya *et al.* reported on a case of a child with an acute apical abscess in a mandibular bicuspid with a necrotic and immature apex that had an apparent fractured occlusal dental tubercle (Iwaya *et al.* 2001). Purulent exudate was found upon initial access. The tooth was managed over multiple visits with sodium hypochlorite,

(A)　　　　　　　　(B)　　　　　　　　(C)

(D)　　　　(E)　　　　(F)　　　　(G)

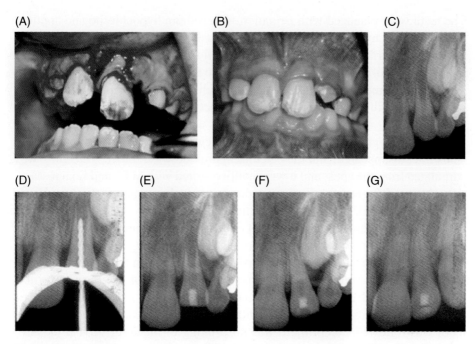

Fig. 6.5 (A) During an accident, a child developed an intruded maxillary lateral incisor. (B) Eight weeks after the tooth re-erupted. (C) Developed symptoms of irreversible pulpitis and apical periodontitis. (D) The tooth was instrumented. (E) The collagen-calcium phosphate gel was placed in the canal. (F) and (G) A radiograph taken 1 year and 3 years later shows closure of the apex and thickening of the tooth walls. Courtesy of Dr. Alan Nevins.

hydrogen peroxide, and intracanal placement of antibiotics. When vital tissue was observed 5 mm apical to the orifice, the coronal access was sealed with calcium hydroxide and a bonded restoration. Healing of the periapical abscess and complete closure of the apex were observed 2.5 years postoperatively.

Banchs and Trope presented a similar case of a child with a necrotic immature lower premolar secondary to an apparent broken dental tubercle (Banchs & Trope 2004). Associated swelling and sinus tract were observed, and purulent exudate was discovered upon entry into the pulp. They irrigated the canal with sodium hypochlorite and Peridex, without any attempt to mechanically clean the walls. A triple antibiotic paste was placed into the canal for 1 month. After removing the paste 1 month later, a blood clot was induced in the canal and the access was closed with MTA and a resin restoration. The patient was recalled periodically over 2 years. The tooth showed continued development radiographically and was responsive to cold at the 2-year recall.

Chueh and Huang presented four similar cases of children with necrotic mandibular premolars with broken dental tubercles (Chueh & Huang 2006).

The teeth were managed with irrigation with sodium hypochlorite and application of calcium hydroxide. All four cases showed continued apical development. The authors attributed lack of coronal deposition of hard tissue in these cases to the placement of calcium hydroxide deep into the canals.

Cotti *et al.* reported a case of a child with traumatized immature necrotic permanent maxillary incisor with a sinus tract (Cotti *et al.* 2008). Upon entry, necrotic tissue was debrided from the canal with a spoon excavator, irrigated with sodium hypochlorite, and filled with calcium hydroxide. After 15 days, the sinus tract disappeared, and the calcium hydroxide was removed, bleeding was stimulated from the apex, and it was finally restored with MTA and final restoration. At the 2.5 year recall, there were radiographic signs of continual root development and dentinal wall thickening.

Jung *et al.* presented a case series of children with immature permanent teeth having necrotic pulps and apical periodontitis (Jung *et al.* 2008). In four teeth with necrotic pulps, the canals were irrigated with sodium hypochlorite, medicated with triple antibiotic paste, followed by evoking of bleeding to form a blood clot, sealed with MTA, and final restoration was placed. In five other cases where there were remnants of vital tissue inside the canal, the same protocol was followed except there was no evoking of bleeding. Apical closure, dentinal wall thickening, and increase in root lengths were observed in all of the cases.

In a case series conducted by Shah *et al.*, 14 nonvital, immature teeth with periapical periodontitis were followed up to three and a half years after attempting revitalization procedures (Shah *et al.* 2008). Teeth were accessed, irrigated (after minimal filing) with hydrogen peroxide and sodium hypochlorite, and dressed with intracanal formocresol. Subsequently, bleeding was initiated from the periapical tissue, and the tooth was restored with glass ionomer cement with no MTA. They reported no signs and/or symptoms of pathosis in 11 out of 14 cases, periapical healing in 8 out 14 cases with thickening in dentinal wall, and an increase in root length in 10 out of 14 cases.

Ding *et al.* followed 12 cases of children having necrotic, immature teeth with or without clinical signs of periapical pathology (Ding *et al.* 2009). The root canals were irrigated with sodium hypochlorite and triple antibiotic paste was used as intracanal medication. After 1 week, bleeding was induced by manipulation with endodontic file, and the teeth were restored with MTA and composite restoration. Due to unresolved symptoms at recall, six teeth required further treatment using an apexification procecure. Three patients were not available for recall. Only three remaining teeth became symptom-free, showed complete root development, and tested positively to vital pulp testing after 15 months after treatment. The authors mention that one of the reasons for failure was inability to induce bleeding after canal disinfection.

Bose *et al.* compared the degree of continual root development and dentinal wall thickening between 48 teeth that underwent revitalization procedures with 40 teeth that underwent either apexification or regular nonsurgical root canal treatment (Bose *et al.* 2009). Those that went through revitalization were necrotic, immature permanent teeth with or without evidence of periapical pathology. The canal infections were managed by triple antibiotic paste, calcium hydroxide, or formocresol. The findings from the study demonstrated that revitalization using triple antibiotic paste or calcium hydroxide produced significantly greater increases in root length than either the apexification or nonsurgical root canal treatment. They also found out that the triple antibiotic paste group resulted in greater dentinal wall thickness than the calcium hydroxide group. The authors concluded that when calcium hydroxide is used as an intracanal dressing as part of the revitalization procedure, it is best to confine the medication to the coronal half of the root.

In a case report by Reynolds *et al.*, two immature mandibular premolars with necrotic pulps and chronic apical periodontitis were treated with revitalization procedures involving the use of sodium hypochlorite, saline, and chlorhexidine gluconate (Reynolds *et al.* 2009). Prior to placement of triple antibiotic paste, a bonding agent was applied to the inner surfaces of the coronal accesses to prevent crown discoloration from the use of the triple antibiotic. Bleeding was initiated from the apex and the canals were sealed with MTA and composite restoration. Within 18 months, the teeth responded normally to cold testing, were asymptomatic, had no coronal discoloration, and exhibited continual root development.

Shin *et al.* reported a case of a child with a partially necrotic and immature lower premolar with a chronic apical abscess (Shin *et al.* 2009). They performed the revitalization procedure in a single visit by irrigating the canal with sodium hypochlorite, saline, and then chlorhexidine gluconate. No instrumentation was attempted, and only the coronal half of the canal was dried and sealed with MTA. The sinus tract was also irrigated with chlorhexidine gluconate. Signs of continual root development and thickening of dentinal walls were noticed at the seven month recall period. Despite radiographic evidence of periapical healing and root wall thickening, the pulpal response remained negative at 19 months.

Mendoza and colleagues published a report of 28 necrotic immature permanent teeth in 21 children that were irrigated with sodium hypochlorite, filled with calcium hydroxide paste, and later restored with IRM and a glass ionomer restoration as part of a revitalization procedure (Mendoza *et al.* 2010). They reported signs of increase of root length and apical closure in almost 85 percent of their cases as well as formation of cementoid tissue in approximately 15% of these cases over the period of 2 years.

Petrino *et al.* presented a series of cases consisting of six necrotic immature teeth in three children with either apical periodontitis or chronic apical abscess

(Petrino *et al.* 2010). The protocol involved the use of sodium hypochlorite, saline, and chlorhexidine irrigation, before the placement of triple antibiotic paste. After 3 weeks, bleeding was induced and then the canals were sealed with MTA and composite restoration. After follow-up of 1 year, all the teeth showed resolution of periapical pathosis, three teeth showed continual root development, and two teeth demonstrated evidence of regained vitality.

Thomson and Kahler reported a similar case of a child with necrotic immature mandibular premolar with chronic apical abscess (Thomson & Kahler 2010). A decision was made to perform a revitalization procedure in which they irrigated the canals with sodium hypochlorite without instrumentation and placed a triple antibiotic paste into the canal for 2 appointments due to unresolved signs and symptoms. After 6 weeks when the patient become asymptomatic, the canal was irrigated with sodium hypochlorite, bleeding was induced, and then the canal was restored with MTA, glass ionomer, and composite. The tooth responded normally to vitality testing and showed signs of continual root development after the 18-month follow-up period.

Nosrat *et al.* presented two cases of children with necrotic immature lower molars with apical periodontitis and chronic apical abscess (Nosrat *et al.* 2011). The canals were managed similarly as in previous reports, in which they irrigated the canals with sodium hypochlorite and then dressed with triple antibiotic paste. After 3 weeks, bleeding was induced and then sealed with calcium enriched mixture (CEM) and amalgam restoration. Both teeth showed continued root development despite negative pulpal response to vitality testing after 15 to 18 months.

In a case series by Cehreli *et al.*, six immature molars that had a nonvital pulp and chronic periodontitis affecting at least one of the roots underwent treatment with revitalization. (Cehreli *et al.* 2011). Four of the molars had previously been instrumented. The orifices were initially irrigated with sodium hypochlorite followed by calcium hydroxide dressing as a first step. After 3 weeks, the canals were irrigated with sodium hypochlorite, bleeding was initiated, and the orifices were restored with MTA and glass ionomer. Final restoration was completed 3 weeks later. After 10 months, all of the teeth were asymptomatic, showed radiographic signs of dentinal thickening, and either complete or advanced apical closure. Two instrumented teeth responded to vitality tests.

Chen *et al.* reported a case series of 20 necrotic immature teeth with either apical periodontitis or abscess (Chen *et al.* 2011). The protocol involved irrigation of the canals with sodium hypochlorite with minimal intracanal instrumentation, followed by calcium hydroxide as an intracanal medicament. After resolution of clinical signs and symptoms, bleeding was initiated and MTA was placed followed by composite restoration. After a recall rate of 6 to 26 months, all of the teeth showed resolution of periapical pathosis, along with dentinal wall thickening, continuation of root development, pulp canal obliteration, calcific barrier under the MTA, and/or apical closure.

Jung *et al*. reported on two immature mandibular second premolars with infected pulps and periapical radiolucencies (Jung *et al*. 2011), The first case was treated with Vitapex for an apexification procedure and whereas the second case was treated with revitalization. A root tip separated from the main root was observed in the second case. For the revitalization procedure, the canal was irrigated with 2.5% NaOCl and then filled with a triple antibiotic paste for 2 weeks. The patient returned and the triple antibiotic paste was rinsed with 2.5% NaOCl, bleeding was induced, MTA was placed in the access, and a composite restoration was placed 2 weeks later. At a 31-month follow up, complete resolution of the periapical radiolucency was observed but the main root did not gain thickness or length. However, an interesting finding in this case was that the separated apical third of the root displayed continued dentinal wall thickening and apical closure.

Kim *et al*. reported on three cases of necrotic teeth which had undergone a revitalization procedure (Kim *et al*. 2012). Three percent NaOCl was used to disinfect the canal and dried with paper points. A triple antibiotic mixture of ciprofloxacin, metronidazole, and cefaclor was placed in the canal for 2 weeks with a cavit filling the access. The antibiotics mixture was removed with 3% NaOCl and saline, bleeding was induced with a K file, MTA placed, then a gutta-percha and composite restoration placed above the set MTA. After a 2-year follow-up periapical healing, an increase in both wall and root length, and complete apical closure was observed. The second and third cases used the same revitalization treatment and after a 4-year follow-up, complete periapical healing and an increase in root thickness was observed in both teeth.

Aggarwal *et al*. compared calcium hydroxide apexification and revitalization procedures on two necrotic teeth in the same patient (Aggarwal *et al*. 2012). The right central incisor was treated with apexification. The left maxillary central was treated with a revitalization procedure which consisted of irrigation with 5.25% NaOCl, saline, and 2% chlorhexidine with minimal instrumentation. The subsequent appointments consisted of placement of triple antibiotic for 1 week followed by removal of antibiotic, induction of bleeding, MTA placement, and a final composite restoration. After 2 years, the revitalization tooth showed complete periapical healing and an increase in both root wall and length. In comparison, the right central incisor showed no change in root length or thickness.

Miller *et al*. reported on a case of an avulsed central incisor that underwent revitalization procedures after eight weeks post-re-plantation (Miller *et al*. 2012). Upon access, the apical third of the canal was found to contain vital tissue. The tooth was disinfected with 2% chlorhexidine and EDTA was used as a final rinse. After drying the canal with paper points, a triple antibiotic paste was placed into the canal and temporized with glass ionomer. After 6 weeks, the triple antibiotic paste was removed with 2% chlorhexidine and 17% EDTA, dried with paper points, and bleeding was induced. Above the established blood clot, MTA was placed followed by glass ionomer and a final restoration with

Geristore. At the 18-month follow-up, the patient was asymptomatic, the tooth responded to CO_2 ice, apical closure, and root development was observed.

Lenzi and Trope reported on the treatment of two traumatized immature central incisors (Lenzi & Trope 2012). Both canals were irrigated with 2.5% sodium hypochlorite followed by intracanal medicament with a triple antibiotic solution. The canals were dried with paper points and a thicker mix of the same triple antibiotic paste was placed into the canals with a lentulo spiral filler and glass ionomer placed as a temporary restoration. After 35 days, the canals were irrigated with sterile saline and a blood clot was provoked by over instrumentation. MTA and a composite restoration was placed as a final restoration. At 21 months, the investigators observed thickening of dentinal walls, apical closure, and resolution of the periapical radiolucency on the upper right incisor. However, the upper left incisor exhibited a lack of dentinal thickening and presence of apical healing and hard tissue barrier after 21 months.

Cehreli *et al.* presented a case with two avulsed central incisors that underwent revitalization therapy (Cehreli *et al.* 2012). One week after replantation, calcium hydroxide was placed as an intracanal mediation. After 3 weeks, apical bleeding was provoked and MTA was placed over the clot. At 18 months, the teeth responded positively to cold test and showed increased root length and width.

Torabinejad and Turman presented a case of a child with a maxillary second premolar with necrotic pulp and an open apex (Torabinejad & Turman 2011). The pulp ultimately became necrotic with concomitant development of symptomatic apical periodontitis (Fig. 6.6). The canal was accessed, irrigated with sodium hypochlorite, and treated with triple antibiotic paste. After three weeks, PRP was processed from the patient's own blood and was injected into the canal space. The canal was then sealed with MTA, Cavit, and an amalgam restoration. After five and a half months there was radiographic evidence of resolution of the periapical lesion, continual root development, and canal wall thickening. Clinically, the tooth responded positively to vitality testing. The authors suggested that PRP can be an ideal scaffold for revitalization procedures. Despite apparently successful revitalization of the pulp space, the patient complained that the tooth had become sensitive, and therefore root canal treatment was performed. The previously revitalization tissue was removed and was processed for histological evaluation. Examination of the recovered tissue revealed presence of vital connective tissue similar to that of a normal dental pulp (Fig. 6.6E). This is the first indication in the dental literature that pulp tissue may be regenerated in a human tooth with the use of PRP.

These clinical cases of revitalization demonstrate that continued hard tissue deposition inside the canals of previously infected and necrotic human teeth can occur under certain conditions. These clinical cases also represent the lack of standardization of revitalization procedures. A variety of scaffolds, medicaments,

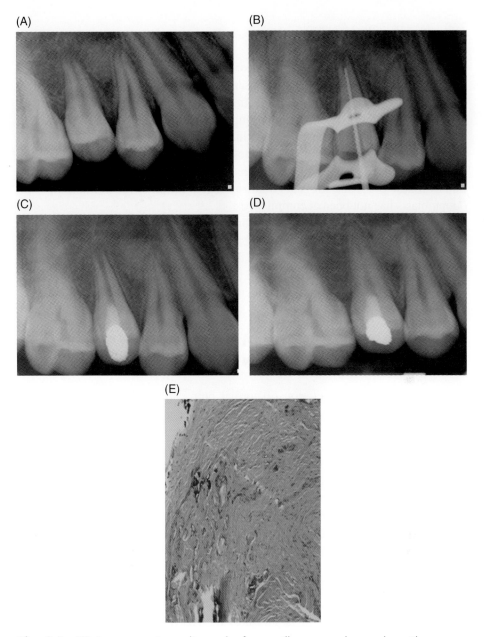

Fig. 6.6 (A) A preoperative radiograph of a maxillary second premolar with an open apex, necrotic pulp, and a periapical lesion. (B) After making an access cavity into the root canal of this tooth, its canal was cleaned and disinfected using triple antibiotics. (C) Three weeks later, PRP was placed inside the canal, which was sealed with a layer of MTA and Cavit. A week later, a permanent filling was placed in the access cavity. (D) A radiograph taken 15 months later shows resolution of the periapical lesion and thickening of the root canal walls. The tooth was sensitive to both cold and electricity. Because of its sensitivity, a root canal was performed on this tooth. (E) Examination of the content of the canal shows presence of connective tissue without any inflammation.

debridement techniques, and final restorations are used. These techniques will continue to develop over time. More research must be done in order to determine the best possible combination of treatments in order to produce consistently favorable results. Currently, there is limited evidence from humans to describe what events are in fact occurring at the histological level under these conditions. In order to definitively establish the type of tissues that have revitalized the pulp space, more histological evidence is needed using current techniques. The limited available evidence suggests that true regeneration of the dental pulp with odontoblasts has not been accomplished.

Three components have been mentioned in the literature to contribute to the success of this procedure (Hargreaves *et al.* 2007). They include stem cells that are capable of hard tissue formation, a three-dimensional physical scaffold that can support differentiation and growth of cells and finally signaling molecules for cellular stimulation, proliferation, and differentiation.

POTENTIAL ROLE OF STEM CELLS IN CANAL TISSUE GENERATION AND REGENERATION

The possibility for regeneration of normal pulp capable of dentin production requires the potential for undifferentiated cells to generate new odontoblasts. The presence of human dental pulp stem cells (DPSCs) was reported by Gronthos *et al.* (2000). DPSCs are a subpopulation of mesenchymal stem cells (MSCs) and they behave differently from the best known MSCs from bone marrow, normally termed bone marrow-derived MSCs (BMMSCs) or BM-derived stromal cells (BMSCs). DPSCs and BMMSCs have different gene expression profiles and differentiation potentials. When mixed with hydroxyapaptite/tricalcium phosphate and transplanted into an *in vivo* environment, BMMSCs form ectopic ossicles containing bone trabeculae and marrow, whereas DPSCs form a pulp/dentin complex and do not form marrow tissues (Huang *et al.* 2009).

DPSCs cells have subsequently been shown to be associated with the microvasculature of the pulp tissue (Shi & Gronthos 2003). Immunoselection procedures have allowed for isolation of DPSCs for investigation (Gronthos *et al.* 2002). Gronthos *et al.* isolated DPSCs and transplanted them into the subcutaneous tissues of immunocompromised mice (Gronthos *et al.* 2002). They found that the regenerated connective tissue formed was a dentin-pulp-like structure, providing evidence that stem cells are present in the pulps and are capable of differentiation. After recovering the transplants three months postoperatively, they found that 15% of the cells were of host origin, demonstrating the self-renewal capacity of the donor stem cells.

Similar findings have been reported in other investigations. Batouli *et al.* isolated human DPSCs and transplanted the cells, with or without associated dentin from the host tooth, into the subcutaneous tissues of mice (Batouli *et al.* 2003). The DPSCs differentiated into odontoblasts at four weeks and generated hard tissue identified as dentin by immunohistochemical staining. Eight weeks post-transplant, a dentin–pulp complex was observed, with pulp-like tissue containing connective tissue, blood vessels, and odontoblasts associated with the newly formed dentin. Reparative dentin was found on the transplanted dentin. A mature dentin–pulp complex was observed at 16 weeks. The authors concluded that DPSCs are not only capable of differentiation into odontoblasts, but that they also have the potential to recruit other host cells to form the pulp-like complex.

Huang and colleagues studied DPSCs *in vitro*, and confirmed that the stem cells in contact with a dentin surface are capable of differentiating into cells of odontoblast morphology with a process extending into existing dentinal tubules (Huang *et al.* 2006; Zhao *et al.* 2007). They theorized that acid treatment of dentin may solubilize various noncollagenous matrix components and growth factors which might have an inductive effect on the differentiation of odontoblast progenitor cells.

Another type of human stem cells similar to DPSCs was discovered and reported by Sonoyama *et al.*, termed stem cells from the apical papilla (SCAP). These stem cells reside in the apical papilla, which is located at the apical end of the developing roots (Sonoyama *et al.* 2006, 2008). Stem cells from the apical papilla are slightly different from DPSCs in several ways: (i) SCAP express CD24 and survivin (while DPSCs do not), and (ii) SCAP have greater population doubling, telomerase activities, migration ability, a higher proliferation rate and dentin regeneration capacities in comparison to DPSCs (Sonoyama *et al.* 2006). Based on these features, SCAP are considered to be more immature type of stem cells than DPSCs and are likely to be responsible for giving rise to root odontoblasts and, therefore, the formation of root.

Subsequently, Huang and colleagues demonstrated the *de novo* regeneration of pulp in an emptied root canal space using SCAP and DPSCs (Huang *et al.* 2010a). They not only showed that pulp tissue can be regenerated, but also that the deposition of newly formed dentin-like mineral tissue on the root canal walls does occur. This finding suggests that these DPSCs and SCAP are capable of reconstituting lost pulp tissue and can differentiate into odontoblast-like cells to form new dentin against the existing dentin walls.

Role of DPSCs and SCAP in revitalization and regenerative endodontic treatments

The aforementioned studies demonstrate that the presence of stem cells in the pulp and apical papilla are capable of self-renewal (with the potential to differentiate into odontoblasts). It logically follows that if enough DPSCs and/or

SCAP are able to survive after infection and if these cells can be preserved during the treatment of that infection, that in sufficient numbers they might be capable of contributing to the regeneration of a functional pulp tissue capable of dentin deposition and completion of root formation.

Lin and colleagues demonstrated that portions of vital pulp with structurally intact and functioning tissue may persist in the presence of apical periodontitis (Lin *et al.* 1984). The investigators extirpated and histologically examined the pulps from teeth demonstrating periapical radiolucencies and found that many of the teeth showed normal, healthy pulp remaining in the apical region. It is possible that the presence of this remaining pulp tissue might have the potential to repopulate the pulp space with normal pulp tissue (Huang *et al.* 2008).

Lovelace *et al.* compared the amount of stem cells from pulpal origin with the amount in the systemic blood of humans (Lovelace *et al.* 2011). They collected samples of blood after being stimulated from the periapical tissues of necrotic immature teeth and examined MSC markers (CD73, CD105, and STRO-1) by means of molecular techniques and compared them to samples from the systemic circulation. It was found that there were 600 times more stem cell markers from periapical samples than from systemic circulation. The pitfall of this finding is two-fold. First, there are no specific stem cell markers for different MSCs such as BMMSCs vs. DPSCs/SCAP. SCAP may have a somewhat unique marker, such as CD24, which is not expressed by DPSCs or BMMSCs (Sonoyama *et al.* 2006). Therefore, detection of the cell surface MSC markers does not mean they are DPSCs or SCAP. Expression of DPSC markers are also nonspecific as it may be expressed by osteoblastic cells. Second, the collected blood sample from the canal obviously should contain more MSCs than that from the systemic blood. Over-instrumentation 3–5 mm beyond the apex for collection of blood could easily breakdown periapical tissues that contain osteoblastic cells and MSCs located on blood vessels, which are then to be collected in the blood via root canals. Therefore, detecting those cells expressing CD105, CD73, and STRO-1 should have been anticipated. On the other hand, it is known that BMMSCs are rarely detected in systemic blood (Kuznetsov *et al.* 2007).

Whether we can anticipate pulp regeneration appears to be dependent upon the presence of survived pulp and apical papilla tissues after the disinfection of the immature teeth. For cases that have completely lost pulp and apical papilla to infection, it is unlikely that pulp would be regenerated. At best, periodontal tissues including cementum, bone, and PDL in the canal (Figs 6.7 and 6.8) may be regenerated (Huang *et al.* 2008; Huang 2009). On the other hand, if pulp and apical papilla have survived, revitalization/regenerative procedures may be able to promote regeneration of the entire pulp and the deposition of new dentin on the canal walls.

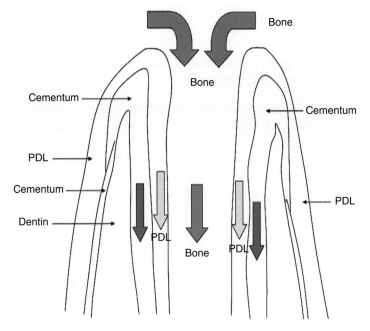

Fig. 6.7 In-growth of periodontal tissue into pulp space, including bone, PDL, and cementum.

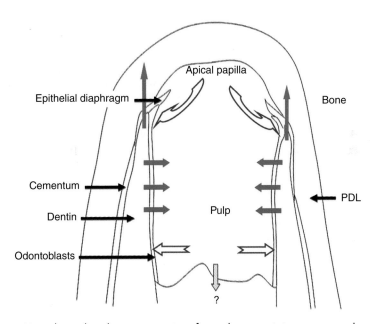

Fig. 6.8 Hypothetical pulp regeneration from the remaining recovered pulp. The question mark indicates that the regeneration of pulp into the empty pulp space is uncertain at present.

Scaffolds and growth factors for regenerative endodontics (Revitalization)

There is evidence showing that what remains in the canal affects the revitalization. The absence of a scaffold does not appear to promote revitalization. England and Best extirpated the pulps of 40 immature teeth in dogs, leaving half of them open and the other half closed with Cavit (England & Best 1977). The authors reported a high incidence of apical closure, observed as apparent cementum deposition at the apex. It did not appear, however, that the pulp space had revitalized, or that there was evidence of continued root thickening.

Ostby (1961) suggested blood as a matrix for revitalization. Myers and Fountain reported in their study that the blood clot was not resorbed, but instead appeared to serve as a matrix for the in-growth of tissue (Myers & Fountain 1974). Thibodeau *et al.* reported that the inclusion of blood as a matrix material was better than no matrix or a collagen matrix (Thibodeau *et al.* 2007). Chang *et al.* determined *in vitro* that collagen is not a favorable medium for regeneration due to contraction (Chang *et al.* 1998).

Platelet-rich plasma (PRP) is an autologous blood source that contains more than 3.5 times the platelets normally found in a regular blood sample (Lindeboom *et al.* 2007). These platelets are considered to be a source of a vast amount of certain growth factors that improve and increase wound healing through various mechanisms. These growth factors include platelet-derived growth factor (PDGF), transforming growth factor (TGF), vascular endothelial growth factor (VEGF), fibroblast growth factor (FGF), osteonectin and osteocalcin, and interleukin-1 (IL-1) (Loe 1967; Broughton *et al.* 2006; Graziani *et al.* 2006). PDGF has been shown to accelerate deposition of wound matrix, promote chemotaxis of PMNs, macrophages, fibroblasts, and smooth muscle cells, and enhance angiogenesis (Senior *et al.* 1983; Graziani *et al.* 2006). TGF is involved in promoting chemotaxis of macrophages and fibroblasts, accelerating deposition and maturation of collagen, angiogenesis, and inhibition of collagen degradation (Marx *et al.* 1998; Graziani *et al.* 2006). VEGF has a leading role in angiogenesis and vasculogenesis (Knighton *et al.* 1983; Graziani *et al.* 2006).

PRP is prepared by withdrawing a venous blood sample. The amount varies between different manufacturers. The withdrawn blood has to come in contact with an anti-coagulant agent that contains citrate and dextrose which binds to the blood calcium to prevent clotting before the PRP is prepared. The whole sample is centrifuged in order to separate the blood into components by means of gradient densities. The resultant centrifuged blood sample will have three fractions: the red blood cell (RBC) layer (containing RBC), the PRP layer, and the PPP layer (platelet-poor plasma). The PRP layer contains the highest amount of platelets, which will be withdrawn separately and mixed with coagulant agent, such as calcium chloride thrombin solution, leading to the formation of a gel-like solution that is ready to be used for various surgical procedures (Harnack *et al.* 2009; Rutkowski *et al.* 2010).

PRP has been used in different dental procedures such as oral surgery and periodontal soft tissue procedures (Marx *et al.* 1998; Anitua 2001; Camargo *et al.* 2002, 2005; Kim *et al.* 2002; Lekovic *et al.* 2002; Nikolidakis & Jansen 2008). In regards to postoperative complications and bone healing following third molar extractions, Rutkowski *et al.* showed that when PRP is applied on extraction sites, early and significant radiographic increase of bone density is observed when compared with extraction sites that have not been treated with PRP (Rutkowski *et al.* 2010). Furthermore, PRP has been shown to enhance osteogenesis in bone grafts and has decreased post-operative bone resorption in alveolar cleft patients receiving iliac bone grafting when assessed by computed tomography scan (Oyama *et al.* 2004). The accelerated bone regenerative effect was also shown by Marx *et al.* (1998).

Mechanisms by which PRP may enhance soft tissue healing include: stimulation of granulation tissue, decrease of inflammation, increase collagen content, and increase early wound strength (Pierce *et al.* 1992; Bashutski & Wang 2008). While assessing the microvascular capillary densities of the mucosa after sinus lift surgeries in 10 patients, Lindeboom *et al.* reported a significant accelerated effect of PRP-treated mucosal wounds during the first 10 postoperative days compared to those that had not been treated with PRP (Lindeboom *et al.* 2007). Other studies have found similar accelerated results of wound healing when different growth factors were examined (Pierce *et al.* 1988; Wieman *et al.* 1998; Smiell *et al.* 1999).

Zhu and associates used PRP and DPSCs for pulp revitalization in a dog study model. They found that PRP alone or DPSCs plus PRP do not appear to help regenerate dental pulp in mature or immature permanent teeth (Zhu *et al* 2012, 2013). Instead, only cementum-like, periodontal-like and bone tissues were formed in the canal space (Fig. 6.9). It is not clear why PRP does not enhance pulp regeneration when mixed with DPSCs. Because DPSCs alone did not produce pulp regeneration in these studies, the effect of PRP cannot be clearly defined.

Platelet-rich fibrin (PRF), a second-generation platelet concentrate, is prepared by centrifuging blood without any addition of chemical agents. PRF does not use anticoagulants, bovine thrombin, calcium chloride, or other exogenous activators in the preparation process (unlike PRP). Therefore, the chair-side preparation of PRF is simple, fast, and easy compared to PRP preparation. PRF produces an inexpensive autologous fibrin membrane and can be used as a fibrin bandage that serves as a matrix to accelerate the healing of wounds while PRP is a gel-like substance (Dohan *et al.* 2006).

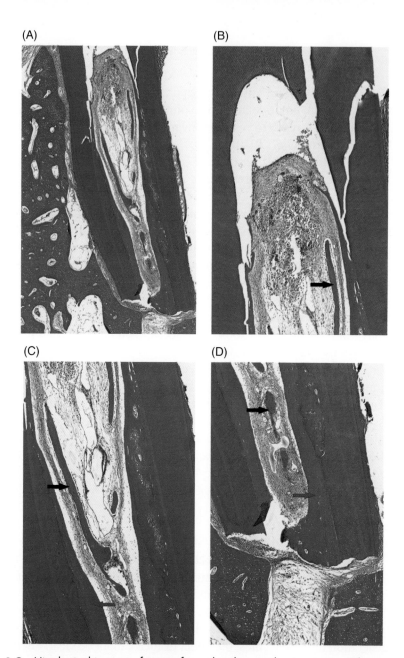

Fig. 6.9 Histological images of tissues formed in the canal space in vivo. The root canals of dog teeth were infected and disinfected followed by transplantation of dental pulp cells plus platelet-rich plasma. At 90 days, the animals were euthanized and the teeth processed for histological analysis. (A) Longitudinal section of a tooth showing the pulp space filled with vital tissues. (B) Closer view of the coronal third of the canal space showing vascular fibrous tissue with some inflammatory infiltrates. Ingrown bone trabeculae-like tissue (arrow) in the pulp space and a layer of cementum-like tissue along the canal wall can be seen. (C) Magnified view of the middle third of the canal space showing bone-like tissue (black arrow) and cementum-like tissue on the canal wall (blue arrow). (D) Magnified view of apical third of the canal showing bone-like islands (black arrow) and a thick layer of cementum-like tissue (blue arrow) containing cells in it. (Adapted from Zhu *et al.* 2013 with permission.)

PRP undergoes a more rapid artificial clinical polymerization while PRF undergoes slow polymerization with the natural thrombin found in the blood sample. This slow polymerization produces a three-dimensional fibrin architecture, very similar to the natural fibrin matrix, leading to more efficient cell migration and proliferation. The difference in polymerization modes affects the structure and biological properties of each substance. There are two different architectures that fibrin can be assembled as: bilateral or equilateral junctions. Bilateral junctions are formed with strong thrombin concentrations such as those used in PRP formation. This leads to thickening of fibrin polymers, which is not favorable to cytokine enmeshment and cellular migration. Weak thrombin concentrations in PRF form equilateral junctions, which cause a fine network that allows cytokine enmeshment, cellular migration, and greater elasticity while still maintaining strength. Therefore, the PRF membrane has a more favorable physiologic architecture to support healing. The PRF preparation process creates a matrix that contains high concentrations of nonactivated, functional, intact platelets, contained within a fibrin matrix, that release a constant concentration of growth factors over a period of seven days (Carroll *et al.* 2005). PRF consists of cytokines, glycanic chains, and structural glycoproteins enmeshed within a slowly polymerized fibrin network (Pradeep *et al.* 2012).

Beneficial effects of PRF have been studied in various procedures, such as facial plastic surgery, sinus-lift procedures, and periodontal defects. It also serves as a suitable scaffold for breeding human periosteal cells *in vitro* (Pradeep *et al.* 2012). However, more studies are needed to fully understand the components of this material.

The limitations of the PRF technique, as compared to other methods for obtaining platelet concentrates, is that quick handling of the blood through immediate centrifugation is the key to obtaining a usable PRF clot. If the duration between blood collection and centrifugation is too long, failure will occur through diffuse polymerization. PRF must be used immediately after blood drawing and centrifugation, while PRP can be activated on demand a few minutes before use (Pradeep *et al.* 2012).

Huang *et al.* (2010b) published a study examining the biological effects of PRF on dental pulp cells (DPCs). PRF samples were obtained from six healthy volunteers and human DPCs were derived from healthy individuals undergoing extraction for third molars. Cell proliferation, the expression of osteoprotegerin (OPG), and alkaline phosphatase (ALP) activity were examined. This study found that PRF did not interfere with the cell viability of DPCs and were observed to attach at the edges of PRF by phase-contrast microscopy. PRF was found to increase DPC proliferation, OPG expression and up-regulate ALP activity significantly. These findings show that PRF may be a potential bioactive scaffold to use in pulp regeneration.

Research has shown that immature stem cells such as DPSCs require growth factors to be able to differentiate (Friedlander *et al.* 2009). Such growth factors that are capable of inducing signals (like PDGF and TGF) can be found in PRP (Graziani *et al.* 2006). Kim and associates have discussed the efficacy of cytokines such as PDGF, VEGF, bFGF, and BMP in attracting pulpal cells into teeth filled with these types of cytokines (Kim *et al.* 2010). After pulpal debridement and delivery of cytokines into extracted human teeth, the samples were embedded into mice dorsa and left alone for 3 weeks. The use of these growth factors resulted in the attraction of stem cells leading to formation of new pulp-like tissue inside the teeth. The potential for pulpal regeneration has been demonstrated through the application of PDGF and IGF, which promoted the differentiation of immature stem cells into pulp tissue phenotypes (Howell *et al.* 1997; Denholm *et al.* 1998).

CLINICAL PROCEDURES FOR PULP REVITALIZATION

The following are modified clinical procedures for pulp revitalization recommended by the American Association of Endodontists.

First appointment

After administration of local anesthetic and placement of rubber dam, an access cavity should be prepared in the affected tooth. Gently but thoroughly irrigate the canal(s) with copious amounts of 1.5% NaOCl using an irrigation system that minimizes the possibility of extrusion of irrigants into the periapical tissues. Dry the canal(s) and place either antibiotic paste or calcium hydroxide to disinfect the root canal system. If you decide to use the triple antibiotic paste, consider sealing the pulp chamber with a dentin bonding agent to reduce the risk of staining. If you plan to use the triple antibiotic paste, mix 1:1:1 ciprofloxacin:metronidazole:minocycline in a lower concentration (0.01–0.1 mg/mL) to reduce toxicity. Place the triple antibiotic paste into the canal system using a lentulo spiral, MAP system, or syringe and ensure the paste remains below the cemenol enamel junction (CEJ) to minimize crown staining. Seal the access cavity with 3–4 mm of Cavit followed by glass ionomer cement (Fig. 6.10A–C).

Second appointment

Evaluate the response of your initial treatment 3–4 weeks later. If there are signs of persistent infection, consider additional antimicrobial treatment with the same antibacterial material or disinfect the canal(s) with an alternative antimicrobial

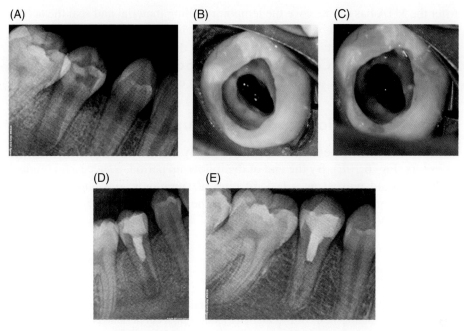

Fig. 6.10 (A) A preoperative radiograph of a mandibular second premolar with an open apex, necrotic pulp, and a periapical lesion. (B) An access cavity is made into the root canal of this tooth, which contains a necrotic pulp. (C) After cleaning and disinfecting the canal, bleeding is generated inside the canal. (D) A layer of MTA is placed over the blood clot. (E) A radiograph taken 15 months later shows resolution of the periapical lesion and thickening of the root canal walls. Courtesy of Dr Debby Knaup.

agent and see the patient again in an additional 3–4 weeks. If there are no signs or symptoms of persistent infection, continue with the second phase of the revascularization procedure.

After administration of 3% mepivacaine without vasoconstrictor (to allow for better induction of apical bleeding), place the dental dam and remove the temporary filling materials. Irrigate the canal(s) with copious amounts of 1.5% NaOCl followed by 20 ml of 17% EDTA. A final rinse with normal saline is done using an irrigation system that minimizes the possibility of extrusion of irrigants into the periapical tissues. Dry the canal(s) with paper points. Create bleeding in the canal(s) by over-instrumenting with endodontic files (#10–15). Keep the level of bleeding 3 mm from the CEJ. Allow the blood to clot for 10 minutes. Alternatively, a scaffold of PRP or PRF can be placed in the canal(s). Some clinicians suggest placing a CollaPlug/Collacote over the scaffold to control the level of MTA. After placing 3–4 mm of MTA, apply a wet cotton pellet to encourage complete setting of the MTA and then place your temporary filling material (Fig. 6.10D).

After the MTA has set, remove the temporary filling material and seal the access cavity with a definitive restorative material such as composite. An alternative procedure is to place reinforced glass ionomer directly over MTA and place a permanent restoration. Consider sealing the pulp chamber with a dentin bonding agent to reduce the risk of staining with MTA in esthetic areas.

Clinical and radiographic follow-up

The patient should be examined postoperatively every 3–6 months for at least 1–2 years (Fig. 6.10E). By the end of the follow-up period, a successful clinical outcome would present as a lack of clinical symptoms, resolution of apical lesions radiographically, and thickening of the root canal walls with extended root length. (Video).

REFERENCES

Aggarwal, V., Miglani, S., Singla, M. (2012) Conventional apexification and revascularization induced maturogenesis of two non-vital, immature teeth in same patient: 24 months follow up of a case. *Journal of Conservation Dentistry* **15**(1), 68–72.

Alsousou, J., Thompson, M., Hulley, P., *et al.* (2009) The biology of platelet-rich plasma and its application in trauma and orthopaedic surgery: a review of the literature. *Journal of Bone and Joint Surgery of Britain* **91**(8), 987–96.

American Association of Endodontists. Considerations for Regenerative Procedures. Available at: http://www.aae.org/uploadedfiles/clinical_resources/regenerative_endodontics/considerationsregendo7-31-13.pdf

Andreasen, J.O., Borum, M.K., Jacobsen, H.L., *et al.* (1995) Replantation of 400 avulsed permanent incisors. 2. Factors related to pulpal healing. *Endodontics and Dental Traumatology* **11**(2), 59–68.

Anitua, E. (2011) The use of plasma-rich growth factors (PRGF) in oral surgery. Practical Procedures in Aesthetic Dentistry **13**(6), 487–93; quiz 487–93.

Banchs, F., Trope, M. (2004) Revascularization of immature permanent teeth with apical periodontitis: new treatment protocol? *Journal of Endodontics* **30**(4), 196–200.

Barrett, A.P., Reade, P.C. (1981) Revascularization of mouse tooth isografts and allografts using autoradiography and carbon-perfusion. *Archives of Oral Biology* **26**(7), 541–5.

Bashutski, J.D., Wang, H.L. (2008) Role of platelet-rich plasma in soft tissue root-coverage procedures: a review. *Quintessence International* **39**(6), 473–83.

Batouli, S., Miura, M., Brahim, J., *et al.* Comparison of stem-cell-mediated osteogenesis and dentinogenesis. *Journal of Dental Research* **82**(12), 976–81.

Bauss, O., Schilke, R., Fenske, C., *et al.* (2002) Autotransplantation of immature third molars: influence of different splinting methods and fixation periods. *Dental Traumatology* **18**(6), 322–8.

Bose, R., Nummikoski, P., Hargreaves, K. (2009) A retrospective evaluation of radiographic outcomes in immature teeth with necrotic root canal systems treated with regenerative endodontic procedures. *Journal of Endodontics* **35**(10), 1343–9.

Broughton, G., 2nd, Janis, J.E., Attinger, C.E. (2006) Wound healing: an overview. *Plastic and Reconstructive Surgery* **117**(7 Suppl), 1e-S–32e-S.

Buhrley, M.R., Corr, R., Shabahang, S., *et al.* (2011) Identification of tissues formed after pulp revascularization in a Ferret model. *Journal of Endodontics* **37**(3), 29.

Camargo, P.M., Lekovic, V., Weinlaender, M., *et al.* (2002) Platelet-rich plasma and bovine porous bone mineral combined with guided tissue regeneration in the treatment of intrabony defects in humans. *Journal of Periodontal Research* **37**(4), 300–6.

Camargo, P.M., Lekovic, V., Weinlaender, M., (2005) A reentry study on the use of bovine porous bone mineral, GTR, and platelet-rich plasma in the regenerative treatment of intrabony defects in humans. *International Journal of Periodontics and Restorative Dentistry* **25**(1), 49–59.

Carroll, R., Amoczky, S., Graham, S., *et al.* (2005) *Characterization of Autologous Growth Factors in Cascade Platelet Rich Fibrin Matrix (PRFM).* Musculoskeletal Transplant Foundation, Edison, NJ.

Cehreli, Z.C., Isbitiren, B., Sara, S., *et al.* (2011) Regenerative endodontic treatment (revascularization) of immature necrotic molars medicated with calcium hydroxide: a case series. *Journal of Endodontics* **37**(9), 1327–30.

Cehreli, Z.C., Sara, S., Aksoy, B. (2012) Revascularization of immature permanent incisors after severe extrusive luxation injury. *Journal of the Canadian Dental Association* **78**, c4.

Chang, M.C., Lin, C.P., Huang, T.F., *et al.* (1998) Thrombin-induced DNA synthesis of cultured human dental pulp cells is dependent on its proteolytic activity and modulated by prostaglandin E2. *Journal of Endodontics* **24**(11), 709–13.

Chen, M.Y., Chen, K.L., Chen, C.A., *et al.* (2012) Responses of immature permanent teeth with infected necrotic pulp tissue and apical periodontitis/abscess to revascularization procedures. *International Endodontics Journal* **45**(3), 294–305.

Chen, X., Bao, Z.F., Liu, Y., *et al.* (2013) Regenerative endodontic treatment of an immature permanent tooth at an early stage of root development: a case report. *Journal of Endodontics* **39**(5), 719–22.

Chueh, L.H., Huang, G.T. (2006) Immature teeth with periradicular periodontitis or abscess undergoing apexogenesis: a paradigm shift. *Journal of Endodontics* **32**(12), 1205–13.

Cotti, E., Mereu, M., Lusso, D. (2008) Regenerative treatment of an immature, traumatized tooth with apical periodontitis: report of a case. *Journal of Endodontics* **34**(5), 611–16.

Cvek, M., Cleaton-Jones, P., Austin, J., *et al.* (1990a) Effect of topical application of doxycycline on pulp revascularization and periodontal healing in reimplanted monkey incisors. *Endodontics and Dental Traumatology* **6**(4), 170–6.

Cvek, M., Cleaton-Jones, P., Austin, J., *et al.* (1990b) Pulp revascularization in reimplanted immature monkey incisors– predictability and the effect of antibiotic systemic prophylaxis. *Endodontics and Dental Traumatology* **6**(4), 157–69.

da Silva, L.A., Nelson-Filho, P., da Silva, R.A., *et al.* (2010) Revascularization and periapical repair after endodontic treatment using apical negative pressure irrigation versus conventional irrigation plus triantibiotic intracanal dressing in dogs' teeth with apical periodontitis. *Oral surgery, Oral Medicine, Oral Pathology, Oral Radiology, and Endodontics* **109**(5), 779–87.

Das, S., Das, A.K., Murphy, R.A. (1997) Experimental apexigenesis in baboons. *Endodontics and Dental Traumatology* **13**(1), 31–5.

Denholm, I.A., Moule, A.J., Bartold, P.M. (1998) The behaviour and proliferation of human dental pulp cell strains in vitro, and their response to the application of platelet-derived growth factorBB and insulin-like growth factor-1. *International Endodontics Journal* **31**(4), 251–8.

Ding, R.Y., Cheung, G.S., Chen, J., *et al.* (2009) Pulp revascularization of immature teeth with apical periodontitis: a clinical study. *Journal of Endodontics* **35**(5), 745–9.

Dohan, D.M., Choukroun, J., Diss, A., *et al.* (2006) Platelet-rich fibrin (PRF): a second-generation platelet concentrate. Part I: technological concepts and evolution. *Oral Surgery, Oral Medicine, Oral Pathology, Oral Radiology, and Endodontics* **101**(3), e37–44.

England, M.C., Best, E. (1977) Noninduced apical closure in immature roots of dogs' teeth. *Journal of Endodontics* **3**(11), 411–17.

Friedlander, L.T., Cullinan, M.P., Love, R.M. (2009) Dental stem cells and their potential role in apexogenesis and apexification. *International Endodontics Journal* **42**(11), 955–62.

Fuss, Z. (1985) Successful self-replantation of avulsed tooth with 42-year follow-up. *Endodontics and Dental Traumatology* **1**(3), 120–2.

Goncalves, S.B., Dong, Z., Bramante, C.M., *et al.* (2007) Tooth slicebased models for the study of human dental pulp angiogenesis. *Journal of Endodontics* **33**(7), 811–14.

Graziani, F., Ivanovski, S., Cei, S., *et al.* (2006) The in vitro effect of different PRP concentrations on osteoblasts and fibroblasts. *Clinical Oral Implants Research* **17**(2), 212–19.

Gronthos, S., Brahim, J., Li, W., *et al.* Stem cell properties of human dental pulp stem cells. *Journal of Dental Research* **81**(8), 531–35.

Gronthos, S., Mankani, M., Brahim, J., *et al.* (2000) Postnatal human dental pulp stem cells (DPSCs) in vitro and in vivo. *Proceedings of the National Academy of Sciences of the U S A* **97**(25), 13625–30.

Ham, J.W., Patterson, S.S., Mitchell, D.F. (1972) Induced apical closure of immature pulpless teeth in monkeys. *Oral Surgery, Oral Medicine, Oral Pathology* **33**(3), 438–49.

Hargreaves, K.M., Giesler, T., Henry, M., *et al.* (2008) Regeneration potential of the young permanent tooth: what does the future hold? *Journal of Endodontics* **34**(7 Suppl), S51–6.

Harnack, L., Boedeker, R.H., Kurtulus, I., *et al.* (2009) Use of platelet-rich plasma in periodontal surgery – a prospective randomised double blind clinical trial. *Clinical Oral Investigations* **13**(2), 179–87.

Hiremath, H., Gada, N., Kini, Y., *et al.* (2008) Single-step apical barrier placement in immature teeth using mineral trioxide aggregate and management of periapical inflammatory lesion using platelet-rich plasma and hydroxyapatite. *Journal of Endodontics* **34**(8), 1020–4.

Howell, T.H., Fiorellini, J.P., Paquette, D.W., *et al.* (1997) A phase I/II clinical trial to evaluate a combination of recombinant human platelet-derived growth factor-BB and recombinant human insulin-like growth factor-I in patients with periodontal disease. *Journal of Periodontology* **68**(12), 1186–93.

Huang, G.T. (2009) Apexification: the beginning of its end. *International Endodontics Journal* **42**(10), 855–66.

Huang, G.T., Sonoyama, W., Chen, J., *et al.* (2006) In vitro characterization of human dental pulp cells: various isolation methods and culturing environments. *Cell and Tissue Research* **324**(2), 225–36.

Huang, G.T., Sonoyama, W., Liu, Y., *et al.* (2008) The hidden treasure in apical papilla: the potential role in pulp/dentin regeneration and bioroot engineering. *Journal of Endodontics* **34**(6), 645–51.

Huang, G.T., Gronthos, S., Shi, S. (2009) Mesenchymal stem cells derived from dental tissues vs. those from other sources: their biology and role in regenerative medicine. *Journal of Dental Research* **88**(9), 792–806.

Huang, G.T., Yamaza, T., Shea, L.D., *et al.* (2010a) Stem/progenitor cell-mediated de novo regeneration of dental pulp with newly deposited continuous layer of dentin in an in vivo model. *Tissue Engineering Part A* **16**(2), 605–15.

Huang, F.M., Yang, S.F., Zhao, J.H., *et al.* (2010b) Platelet-rich fibrin increases proliferation and differentiation of human dental pulp cells. *Journal of Endodontics* **36**(10), 1628–32.

Iwaya, S.I., Ikawa, M., Kubota, M. (2001) Revascularization of an immature permanent tooth with apical periodontitis and sinus tract. *Dental Traumatology* **17**(4), 185–7.

Jadhav, G., Shah, N., Logani, A. (2012) Revascularization with and without platelet-rich plasma in nonvital, immature, anterior teeth: a pilot clinical study. *Journal of Endodontics* **38**(12), 1581–7.

Jeeruphan, T., Jantarat, J., Yanpiset, K., *et al.* (2012) Mahidol study 1: comparison of radiographic and survival outcomes of immature teeth treated with either regenerative endodontic or apexification methods: a retrospective study. *Journal of Endodontics* **38**(10), 1330–6.

Johnson, W.T., Goodrich, J.L., James, G.A. (1985) Replantation of avulsed teeth with immature root development. *Oral Surgery, Oral Medicine, Oral Pathology* **60**(4), 420–27.

Jung, I.Y., Lee, S.J., Hargreaves, K.M. (2008) Biologically based treatment of immature permanent teeth with pulpal necrosis: a case series. *Journal of Endodontics* **34**(7), 876–87.

Jung, I.Y., Kim, E.S., Lee, C.Y., *et al.* (2011) Continued development of the root separated from the main root. *Journal of Endodontics* **37**(5), 711–14.

Kakehashi, S., Stanley, H.R., Fitzgerald, R.J. (1965) The effects of surgical exposures of dental pulps in germ-free and conventional laboratory rats. *Oral Surgery, Oral Medicine, Oral Pathology* **20**, 340–9.

Kerekes, K., Heide, S., Jacobsen, I. (1980) Follow-up examination of endodontic treatment in traumatized juvenile incisors. *Journal of Endodontics* **6**(9), 744–8.

Keswani, D., Pandey, R.K. (2013) Revascularization of an immature tooth with a necrotic pulp using platelet-rich fibrin: a case report. *International Endodontics Journal* **46**(11), 1096–104.

Kim, S.G., Kim, W.K., Park, J.C., *et al.* (2002) A comparative study of osseointegration of Avana implants in a demineralized freeze-dried bone alone or with platelet-rich plasma. *Journal of Oral and Maxillofacial Surgery* **60**(9), 1018–25.

Kim, D.S., Park, H.J., Yeom, J.H., *et al.* (2012) Long-term follow-ups of revascularizedimmature necrotic teeth: three case reports. *International Journal of Oral Science* **4**(2), 109–13.

Kim, J.Y., Xin, X., Moioli, E.K., *et al.* (2010) Regeneration of dental pulp-like tissue by chemotaxis-induced cell homing. *Tissue Engineering Part A* **16**(10), 3023–31.

Kling, M., Cvek, M., Mejare, I. (1986) Rate and predictability of pulp revascularization in therapeutically reimplanted permanent incisors. *Endodontics and Dental Traumatology* **2**(3), 83–9.

Knighton, D.R., Hunt, T.K., Scheuenstuhl, H., *et al.* (1983) Oxygen tension regulates the expression of angiogenesis factor by macrophages. *Science* **221**(4617), 1283–5.

Kuznetsov, S.A., Mankani, M.H., Leet, A.I., *et al.* (2007) Circulating connective tissue precursors: extreme rarity in humans and chondrogenic potential in guinea pigs. *Stem Cells* **25**(7), 1830–9.

Kvinnsland, I., Heyeraas, K.J. (1989) Dentin and osteodentin matrix formation in apicoectomized replanted incisors in cats. *Acta Odontologica Scandinavica* **47**(1), 41–52.

Lekovic, V., Camargo, P.M., Weinlaender, M., *et al.* (2002) Comparison of platelet-rich plasma, bovine porous bone mineral, and guided tissue regeneration versus plateletrich plasma and bovine porous bone mineral in the treatment of intrabony defects: a reentry study. *Journal of Periodontology* **73**(2), 198–205.

Lenzi, R., Trope, M. (2012) Revitalization procedures in two traumatized incisors with different biological outcomes. *Journal of Endodontics* **38**(3), 411–14.

Lin, L., Shovlin, F., Skribner, J., *et al.* (1984) Pulp biopsies from the teeth associated with periapical radiolucency. *Journal of Endodontics* **10**(9), 436–48.

Lindeboom, J.A., Mathura, K.R., Aartman, I.H., *et al.* (2007) Influence of the application of platelet-enriched plasma in oral mucosal wound healing. *Clinical Oral Implants Research* **18**(1), 133–9.

Loe, H. (1967) The Gingival Index, the Plaque Index and the Retention Index Systems. *Journal of Periodontology* **38**(6):Suppl, 610–16.

Love, R.M. (1996) Bacterial penetration of the root canal of intact incisor teeth after a simulated traumatic injury. *Endodontics and Dental Traumatology* **12**(6), 289–93.

Lovelace, T.W., Henry, M.A., Hargreaves, K.M., *et al.* (2011) Evaluation of the delivery of mesenchymal stem cells into the root canal space of necrotic immature teeth after clinical regenerative endodontic procedure. *Journal of Endodontics* **37**(2), 133–38.

Marx, R.E., Carlson, E.R., Eichstaedt, R.M., *et al.* (1998) Plateletrich plasma: Growth factor enhancement for bone grafts. *Oral Surgery, Oral Medicine, Oral Pathology, Oral Radiology, and Endodontics* **85**(6), 638–46.

Mendoza, A.M., Reina, E.S., Garcia-Godoy, F. (2010) Evolution of apical formation on immature necrotic permanent teeth. *American Journal of Dentistry* **23**(5), 269–74.

Mesaros, S.V., Trope, M. (1997) Revascularization of traumatized teeth assessed by laser Doppler flowmetry: case report. *Endodontics and Dental Traumatology* **13**(1), 24–30.

Miller, E.K., Lee, J.Y., Tawil, P.Z., *et al.* (2012) Emerging therapies for the management of traumatized immature permanent incisors. *Pediatric Dentistry* **34**(1), 66–69.

Monsour, F.N. (1971) Pulpal changes following the reimplantation of teeth in dogs: a histological study. *Australian Dental Journal* **16**(4), 227–31.

Myers, W.C., Fountain, S.B. (1974) Dental pulp regeneration aided by blood and blood substitutes after experimentally induced periapical infection. *Oral Surgery, Oral Medicine, Oral Pathology* **37**(3), 441–50.

Nevins, A.J., Finkelstein, F., Borden, B.G., *et al.* (1976) Revitalization of pulpless open apex teeth in rhesus monkeys, using collagen-calcium phosphate gel. *Journal of Endodontics* **2**(6), 159–65.

Nevins, A., Wrobel, W., Valachovic, R., *et al.* (1977) Hard tissue induction into pulpless open-apex teeth using collagen-calcium phosphate gel. *Journal of Endodontics* **3**(11), 431–3.

Nevins, A., Finkelstein, F., Laporta, R., *et al.* (1978) Induction of hard tissue into pulpless open-apex teeth using collagen-calcium phosphate gel. *Journal of Endodontics* **4**(3), 76–81.

Nikolidakis, D., Jansen, J.A. (2008) The biology of platelet-rich plasma and its application in oral surgery: literature review. *Tissue Engineering. Part B, Reviews* **14**(3), 249–58.

Nosrat, A., Seifi, A., Asgary, S. (2011) Regenerative endodontic treatment (revascularization) for necrotic immature permanent molars: a review and report of two cases with a new biomaterial. *Journal of Endodontics* **37**(4), 562–7.

Ostby, B.N. (1961) The role of the blood clot in endodontic therapy. An experimental histologic study. *Acta Odontologica Scandinavica* **19**, 324–53.

Oyama, T., Nishimoto, S., Tsugawa, T., *et al.* (2004) Efficacy of platelet-rich plasma in alveolar bone grafting. *Journal of Oral Maxillofacial Surgery* **62**(5), 555–8.

Petrino, J.A., Boda, K.K., Shambarger, S., *et al.* (2010) Challenges in regenerative endodontics: a case series. *Journal of Endodontics* **36**(3), 536–41.

Pierce, G.F., Mustoe, T.A., Senior, R.M., *et al.* (1988) In vivo incisional wound healing augmented by platelet-derived growth factor and recombinant c-sis gene homodimeric proteins. *Journal of Experimental Medicine* **167**(3), 974–87.

Pierce, G.F., Tarpley, J.E., Yanagihara, D., *et al.* (1992) Plateletderived growth factor (BB homodimer), transforming growth factor-beta 1, and basic fibroblast growth factor in dermal wound healing. *Neovessel and matrix formation and cessation of repair. American Journal of Pathology* **140**(6), 1375–88.

Pradeep, A.R., Rao, N.S., Agarwal, E., *et al.* (2012) Comparative evaluation of autologous platelet-rich fibrin and platelet-rich plasma in the treatment of 3-wall intrabony defects in chronic periodontitis: a randomized controlled clinical trial. *Journal of Periodontology* **83**(12), 1499–1507.

Reynolds, K., Johnson, J.D., Cohenca, N. (2009) Pulp revascularization of necrotic bilateral bicuspids using a modified novel technique to eliminate potential coronal discolouration: a case report. *International Endodontics Journal* **42**(1), 84–92.

Ritter, A.L., Ritter, A.V., Murrah, V., *et al.* (2004) Pulp revascularization of replanted immature dog teeth after treatment with minocycline and doxycycline assessed by laser Doppler flowmetry, radiography, and histology. *Dental Traumatology* **20**(2), 75–84.

Rule, D.C., Winter, G.B. (1966) Root growth and apical repair subsequent to pulpal necrosis in children. *British Dental Journal* **120**(12), 586–90.

Rutkowski, J.L., Johnson, D.A., Radio, N.M., *et al.* (2010) Platelet rich plasma to facilitate wound healing following tooth extraction. *Journal of Oral Implantology* **36**(1), 11–23.

Scarparo, R.K., Dondoni, L., Bottcher, D.E., *et al.* (2011) Response to intracanal medication in immature teeth with pulp necrosis: an experimental model in rat molars. *Journal of Endodontics* **37**(8), 1069–73.

Schilder, H. (1967) Filling root canals in three dimensions. *Dental Clinics of North America* Nov: 723–44.

Senior, R.M., Griffin, G.L., Huang, J.S., *et al.* (1983) Chemotactic activity of platel*et al*pha granule proteins for fibroblasts. *Journal of Cell Biology* **96**(2), 382–5.

Shah, N., Logani, A., Bhaskar, U., *et al.* (2008) Efficacy of revascularization to induce apexification/apexogensis in infected, nonvital, immature teeth: a pilot clinical study. *Journal of Endodontics* **34**(8), 919–25; Discussion 1157.

Sheppard, P.R., Burich, R.L. (1980) Effects of extra-oral exposure and multiple avulsions on revascularization of reimplanted teeth in dogs. *Journal of Dental Research* **59**(2), 140.

Shi, S., Gronthos, S. (2003) Perivascular niche of postnatal mesenchymal stem cells in human bone marrow and dental pulp. *Journal of Bone and Mineral Research* **18**(4), 696–704.

Shin, S.Y., Albert, J.S., Mortman, R.E. (2009) One step pulp revascularization treatment of an immature permanent tooth with chronic apical abscess: a case report. *International Endodontics Journal* **42**(12), 1118–26.

Skoglund, A. (1981) Vascular changes in replanted and autotransplanted apicoectomized mature teeth of dogs. *International Journal of Oral Surgery* **10**(2), 100–10.

Skoglund, A., Tronstad, L. (1981) Pulpal changes in replanted and autotransplanted immature teeth of dogs. *Journal of Endodontics* **7**(7), 309–16.

Smiell, J.M., Wieman, T.J., Steed, D.L., *et al.* (1999) Efficacy and safety of becaplermin (recombinant human platelet-derived growth factor-BB) in patients with nonhealing, lower extremity diabetic ulcers: a combined analysis of four randomized studies. *Wound Repair and Regeneration* **7**(5), 335–46.

Soares Ade, J., Lins, F.F., Nagata, J.Y, *et al.* (2013) Pulp revascularization after root canal decontamination with calcium hydroxide and 2% chlorhexidine gel. *Journal of Endodontics***39**(3), 417–20.

Sonoyama, W., Liu, Y., Fang, D., *et al.* (2006) Mesenchymal stem cell-mediated functional tooth regeneration in swine. *PLoS One* **1**, e79.

Sonoyama, W., Liu, Y., Yamaza, T., *et al.* (2008) Characterization of the apical papilla and its residing stem cells from human immature permanent teeth: a pilot study. *Journal of Endodontics* **34**(2), 166–71.

Thibodeau, B., Teixeira, F., Yamauchi, M., *et al.* (2007) Pulp revascularization of immature dog teeth with apical periodontitis. *Journal of Endodontics* **33**(6), 680–9.

Thomson, A., Kahler, B. (2010) Regenerative endodontics – biologically-based treatment for immature permanent teeth: a case report and review of the literature. *Australian Dental Journal* **55**(4), 446–52.

Torabinejad, M., Turman, M. (2011) Revitalization of tooth with necrotic pulp and open apex by using platelet-rich plasma: a case report. *Journal of Endodontics* **37**(2), 265–8.

Torabinejad, M., Anderson, P., Bader, J., *et al.* (2007) Outcomes of root canal treatment and restoration, implant-supported single crowns, fixed partial dentures, and extraction without replacement: A systematic review. *Journal of Prosthetic Dentistry* **98**(4), 285–311.

Torneck, C.D., Smith, J.S., Grindall, P. (1973) Biologic effects of endodontic procedures on developing incisor teeth. 3. Effect of debridement and disinfection procedures in the treatment of experimentally induced pulp and periapical disease. *Oral Surgery, Oral Medicine, Oral Pathology* **35**(4), 532–40.

Tsukamoto-Tanaka, H., Ikegame, M., Takagi, R., *et al.* (2006) Histochemical and immunocytochemical study of hard tissue formation in dental pulp during the healing process in rat molars after tooth replantation. *Cell and Tissue Research* **325**(2), 219–229.

Wang, X., Thibodeau, B., Trope, M., *et al.* (2010) Histologic characterization of regenerated tissues in canal space after the revitalization/revascularization procedure of immature dog teeth with apical periodontitis. *Journal of Endodontics* **36**(1), 56–63.

Wieman, T.J., Smiell, J.M., Su, Y. (1998) Efficacy and safety of a topical gel formulation of recombinant human platelet-derived growth factor-BB (becaplermin) in patients with chronic neuropathic diabetic ulcers. A phase III randomized placebo-controlled double-blind study. *Diabetes Care* **21**(5), 822–7.

Yamauchi, N., Yamauchi, S., Nagaoka, H., *et al.* (2011) Tissue engineering strategies for immature teeth with apical periodontitis. *Journal of Endodontics* **37**(3), 390–97.

Yang, J., Zhao, Y., Qin, M., *et al.* (2013) Pulp revascularization of immature dens invaginatus with periapical periodontitis. *Journal of Endodontics* **39**(2), 288–92.

Yanpiset, K., Trope, M. (2000) Pulp revascularization of replanted immature dog teeth after different treatment methods. *Endodontics and Dental Traumatology* **16**(5), 211–17.

Zhao, C., Hosoya, A., Kurita, H., *et al.* (2007) Immunohistochemical study of hard tissue formation in the rat pulp cavity after tooth replantation. *Archives of Oral Biology* **52**(10), 945–53.

Zhu, X., Zhang, C., Huang, G.T., *et al.* (2012) Transplantation of dental pulp stem cells and platelet-rich plasma for pulp regeneration. *Journal of Endodontics* **38**, 1604–9.

Zhu, W., Zhu, X., Huang, G.T., *et al.* (2013) Regeneration of dental pulp tissue in immature teeth with apical periodontitis using platelet-rich plasma and dental pulp cells. *International Endodontics Journal* **46**(10), 962–70.

Zuong, X.Y., Yang, Y.P., Chen, W.X., *et al.* (2010) [Pulp revascularization of immature anterior teeth with apical periodontitis]. *Hua Xi Kou Qiang Yi Xue Za Zhi* **28**(6), 672–4.

7 Use of MTA as Root Perforation Repair

Mahmoud Torabinejad[1] and Ron Lemon[2]

[1] Department of Endodontics, Loma Linda University
School of Dentistry, USA
[2] UNLV, School of Dental Medicine, USA

Mineral Trioxide Aggregate: Properties and Clinical Applications, First Edition.
Edited by Mahmoud Torabinejad.

INTRODUCTION

The decision of the clinician and patient with respect to the attempt to repair perforation by any cause requires the consideration of many factors. Iatrogenic perforation should be a rare event. If not, the clinician should review his/her case selection, technical skills, and availability of aids, such as the dental operating microscope (DOM), in order to reduce the incidence of perforation. Prevention is always preferable to repair and the clinician should select cases within his/her skill and experience level and refer challenging cases to an endodontist. Even successfully treated perforations may lower the long-term prognosis for the tooth due to loss of tooth structure and consequential increase in susceptibility to root fracture or periodontal breakdown.

The clinician must understand the important variables affecting the prognosis of perforation repair: time, location, and size of defect (Petersson *et al.* 1985; Fuss & Trope 1996). Many types of perforation can offer a good prognosis for repair if these variables are evaluated. Tooth loss is not inevitable after perforation and the clinician should offer treatment options to the patient prior to a recommendation for extraction. An "Endodontic Informed Consent" document must contain a statement concerning the possibility of perforation and the clinician should not be reluctant to discuss this outcome with the patient.

Important factors concerning the decision for repair or extraction of a perforated tooth include the interest of the patient to retain the tooth, the prognosis

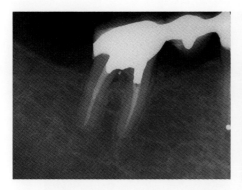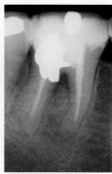

Fig. 7.1   Prior to the introduction of MTA, restorative material such as amalgam was used to seal perforation defects. Failure rate was high due to the presence of moisture and inability to control the placement of the materials. Both of these perforation repairs are failing due to periodontal breakdown.

for repair, and the general condition of the patient's mouth, restoratively and periodontally. Poor periodontal health related to inadequate oral hygiene compromises the prognosis for perforation repair. Additional treatment costs associated with perforation repair may not be advisable if the patient has extensive restorative needs.

Compared to historical treatment approaches, the prognosis for perforation repair has improved. A better understanding of the etiologic factors associated with successful outcomes and recent, biologically active materials, such as mineral trioxide aggregate (MTA; Dentsply Tulsa Dental, Tulsa, OK), have greatly improved repair prognosis. Prior to the era of biologically active materials, restorative materials were used in an attempt to seal the perforation defect. Amalgam, Cavit, Intermediate Restorative Material (IRM), glass ionomer, and composite were used with marginal results (Fig. 7.1). Wet conditions associated with perforation repair negatively affected the sealing properties of many of the materials (Seltzer *et al.* 1970; Alhadainy 1994; Fuss & Trope 1996; Regan *et al.* 2005; Tsesis & Fuss 2006). Controlling the placement of the materials was problematic and often the defect was not sealed adequately or the periodontal support tissues were chronically irritated from uncontrollable overfill of repair material (Fig. 7.2).

To control moisture and to minimize extrusion of the repair material, an "internal matrix" method was developed. A biologically tolerant graft material, such as hydroxyapatite or calcium sulfate, was packed through the perforation to fill the osseous defect. Then, the repair material could be placed so that moisture contamination was reduced and placement of the repair material was more

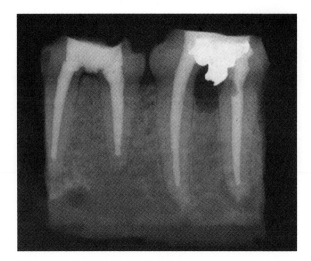

Fig. 7.2 Controlling the placement of amalgam and its lack of seal in experiment has led to the development of a periodontal defect and formation of chronic inflammation in the furcation. In contrast the adjacent tooth repaired with MTA has not led into the same results.

controllable, which reduced the incidence of extrusion of repair material (Lemon 1990, 1992).

When MTA was introduced into the market in 1998, the age of biologic repair began. The unique and desirable properties of MTA have been described earlier in this book. MTA has been shown to induce a biologic repair of the perforation defect. When MTA is hydrated in the presence of a balanced salt solution containing phosphate ions, hydroxyapatite crystals are formed on the surface of the MTA (Sarkar *et al.* 2005). Hydroxyapatite is essential for mineralization. A biologic repair implies that cementum or bone will cover the surface of the set MTA. Most importantly, chronic inflammation is minimal (Fig. 7.3) compared with other repair materials (Pitt Ford *et al.* 1995; Torabinejad *et al.* 1995; Koh *et al.* 1997; Keiser *et al.* 2000; Holland *et al.* 2001; Rafter *et al.* 2002; Camilleri & Pitt Ford 2006; Ribeiro *et al.* 2006; Souza *et al.* 2006; Camilleri 2008; Komabayashi & Spångberg 2008; Wang *et al.* 2009; Brito-Júnior *et al.* 2010; Samiee *et al.* 2010; Silva Neto *et al.* 2010; Fayazi *et al.* 2011). Pitt Ford *et al.* (1995) created furcation perforations in premolars of dogs and repaired them immediately or after a week of contamination with either amalgam or MTA. Their histological findings showed cementum formation underneath MTA in most treated specimens, in contrast to the samples whose furcation perforations

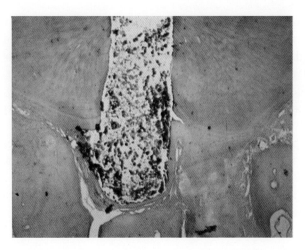

Fig. 7.3 Repair of a furcation perforation in a dog premolar with MTA results in formation of cementum adjacent to the repair material and lack of inflammation in the periodontal ligament.

had been repaired with amalgam. They also reported that when perforations are treated immediately and without contamination, the healing rate after their repair with MTA was significantly better than those contaminated with delayed repair. Yildirim *et al.* (2005) compared the healing of furcation perforations repaired with either MTA or Super EBA in dogs' teeth. Their histological findings showed cementum formation underneath all MTA specimens at the 6-month interval. In contrast their Super EBA specimens showed no cementum formation and they had mild to severe inflammation at the same time interval. Noetzel *et al.* (2006), in another dog study, showed significantly more inflammation in furcation perforation sites repaired with tricalcium phosphate cement compared with those repaired with MTA after 12 weeks. Al-Daafas and Al-Nazhan (2007) compared gray MTA and amalgam as furcation perforation repair materials in dogs' teeth that had been contaminated with bacteria. They also investigated the effect of calcium sulfate as a barrier beneath MTA. As in the previous investigation, the MTA samples showed significantly less inflammation and greater bone formation compared with their amalgam specimens. Their results showed when calcium sulfate was used to prevent MTA extrusion, it caused formation of mild to moderate chronic inflammation and stratified squamous epithelium around the repaired perforation sites. Vladimirov *et al.* (2007) repaired furcation perforations in dogs' teeth with either ProRoot MTA or Titan cement. Their findings after 30 days showed presence of thinner capsules and fewer inflammatory cells in MTA specimens compared with those repaired with Titan cement. Based on available information, it appears that MTA produces better histological results compared with other currently used perforation repair materials. In addition, placement of a barrier beneath MTA has no significant effect on treatment success. Furthermore, repairing the perforation site immediately and avoiding bacterial contamination produces better results than their counterparts.

The formation of hydroxyapatite crystals between the MTA and the tooth interface has been implicated in the excellent sealing properties reported for MTA (Koh *et al.* 1997; Holland *et al.* 1999; Regan *et al.* 2002; Main *et al.* 2004; Juárez Broon *et al.* 2006; Pace *et al.* 2008; Roberts *et al.* 2008; Miranda *et al.* 2009; Mente *et al.* 2010). The treatment outcome for many types of perforation defects has been greatly improved with the proper use of MTA.

TYPES OF PERFORATION DEFECTS

Access preparation-related perforations

Exploration for calcified canals can result in perforation. Perforation coronal to the crestal bone should be repaired with an appropriate restorative material, such as amalgam or composite (Fig. 7.4). Perforation below the crestal bone should be repaired with MTA. Every attempt should be made to avoid access-related perforations. Even with successful repair, the tooth is weakened and more susceptible to fracture. Preventive measures include:

1 Careful evaluation of the preoperative radiograph. Calcification of the coronal chamber, angulation of the long axis of the root(s), and anatomy of the tooth should be considered. Horizontal radiographic angulation (mesial, distal) provides additional information to guide access preparation.
2 Proper outline form for each type of access preparation. An improper design will result in inadequate vision and orientation during the access opening (Fig. 7.5).
3 Magnification and lighting. Adequate vision allows the operator to see the subtle changes in the color and consistency of dentin that can offer clues to orifice location. If the coronal restoration is defective and will be replaced, vision is greatly enhanced if the restoration is removed before starting the access preparation. A microscope should be used for challenging cases, such as calcified canals or endodontic therapy through crowns.
4 Radiographs taken during preparation. Metal clamps may prevent visualization of the access opening. Placement of the clamp on a distal or

(A) (B)

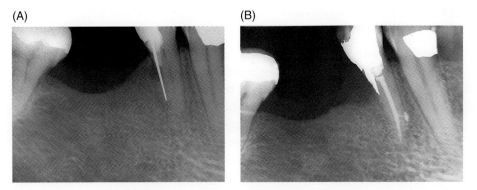

Fig. 7.4 (A) An accidental procedure has resulted in coronal perforation and development of a lesion on the distal of second mandibular premolar. (B) After finding the canal and its cleaning, as well as its obturation, the defect was repaired with amalgam.

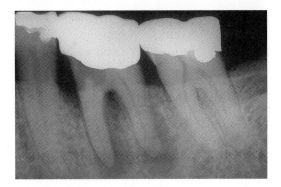

Fig. 7.5 An improper design has resulted in inadequate vision and orientation and lateral crown perforation during access preparation.

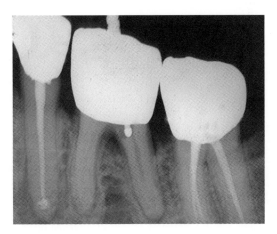

Fig. 7.6 Placement of a small bur at the bottom of the access preparation and taking a radiograph is extremely helpful to locate calcified canals.

proximal tooth and placement of a "split dam" may prevent this problem. In some cases, location of the canal or chamber prior to placement of the rubber dam is recommended. The preoperative radiograph should be measured to determine the depth of preparation required to locate the chamber or canal. If this depth is approached and the chamber or canal is not located, a radiograph should be taken to evaluate orientation of the preparation (Fig. 7.6).

Cleaning and shaping related ("strip") perforations

Most perforations of this type can be avoided by utilization of proper endodontic technique. Knowledge of root anatomy for each type of tooth and study of the preoperative and working length radiographs for canal curvatures are essential in the prevention of perforation (Fig. 7.7). Perforation repair with MTA is more difficult in the coronal area of the root compared to the apical portion of the canal. Using cleaning and shaping instruments too large for a given canal and failure to recognize the proximity of canals to the furcation in multi-rooted teeth are the most frequent causes of this type of perforation (Fig. 7.8).

Resorption-related perforations (internal/external)

Internal resorption has a pulpal etiology. Routine endodontic therapy will prevent progression of the resorption, and the prognosis is excellent if the treatment is performed prior to perforation into the periradicular tissues. MTA repair is not necessary if the resorption is intercepted prior to perforation.

(A)   (B)

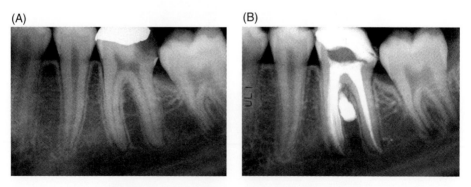

Fig. 7.7 Lack of attention to the anatomy of mesial roots (A) has resulted in severe strip perforation (B) in the mandibular molar.

(A)

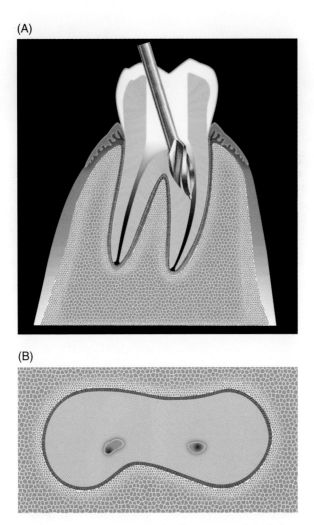

(B)

Fig. 7.8   (A) Using large rotary instruments for thin roots and (B) failure to recognize the proximity of canals to the furcation in multi-rooted teeth are the most frequent causes of strip perforation.

However, MTA may be the obturation material of choice if perforation is detected (Fig. 7.9).

Inflammatory external resorption may perforate into the pulp canal space (Fig. 7.10). The prognosis depends on the etiology of the resorption and the amount of dentin loss. Replacement resorption (ankylosis) is caused by loss of the cementum barrier. Most commonly, this phenomenon is associated with

(A) (B) (C)

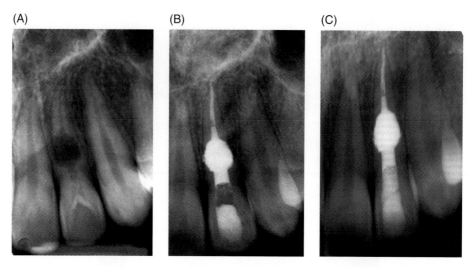

Fig. 7.9 (A) Internal resorption of pulpal origin. (B) Routine endodontic therapy was performed in the apical portion of the root using gutta-percha and sealer. MTA was used to fill the defect as obturation material. (C) A radiograph taken 1 year later shows excellent results.

(A) (B)

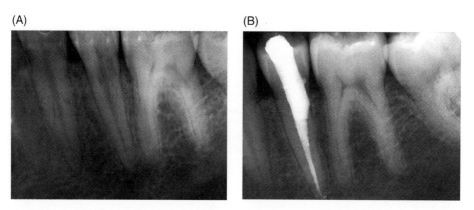

Fig. 7.10 (A) An extracanal invasive root resorption is present in the mandibular second premolar. After root canal cleaning and identifying the portal of entry into the root canal, the entire root canal was filled. (B) A radiograph taken 2 years later shows this procedure has stopped the root resorption.

the replantation of avulsed teeth. MTA is of questionable value for stopping this process. Inflammatory resorption may be arrested with MTA obturation if the etiology is associated with a necrotic pulp. However, the prognosis is guarded.

FACTORS INFLUENCING PROGNOSIS FOR REPAIR (TABLE 7.1)

Size of perforation

The larger the perforation, the greater the potential damage to the periradicular tissues. Repair of a large perforation is more complex. Hemorrhage is more difficult to control and placement of an internal matrix is usually necessary. The matrix material recommended for very large perforations is Collatape (Zimmer Dental, Carlsbad, CA). This material is composed of collagen fibers that promote hemostasis but remain wet and provide the additional moisture MTA requires to set. The collagen fibers will resorb a few weeks after placement.

Location of the perforation

Root perforations may occur at different locations during access preparation, cleaning and shaping, and post space preparation (Fig. 7.11). The anatomy of the tooth and the location of the perforation will affect the difficulty of repair of the defect and the prognosis for the mishap (Tables 7.1 and 7.2).

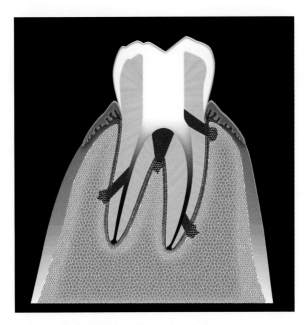

Fig. 7.11   Roots can be perforated at different levels during access preparation, cleaning and shaping, and post space preparation. Larger perforations are more difficult to seal and to control placement of the repair material.

Table 7.1 Perforation location: single-rooted teeth.

Location	Repair material	Considerations
Coronal to crestal bone	Geristore, amalgam, composite, glass ionomer cement	Difficult to control placement of repair material May require surgery May compromise esthetic result
Cervical third of root apical to crestal bone	MTA ± collagen matrix	Decreased prognosis if periodontal pocket communicates with perforation Canal patency difficult to maintain MTA must set (1 week) prior to obturation
Middle/apical third of root	MTA ± collagen matrix	Difficult to visualize Obturate canal with MTA coronal to level of perforation Hydrate MTA (1 week with wet cotton)

Table 7.2 Perforation location: multi-rooted teeth (furcation) – see diagram.

Location	Repair material	Considerations
Coronal to crestal bone (external root surface)	Geristore, amalgam, composite, glass ionomer cement	Difficult to control placement of repair material May require surgical repair May compromise periodontal health
Furcation (floor of chamber)	MTA ± collagen matrix	Decreased prognosis if periodontal pocket communicates with perforation Perforation is repaired prior to cleaning & shaping
Strip perforation (furcation)	MTA ± collagen matrix	Difficult to visualize. Repair perforation first, then establish patency; place gutta-percha cone without sealer to maintain patency (1 week) Hydrate MTA with wet cotton
Middle/apical third of root	MTA ± collagen matrix	Difficult to visualize Obturate canal with MTA coronal to level of perforation Hydrate MTA (1 week with wet cotton) If post space is necessary, remove MTA to desired level before set of MTA

PULP CHAMBER PERFORATIONS

Etiologies

Searching for the pulp chamber or the orifices of root canals of calcified chambers or calcified roots can result in pulp chamber perforations. Failure to recognize when the bur has passed through a calcified pulp chamber in multi-rooted teeth can cause gouging or perforation in the furcation (Fig. 7.12). Lack of alignment between a cemented crown and the long axis of the root may also result in a coronal or radicular perforation.

Prevention

Exposing radiographs from different horizontal angles provides valuable information regarding the location, size and extent of the pulp chamber and the presence of calcification. Using magnification while performing the access preparation in calcified pulp chambers and crowned teeth is essential for locating pulp chambers and orifices of canals. To find the orifice of a calcified canal, a small bur should be placed in the area of the orifice and a radiograph taken (Fig. 7.6). This procedure is very helpful for locating calcified canals.

Recognition and treatment of pulp chamber perforations

The main indicator for pulp chamber perforation during access preparation is the sudden appearance of persistent hemorrhage and radiographic evidence

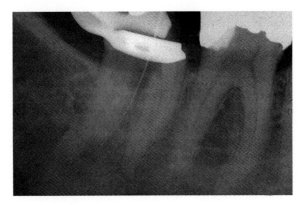

Fig. 7.12 A file passing through the tooth structure and entering into the periodontal ligament or bone is the main sign of root perforation.

of a file passing through the tooth structure and entering into the periodontal ligament or bone (Fig. 7.12). Occasionally, this accident results in pain in a previously asymptomatic patient. Proper use of an electronic apex locator may confirm the presence of perforation.

Gouging of the wall can be repaired by restorative materials such as composite in the anterior teeth and amalgam in the posterior teeth. When the crown of a tooth is excessively weakened, a full crown is recommended.

Lateral surface repairs

If perforation of the crown is above the crestal bone and readily accessible, it should be restored with composite, amalgam, or a crown, depending on the size of the perforation. Subgingival perforations or those slightly apical to the crestal bone are correctable by either extrusion or crown lengthening procedures (Fig. 7.4).

Furcation repairs

Materials such as amalgam, gutta-percha, zinc oxide-eugenol, Cavit, calcium hydroxide, and indium foil have been used clinically or experimentally in animals to repair furcation perforations. Before development of MTA, most clinicians were using amalgam to seal these defects (Fig. 7.1). Because of high failure of these cases and high success rate of perforation repairs with MTA, most furcation perforations are currently repaired with MTA. The furcation perforation should be sealed immediately after the canals have been located. Files should be placed in the canals to prevent blockage of the canals with MTA (Fig. 7.13).

In a case report, Oliveira et al. (2008) demonstrated complete resolution of a furcation lesion and clinical symptoms after a furcation perforation in a primary molar repaired with MTA 20 months after treatment. Pace and associates (Pace et al. 2008) examined ten cases of furcation perforations that had been cleaned with NaOCl, EDTA, and ultrasonic tips and sealed with MTA without internal matrix. The teeth were endodontically treated and coronally restored with permanent restorations. Clinical and radiographic follow-ups were done at 6 months, 1 year, 2 years, and 5 years. After 5 years, 9 out of the 10 teeth were functional and free of radiolucent lesions, pain, and swelling. Based on these observations the authors concluded that MTA without matrix provides an effective seal of root perforations and clinical healing of the surrounding periodontal tissue.

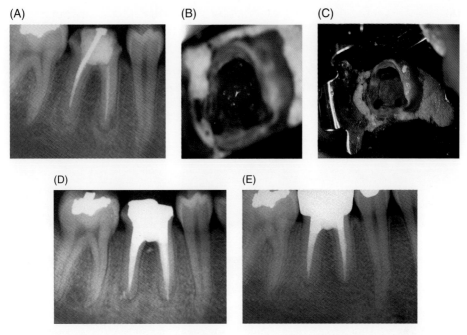

Fig. 7.13 (A) When the perforation is located in the furcation, the patency of the canal must be protected. After the furcation perforation was located (B), files were placed in the canals during perforation repair with MTA (C). No internal matrix was used (D). Twenty-six months later, there was no evidence of periodontal pocket communicating with the perforation site (E). Courtesy of Dr. Mahmoud Torabinejad and Dr. Randy Garland.

ROOT PERFORATIONS DURING CLEANING AND SHAPING

Roots can be perforated at different levels during cleaning and shaping (Fig. 7.11). The level (coronal, mid-root, or apical) at which the perforation has occurred affects treatment planning and prognosis significantly.

Coronal root perforations

Causes, indicators and prevention

Coronal root perforations can occur by over enlarging canals in the cervical portion of a canal by files, Gates–Glidden drills, or Peeso reamers (Fig. 7.14). Straight-line access to the orifice of the root canal, careful exploration for

(A)

(B)

(C)

(D)

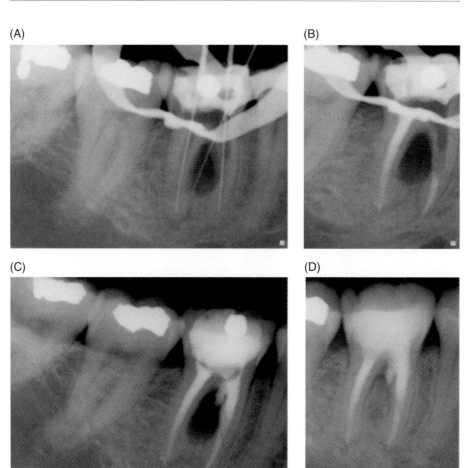

Fig. 7.14 If the perforation is located in the root, the patency of the canal must be protected. After the strip perforation was located (A) and patency established (B), the distal canal and apical portion of the mesial canals were filled with gutta-percha and sealer. (C) The coronal portion of the mesial roots were then obturated with MTA. No internal matrix was used. (D) At 9 months, there was evidence of osseous repair and no periodontal pocket communicating with the perforation site. Courtesy of Dr. Albert G Goerig.

calcified canals, and careful consideration of apical size and canal taper can prevent the majority of root perforations. Like pulp chamber perforations, sudden copious hemorrhage and radiographic evidence of a file passing through the root structure and entering into the periodontal ligament or bone are primary indicators of this procedural accident (Fig. 7.14b).

Treatment

Prevention of communication between the perforation site and the gingival sulcus is very important in prognosis of these accidents. Once a pathway is established, development of a permanent periodontal lesion is inevitable (Fig. 7.15). Repair of a strip perforation in the coronal third of the root has the poorest long-term prognosis of any type of perforation (Lemon 1992). The defect is usually inaccessible for adequate repair. An attempt should be made to clean and obturate the canal apical to the perforation with gutta-percha and sealer, and seal the rest of the canal with MTA. For those clinicians who know how to seal the entire canals with MTA, that approach can be attempted.

Prognosis

The prognosis for coronal perforation is poor because of the predictable development of periodontal defects. When the intracanal treatment fails, other alternative treatment modalities should be considered. If the perforation site can be surgically repaired to leave a collar of bone between the defect and the gingival attachment, the potential for the development of a periodontal lesion is reduced significantly. However, surgical repair of cervical perforations usually results in a periodontal pocket extending at least to the apical base of the perforation. The etiologic factor is the apical proliferation of junctional epithelium and eventual loss of attachment. Therefore, teeth with coronal root perforations close to the crestal bone should be treated with non surgical extrusion or surgical crown lengthening to "externalize" the perforation.

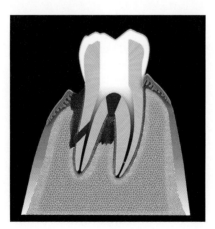

Fig. 7.15   When a perforation is not sealed it can cause development of a pathway to the oral cavity and establish a permanent periodontal lesion.

Lateral perforations

Causes and indicators

Ledge formation and attempts to negotiate ledges and application of misdirected pressure can result in formation of a new canal and eventually a mid-root or an apical perforation (Fig. 7.16). Signs of lateral root perforation are similar to those of other perforations: sudden appearance of fresh blood in the root canal or pulp chamber pain, and radiographic evidence of deviation of intracanal instruments from the original canal.

Treatment of mid-root perforation

Treatment is similar to the treatment of coronal root perforations. An attempt should be made to clean, shape the canal apical to the root perforation. In

(A) (B)

(C)

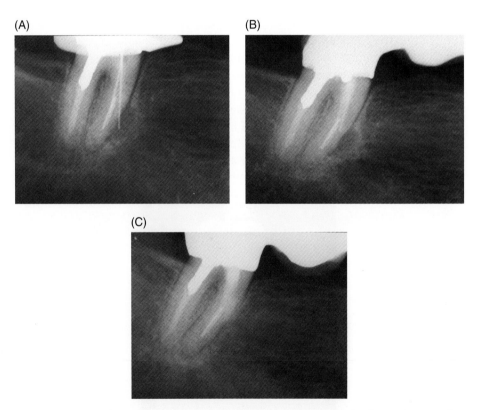

Fig. 7.16 (A) A lateral root perforation is present in the mandibular first molar. (B) After root canal cleaning and identifying the site of perforation, the entire root canal was filled with MTA. (C) A radiograph taken one year later shows this procedure has resulted in healing of the lateral lesion. Courtesy of Dr. Ahmad Fahid.

these perforations an attempt should be made obturate the canal apical to the perforation with gutta-percha and sealer and seal the rest of the canal with MTA. For those clinicians who know how to seal the entire canals with MTA, this method is preferable because of the difficulty of controlling hemorrhage within the canal during obturation. Lee *et al*. (1993), in a dye leakage study, showed the superiority of MTA over IRM and amalgam as an endodontic filling material for repairing lateral root perforations. Holland *et al*. (2001) repaired lateral perforations in dogs with either Sealapex or MTA. After 180 days, most MTA specimens showed cementum deposition around lateral perforations and no sign of inflammation. In contrast, Sealapex samples showed presence of inflammation even after 180 days. The same group of investigators (Holland *et al*. 2007) purposely induced lateral perforations in dogs' teeth and repaired them with MTA, either immediately or 7 days later, with or without pretreatment with calcium hydroxide as a disinfectant. After 90 days, the immediately repaired samples without contamination showed significantly better histologic results than contaminated specimens. The authors concluded that contamination of perforated sites has a deleterious effect on the prognosis of perforated roots and that calcium hydroxide therapy before repairing a contaminated perforation does not improve the healing of a perforation.

Prognosis

The prognosis of teeth with mid root perforations depends on the effectiveness of cleaning and shaping, control of hemorrhage, and the ability to seal the canal apical to the perforation. Root perforations in teeth in which the perforation occurred after complete or partial debridement have better prognosis than those that occur before any cleaning. Perforations located close to the apex have better prognosis that those near the crestal bone. The size and surgical accessibility of perforations also are important variables with respect to long term success. Small perforations are easier to seal than are large ones. Because of surgical accessibility, perforations located on the facial aspect are more easily repaired and therefore have a better prognosis than those in other areas. MTA is the material of choice for surgical and non surgical management of these mishaps.

Apical perforations

Apical perforations can occur either directly through the apical foramen (overinstrumentation) or through the apical portion of root itself (failure to negotiate a curved canal).

Causes and indicators

Overinstrumentation at an incorrect working length through the anatomic apical foramen results in perforation of the apical foramen and "blowing out" the apical foramen (Fig. 7.17A). Ledge formation and application of misdirected pressure can also result in formation of a new canal and eventually an apical perforation.

Presence of fresh bleeding in the canal or on the surface of files or paper points and lack of an apical stop are indicators of perforation of the apical foramen. Penetration of the last file beyond the radiographic apex confirms the presence of this procedural accident.

(A)   (B)

(C)

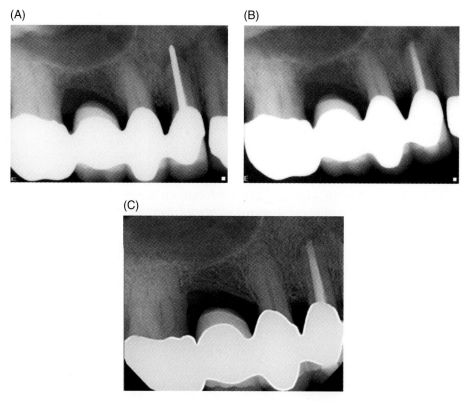

Fig. 7.17 (A) Over-instrumentation at an incorrect working length through the anatomic apical foramen has resulted in "blowing out" the apical foramen and over filling with a silver point. (B) The silver point is removed, the canal is cleaned and the apical 3 mm is filled with MTA. Collacote was used to prevent MTA extrusion. The rest of the canal was filled with gutta-percha and root canal sealer. (C) A radiograph taken 2 years later shows this procedure has resulted in healing of the apical lesion. Courtesy of Dr. Jeffrey Samyn.

Treatment

Establishing a new working length, creating an apical seat, and obturating the canal to its new length are the treatment of choice. Placement of MTA as an apical barrier or filling the entire canal with MTA can prevent extrusion of obturation materials (Fig. 7.17B, C). Placement of an apical barrier of MTA requires obturating the apical 3–4 mm with MTA.

Prognosis

The size, shape and location of the apical perforation are important factors. Large apical perforations are difficult to seal. Placement of an apical plug of MTA improves the prognosis of these cases. In addition, the feasibility of surgically repairing the apical foramen perforation also may influence the final outcome. In general, repair of apical perforations in anterior teeth is easier and more practical than in posterior teeth.

ROOT PERFORATION DURING POST SPACE PREPARATION

The post should be parallel with the long axis of the root. Its width should not exceed a third of the width of the root and its length should not be more than two thirds of the working length (Fig. 1.12).

Causes, indicators and prevention

Creating oversized preparations deviating from the long axis of the tooth with a rotary instrument are the main cause of root perforations (Fig. 7.18A). Appearance of fresh blood in the root canal and/or radiographic evidence of extrusion of post into the periodontium are immediate the sign of a post space perforation. The presence of a sinus tract stoma or probing defects extending to the base of a post are clinical signs of post perforation. (Fig. 7.18a) To prevent root perforation, gutta-percha should be removed to the desired level with heated instruments or devices that create "pilot" post space to receive rotary drills. Post space preparation should NEVER extend apical to any root curvature. The post preparation must be centered within the root in order to reduce the chance of vertical root fracture.

Treatment

If the post can be removed, nonsurgical repair is preferred (Fig. 7.18B). If the post cannot be removed and it is accessible surgically, surgical repair with MTA should be attempted (Fig. 7.19).

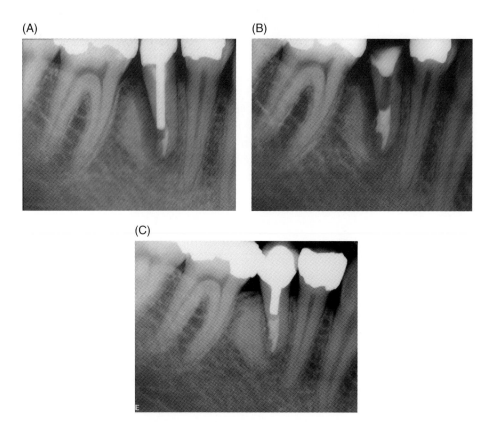

Fig. 7.18 (A) The distal aspect of the root of a mandibular second bicuspid was perforated during preparation for a post. (B) The perforation was repaired with MTA. (C) A radiograph taken 13 years later shows excellent healing of the apical lesion. Courtesy of Dr. Noah Chivian.

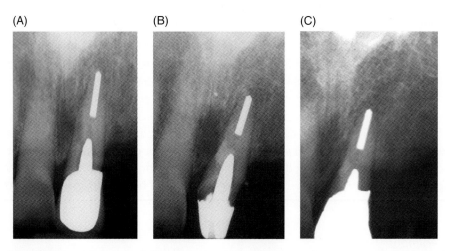

Fig. 7.19 (A) The coronal distolingual aspect of the root of a maxillary lateral incisor was perforated during preparation for a post. (B) The perforation was repaired surgically with intentional replantation using MTA as repair material. (C) A radiograph taken 5 years later shows excellent healing of the lateral lesion.

Prognosis

The prognosis of teeth with root perforation during post space preparation depends on the root size, location relative to epithelial attachment, and accessibility for repair. If the post can be removed, nonsurgical repair is preferred (Fig. 7.18C). Teeth with small root perforations that are located in the apical region and are accessible for surgical repair have a better prognosis than those with large perforations, close to the gingival sulcus, or inaccessible.

Time elapsed since perforation

As a general rule, the prognosis for repair decreases as the time since perforation increases. The inflammatory response associated with perforation results in periodontal breakdown. If a periodontal communication develops, repair and healing are compromised due to the influx of oral bacteria. Therefore, in this situation, the long-term prognosis decreases. Immediate repair of a perforation offers the best prognosis. When a perforation is detected during the process of endodontic therapy, priority should be directed toward repair of the defect instead of continuing with the endodontic procedure.

TECHNIQUES FOR INTERNAL REPAIR USING MTA

MTA is a technique-sensitive material. However, the learning curve for using MTA is low if basic principles are followed. Just enough sterile water should be added to the powder to wet the particles. If the mixture has a "shine" or light reflection, then there is excess water in the mixture. Before placement, blot the mixture with sterile cotton gauze to remove excess water and the mixture will have the proper consistency for delivery with any carrier device.

Method

1   *Site preparation*
    If the perforation occurred prior to the completion of endodontic therapy, repair of the defect must be completed before continuing the endodontic procedure (Fig. 7.14). Protection of canal patency must be maintained during the perforation repair process. Hemorrhage from the perforation site must be controlled and, if indicated, the surrounding dentin must be disinfected. A cotton pellet saturated with sodium hypochlorite can be applied to infected dentin around the perforation for two minutes to provide hemostasis and disinfection. If hemostasis is inadequate or the perforation defect is

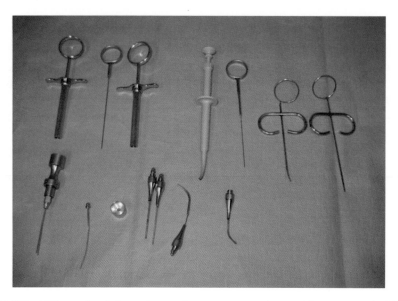

Fig. 7.20 MTA can be delivered to perforation sites and apical locations with different carriers.

large, an internal matrix with Collatape should be placed. The collagen is then packed through the perforation into the bone defect. As mentioned, the collagen provides a soft matrix to minimize overfill while allowing moisture for hardening of the MTA.

2 *MTA delivery*

Just enough sterile water is added to the MTA powder to wet the particles. Lightly blot the mixture with sterile gauze to remove any excess water. When a large volume of MTA is required to repair the perforation, an amalgam carrier can be used to deliver the MTA to the site. For smaller perforations, MTA can be delivered with specially designed micro carriers (Fig. 7.20). After placement, blot the MTA with a sterile cotton pellet. An endodontic plugger is used to gently condense the mixture into the perforation. This process is repeated if necessary to place an adequate thickness of the MTA. Excess material can be removed by carving with an endodontic excavator. A cotton pellet saturated with sterile water should be placed in the chamber over the MTA. The MTA requires additional moisture during the setting process. A temporary restoration is placed over the wet cotton pellet. (Video).

3 *Follow-up Therapy*

Allow 1 week for the MTA to set. Establish access to the perforated area and remove the cotton. Check for set of the MTA. If endodontic therapy

(A)

(B)

(C)

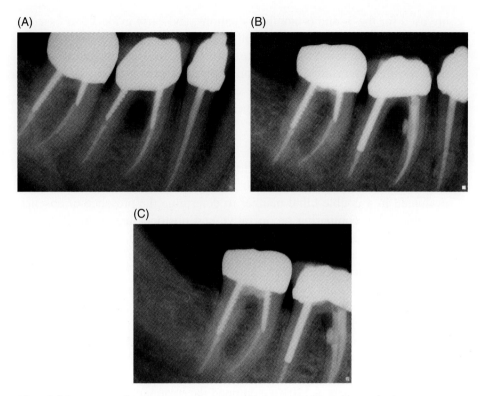

Fig. 7.21 Repair of strip-type perforation. (A) Pretreatment radiograph shows extensive furcation bone loss. (B) Nonsurgical repair with MTA. (C) Six-month recall showing furcation bone fill. Courtesy of Dr. M. Pouresmail.

has not been completed, routine procedures for completion of the non-surgical endodontic therapy can proceed. If canal patency is lost during perforation repair, the treatment prognosis decreases. Therefore, great attention must be given to patency protection during the repair process with MTA.

4   *Recall evaluation*
    Evaluation times should be at 1, 3, and 6 months. Success or failure of the repair can be determined within these time parameters (Fig. 7.21). At 1 month, the patient should be experiencing no discomfort during function. If a preoperative sinus tract was present, healing should be complete with no recurrence. If a periodontal pocket was present preoperatively, reduction in depth would be expected. If no periodontal pocket or sinus tract was present preoperatively, the presence on either of these on recall would indicate fail-ure. There may be no obvious changes radiographically. The same criteria

are used for the 3- and 6-month evaluations, and early evidence of osseous repair should be seen radiographically.

Situations vary with respect to timing of the placement of a new cast restoration. A core restoration should be placed after the perforation repair and completion or the endodontic therapy. A minimum of a favorable one-month recall is suggested prior to placement of a new cast restoration.

5 *Prognosis*

Main *et al.* (2004) examined the long-term outcome of 16 root perforations that had been repaired with MTA. Three independent examiners evaluated in a double-blind manner to determine the presence or absence of pathosis by comparing preoperative and postoperative radiographs. In addition, they performed clinical examinations including periodontal probing at the post operative visits. 5/16 perforations were classified as lateral, 5/16 as strip perforations, 3/16 as furcation perforations, and 3/16 as apical perforations. None of these cases had preoperative periodontal pockets greater than 3 mm. Seven out of 16 cases had radiolucencies prior to repair. The postoperative examination periods ranged from 12 to 45 months. All cases with evidence of pathosis appeared to have healed at the examination time and none of the cases without pathosis developed any pathosis.

Mente and associates (2010) examined the treatment outcome of 26 root perforations repaired with MTA between 2000 and 2006. The treatment was provided by supervised undergraduate students (29%), general dentists (52%), or dentists who had focused on endodontics (19%). The repair was performed under a dental operating microscope. Calibrated examiners assessed clinical and radiographic outcomes 12 to 65 months after treatment. Eighteen of 21 teeth (86%) examined were classified as healed. Based on these findings the authors concluded that MTA provides a biocompatible and favorable long-term results for perforations in all parts of the root.

SUMMARY

The bioactive material MTA has significantly improved the prognosis for repair of perforation defects. Handling characteristics of the material require an understanding of different delivery techniques. However, once mastered, successful repair of perforations that were once considered hopeless will become possible.

REFERENCES

Al-Daafas, A., Al-Nazhan, S. (2007) Histological evaluation of contaminated furcal perforation in dogs' teeth repaired by MTA with or without internal matrix. *Oral Surgery, Oral Medicine, Oral Pathology, Oral Radiology and Endodontics* **103**, e92–9.

Alhadainy, H.A. (1974) Root perforations: A review of literature. *Oral Surgery, Oral Medicine, Oral Pathology* **78**, 368–74.

Brito-Júnior, M., Viana, F.A., Pereira, R.D. *et al.* (2010) Sealing ability of MTA-Angelus with propyleneglycol in furcal perforations. *Acta Odontologica Latinoamerica* **23**, 124–8.

Camilleri, J. (2008) The chemical composition of mineral trioxide aggregate. *Journal of Conservative Dentistry* **11**, 141–3.

Camilleri, J., Pitt Ford, T.R. (2006) Mineral trioxide aggregate: a review of the constituents and biological properties of the material. *International Endodontics Journal* **39**, 747–54.

Fayazi, S., Ostad, S.N., Razmi, H. (2011) Effect of ProRoot MTA, Portland cement, and amalgam on the expression of fibronectin, collagen I, and TGFβ by human periodontal ligament fibroblasts in vitro. *Indian Journal of Dental Research* **22**, 190–4.

Fuss, Z., Trope, M. (1996) Root perforations: Classification and treatment choices based on prognostic factors. *Endodontics and Dental Traumatology* **12**, 55–64.

Holland, R., de Souza, V., Nery, M.J. *et al.* (1999) Reaction of dogs' teeth to root canal filling with mineral trioxide aggregate or a glass ionomer sealer. *Journal of Endodontics* **25**, 728–30.

Holland, R., Filho, J.A., de Souza, V. *et al.* (2001) Mineral trioxide aggregate repair of lateral root perforations. *Journal of Endodontics* **27**, 281–4.

Holland, R., Bisco Ferreira, L., de Souza, V., *et al.* (2007) Reaction of the lateral periodontium of dogs' teeth to contaminated and noncontaminated perforations filled with mineral trioxide aggregate. *Journal of Endodontics* **33**, 1192–7.

Juárez Broon, N., Bramante, C.M., de Assis, G.F. *et al.* (2006) Healing of root perforations treated with Mineral Trioxide Aggregate (MTA) and Portland cement. *Journal of Applied Oral Science* **14**, 305–11.

Keiser, K., Johnson, C.C., Tipton, D.A. (2000) Cytotoxicity of mineral trioxide aggregate using human periodontal ligament fibroblasts. *Journal of Endodontics* **26**, 288–91.

Koh, E.T., Torabinejad, M., Pitt Ford, T.R. (1997) Cellular response to mineral trioxide aggregate. *Journal of Endodontics* **24**, 543–7.

Komabayashi, T., Spångberg, L.S. (2008) Comparative analysis of the particle size and shape of commercially available mineral trioxide aggregates and Portland cement: A study with a flow article image analyzer. *Journal of Endodontics* **34**, 94–8.

Lee, S.J., Monsef, M., Torabinejad, M. (1993) Sealing ability of a mineral trioxide aggregate for repair of lateral root perforations. *Journal of Endodontics* **19**, 541–4.

Lemon, R.R. (1990) Furcation repair management: classic and new concepts. In: *Clark's Clinical Dentistry* (Hardin, J. F., ed.). J B Lippincott Co., Philadelphia, Vol **1**, Chapter 10.

Lemon, R.R. (1992) Nonsurgical repair of perforation defects: internal matrix concept. *Dental Clinics of North America* **36**(2) 439–57.

Main, C., Mirzayan, N., Shabahang, S., *et al.* (2004) Repair of root perforations using mineral trioxide aggregate: a long-term study. *Journal of Endodontics* **30**, 80–3.

Mente, J., Hage, N., Pfefferle, T. *et al.* (2010) Treatment outcome of mineral trioxide aggregate: repair of root perforations. *Journal of Endodontics* **36**, 208–13.

Miranda, R.B., Fidel, S.R., Boller, M.A. (2009) L929 cell response to root perforation repair cements: an in vitro cytotoxicity assay. *Brazilian Dental Journal* **20**, 22–6.

Oliveira, T.M., Sakai, V.T., Silva, T.C. *et al.* Repair of furcal perforation treated with mineral trioxide aggregate in a primary molar tooth: 20-month follow-up. *Journal of Dentistry in Childhood (Chicago)* **75**, 188–91.

Noetzel, J., Ozer, K., Reisshauer, B.H., *et al.* (2006) Tissue responses to an experimental calcium phosphate cement and mineral trioxide aggregate as materials for furcation perforation repair: a histological study in dogs. *Clinical Oral Investigation* **10**, 77–83.

Pace, R., Giuliani, V., Pagavino, G. (2008) Mineral trioxide aggregate as repair material for furcal perforation: case series. *Journal of Endodontics* **34**, 1130–3.

Petersson, K., Hasselgren, G., Tronstad, L. (1985) Endodontic treatment of experimental root perforations in dog teeth. *Endodontics and Dental Traumatology* **1**, 22–8.

Pitt Ford, T.R., Torabinejad, M., McKendry, D.J. *et al.* (1995) Use of mineral trioxide aggregate for repair of furcal perforations. *Oral Surgery, Oral Medicine, Oral Pathology and Endodontics* **79**, 756–63.

Rafter, M., Baker, M., Alves, M. *et al.* (2002) Evaluation of healing with use of an internal matrix to repair furcation perforations. *International Endodontics Journal* **35**, 775–83.

Regan, J.D., Gutmann, J.L., Witherspoon, D.E. (2002) Comparison of Diaket and MTA when used as root-end filling materials to support regeneration of the periradicular tissues. *International Endodontics Journal* **35**, 840–7.

Regan, J.D., Witherspoon, D.E., Foyle, D.M. (2005) Surgical repair of root and tooth perforations. *Endodontic Topics* **11**, 152–78.

Ribeiro, C.S., Kuteken, F.A., Hirata Junior, R., *et al.* (2006) Comparative evaluation of antimicrobial action of MTA, calcium hydroxide and portland cement. *Journal of Applied Oral Science* **14**, 330–3.

Roberts, H.W., Toth, J.M., Berzins, D.W., *et al.* (2008) Mineral trioxide aggregate material use in endodontic treatment: A review of the literature. *Dental Materials* **24**, 149–64.

Samiee, M., Eghbal, M.J., Parirokh, M. *et al.* (2010) Repair of furcal perforation using a new endodontic cement. *Clinical Oral Investigation* **14**, 653–8.

Sarkar, N.K., Caicedo, R., Ritwik, P., *et al.* (2005) Physiochemical basis of the geologic properties of mineral trioxide aggregate. *Journal of Endodontics* **31**(2), 97–100.

Seltzer, S., Sinai, I., August, D. (1970) Periodontal effects of root perforations before and during endodontic procedures. *Journal of Dental Research* **49**, 332–9.

Silva Neto, J.D., Brito, R.H., Schnaider, T.B., *et al.* (2010) Root perforations treatment using mineral trioxide aggregate and Portland cements. *Acta Cirugica Brasilica* **25**, 479–84.

Souza, N.J.A., Justo, G.Z., Oliveira, C.R. *et al.* (2006) Cytotoxicity of materials used in perforation repair tested using the V79 fibroblast cell line and the granulocyte-macrophage progenitor cells. *International Endodontics Journal* **39**, 40–7.

Torabinejad, M., Hong, C.U., Pitt Ford, T.R., *et al.* (1995) Cytotoxicity of four root end filling materials. *Journal of Endodontics* **21**, 489–92.

Tsesis, I., Fuss, Z. (2006) Diagnosis and treatment of accidental root perforations. *Endodontic Topics* **13**, 95–107.

Vladimirov, S.B., Stamatova, I.V., Atanasova, P.K, *et al.* (2007) Early results of the use of ProRoot MT and Titan cement for furcation perforation repair: a comparative experimental study. *Folia Medica (Plovdiv)* **49**, 70–4.

Wang, L., Yin, S.H., Zhong, S.L., *et al.* (2009) Cytotoxicity evaluation of three kinds of perforation repair materials on human periodontal ligament fibroblasts in vitro. *Hua Xi Kou Qiang Yi Xue Za Zhi* **27**, 479–82.

Yildirim, T., Gençoğlu, N., Firat, I., *et al.* (2005) Histologic study of furcation perforation-streated with MTA or Super EBA in dogs' teeth. *Oral Surgery, Oral Medicine, Oral Pathology, Oral Radiology and Endodontics* **100**, 120–4.

8 MTA Root Canal Obturation

George Bogen,[1] Ingrid Lawaty,[2]
and Nicholas Chandler[3]

[1] Private Practice, USA
[2] Private Practice, USA
[3] Faculty of Dentistry, University of Otago, New Zealand

Mineral Trioxide Aggregate: Properties and Clinical Applications, First Edition.
Edited by Mahmoud Torabinejad.
© 2014 John Wiley & Sons, Inc. Published 2014 by John Wiley & Sons, Inc.

INTRODUCTION

Mineral trioxide aggregate (MTA) was originally introduced to dentistry as a root-end filling and perforation repair material (Lee *et al*. 1993; Abedi & Ingle 1995; Torabinejad & Chivian 1999). This hydraulic calcium-silicate based cement has been shown to exhibit excellent biocompatibility and pronounced osteoconductivity. The therapeutic scope of this bioactive cement has expanded to include pulp capping, pulpotomy, apexogenesis, repair of anatomical anomalies, resorptions, regenerative procedures, and recently as a canal obturation material (Torabinejad & Chivian 1999; Koh *et al*. 2001; O'Sullivan & Hartwell 2001; White & Bryant 2002; Branchs & Trope 2004; Aggarwal & Singla 2010; Roig *et al*. 2011; Dreger *et al*. 2012). Since perforation repair, root-end filling and apical plug placement represent a form of partial canal obturation, the complete filling of canal systems with MTA can also be viewed as an advanced clinical concept that provides significant advantages in surgical, conventional or combined therapies.

MTA canal obturation offers an innovative method to approach challenging endodontically involved teeth that may not respond using traditional filling materials and sealers when extensive pathosis is present. Although gutta-percha (GP) is the most universally employed core material in conventional root canal therapy, it is susceptible to bacterial ingress when exposed directly or indirectly to oral fluids (Swanson & Madison 1987; Madison & Wilcox 1988; Khayat *et al*. 1993; Jacobson *et al*. 2002; Yazdi *et al*. 2009). Furthermore, the ability of all obturation materials to maintain a bacteria-tight seal and prevent recontamination is largely dependent on the sealing ability and quality of the provisional and permanent coronal restorations (Saunders & Saunders 1994; Ray & Trope 1995; Uranga *et al*. 1999; Tronstad *et al*. 2000; Siqueira *et al*. 2000; Balto 2002; Weston *et al*. 2008). Many dentists would claim a key advantage of GP is its ease of removal during retreatment. This unusual quality of the material has allowed improved success rates for root canal retreatment along with the evolution of instrumentation and visualization. However, it may be advantageous to use a canal filling material that can overcome the many shortcomings of GP based systems.

In general, the ideal root filling material should preclude reinfection of the root canal system by eliminating the microbial nutrient supply and creating an inhospitable environment for their continued survival (Sundqvist & Figdor 1998; Carrotte 2004). Its ideal requirements therefore include that it be nonirritating to periapical tissues, bacteriostatic, radiopaque, sterile, nonstaining, insoluble, not affected by tissue fluids, dimensionally stable, seal laterally and apically, exhibit biocompatibility, and be easily placed and removed (Grossman 1982). If a material has the ability to completely seal the canal system apically and laterally, then its removal should be difficult or virtually impossible (Torabinejad *et al*. 1993; Boutsioukis *et al*. 2008). Although MTA and all other obturation materials may not be ideal in this regard, MTA can provide important advantages due to its bioactive and bioinductive properties.

Some clinicians view MTA obturation as a relatively new approach to orthograde canal treatment (O'Sullivan & Hartwell 2001; de Leimburg *et al*. 2004; D'Arcangelo & D'Amario 2007; Bogen & Kutler 2009). However, this filling method is an older concept and is antedated by a German publication from the late nineteenth century. During that period, Portland cement, a material very similar to MTA, was not only used to fill root canals but also placed as a pulp capping agent (Witte 1878; Schlenker 1880). In Mayan populations, around 400 CE a related substance was used as an inlay cement (Versiani *et al*. 2011). Interestingly, the early reports of root fillings show that the material was quite successful in curing "apical periostitis", with patients exhibiting diminishing or resolution of pain after treatment and during healing. Both the early Portland cement investigators claimed that they knew of no failures during the observation period, and commented that in replantation cases it also resulted in successful canal closure. They remarked that the material when set produced a "porous" seal, which bound well with other cement filling materials and that the only notable drawback was discoloration of anterior teeth.

Since the nineteenth century, the materials used to obturate the cleaned and shaped root canal space have undergone considerable modification as our understanding of the etiology and microbiology of endodontic disease has expanded. Materials included pastes, cements, plastics and solids (Grossman 1982). Guttapercha transitioned into popularity as the material of choice, based on its ease of delivery, availability and biocompatibility (Weine 1992; Glick & Frank 1986; Seltzer *et al*. 2004). A wide range of core materials have since been introduced that share common properties with GP.

Research investigations have shown a variety of recently developed obturation materials to have acceptable sealability and improved handling properties when used in conjunction with sealers to fill the root canal system. The different compositions of these core materials can include epoxy resin, glass-ionomer, bioceramic, methacrylate, synthetic polyester, and silicone-based substances. Some investigators have recommended filling canals with resin or silicone-based sealers alone rather than a core and sealer combination (Malagnino *et al.* 2001; Tanomaru-Filho *et al.* 2007; Guess 2008; Cotton *et al.* 2008; Ordinola-Zapata *et al.* 2009; Williamson *et al.* 2009; Hammad *et al.* 2009; Ari *et al.* 2010; Kato & Nakagawa 2010; Savariz *et al.* 2010; Pameijer & Zmener 2010; Pawińska *et al.* 2011; Anantula & Ganta 2011; McKissock *et al.* 2011). The current search for new filling materials indicates that even though GP is currently the most widely accepted obturation substance, major advances are needed to satisfy the requirements of the ideal material including MTA.

MTA obturation can offer distinct advantages by promoting the repair of the periodontium and the supporting tissues of the tooth (Pitt Ford *et al.* 1995; Zhu *et al.* 2000; Holland *et al.* 2001; Zhang *et al.* 2009). The induction of cellular repair responses by a filling material that can promote cementum deposition, encourage bone formation and periodontal ligament regeneration must be considered a substantial breakthrough when treating teeth compromised by long-standing disease and failed conventional treatments. The specific characteristics that contribute to the bioactive properties of MTA will be reviewed in order to understand the advantages that this hydraulic tricalcium silicate cement can provide.

CHARACTERTICS/PROPERTIES

Mechanisms of action in obturation

Several key features in the composition of MTA account for its bioactive and bioinductive properties when used as a canal filling cement. These include: the material's particle size, hydration products, sustained pH, interstitial layer formation with dentin, sealing ability, setting expansion, and antimicrobial properties (see Table 8.1).

Table 8.1 Advantages of MTA as a root filling material.

Sustained alkaline pH during slow set
Forms interfacial layer with dentin similar to hydroxyapatite
Seals at zero microns when examined under SEM
Particle size penetrates/occludes dentinal tubules
Setting properties not affected by smear layer
Inhibits growth of *E. faecalis* and *C. albicans*
Promotes cementogenesis and PDL reformation
Promotes bone coupling factors and osteogenesis
Antibacterial effect is enhanced in presence of dentin
Can increase resistance of root to fracture

Particle size

Several investigations have analyzed the particle size and shape of ProRoot MTA, in its gray (GMTA) and white (WMTA) formulations (Lee *et al*. 2004; Dammasckhe *et al*. 2005; Camilleri *et al*. 2005; Camilleri 2007; Asgary *et al*. 2006; Komabayashi & Spångberg 2008a). Overall, it may be said that the particle size of WMTA is finer and more homogeneous than GMTA. Komabayashi and Spångberg reported that the diameter of GMTA particles measured 10.48 ± 5.68 µm in the low-power-field (LPF) mode, and 3.05 ± 2.44 µm at high-power-field (HPF) mode. The diameter of WMTA particles has been measured at 9.86 ± 4.73 µm at LPF mode and 2.96 ± 2.36 µm at the HPF. WMTA therefore contains smaller particles with a narrower range of size distribution. Approximately 70% of both GMTA and WMTA exhibit an average particle size of 1.5 to 3.0 µm. The investigation demonstrated that the small particles permit their entry into open dentin tubules, which average 2–5 µm in diameter (Garberoglio & Brännstrom 1976). This may constitute a mechanism for hydraulic sealing (Komabayashi & Spångberg 2008b). The size and shape of MTA particles may therefore facilitate the occlusion of tubules where microorganisms may persist and otherwise survive following the cleaning and shaping of the root canal system.

Hydration products and pH

MTA releases calcium ions during its setting reaction and more importantly provides an alkaline pH (Holland *et al*. 2002; Lee *et al*. 2004; Santos *et al*. 2005; Bozeman *et al*. 2006; Camilleri 2008a). The sustained alkaline pH of 12.5 is a potent antibacterial and antifungal property (Duarte *et al*. 2003; Al-Nazhan & Al-Judai 2003; Fridland & Rosado 2005; Al-Hezaimi *et al*. 2006a). It has also been demonstrated that MTA leaches calcium ions several days after the initiation of hydration and during setting (Ozdemir *et al*. 2008). A further reaction during hydration produces a high-sulfate calcium sulfoaluminate (Taylor 1997; Budig & Eleazer 2008). The continuous release of calcium from the setting MTA diffuses through dentinal tubules, with increasing calcium ion concentration during the prolonged curing process (Fridland & Rosado 2005; Camilleri 2008a; Ozdemir *et al*. 2008).

It has also been postulated that the biocompatibility of the cement may be attributable to the release of hydroxyl ions and the formation of calcium hydroxide during the course of hydration (Camilleri 2008b). In a further reaction, calcium silicates react with calcium hydroxide to form calcium silicate hydrate gel, producing an alkaline environment unfavorable towards commonly encountered microorganisms such as *Enterococcus faecalis* (Sen *et al*. 1995; Molander *et al*. 1998; Peciuliene *et al*. 2001; Santos *et al*. 2005) and *Candida albicans* (Al-Nazhan & Al-Judai 2003; Mohammadi *et al*. 2006; Al-Hezaimi *et al*.

2006a). MTA has shown to be effective in bacterial elimination and to decrease bacterial viability (Ribeiro *et al.* 2006; Jacobovitz *et al.* 2009).

Formation of interstitial layer

As the setting reaction proceeds, hydroxyapatite is produced, which occurs when the calcium ions released by the MTA come into contact with tissue fluid and culminates in interstitial layer formation (Lee et. 2004; Bozeman *et al.* 2006). During this process, an amorphous calcium phosphate initially forms, which transforms later to an apatite phase. Calcium-deficient B-type carbonated apatite crystallites characterize this latter phase. During the process of skeletal calcification, this weak crystalline amorphous calcium phosphate is recognized as an important intermediate that precedes apatite formation (Tay *et al.* 2007). The spontaneous apatite formation induced through the setting activity of MTA accumulates within collagen fibrils. As the development of the interfacial layer proceeds, apatite deposition promotes mineral nucleation on the dentin surface, which is characterized by tag-like structures extending into the dentinal tubules (Reyes-Carmona *et al.* 2009; Okiji & Yoshiba 2009). Materials characterized by an apatite layer have been shown to form a chemical bond with calcified tissues such as bone (Holland *et al.* 1999a; Reyes-Carmona *et al.* 2009).

The adherent interstitial dentin-MTA interfacial layer that forms in the presence of tissue fluid phosphates shows marginal adaptation superior to amalgam, Intermediate Restorative Material, and Super-EBA under scanning electron microscopy (Torabinejad *et al.* 1993; Sarkar *et al.* 2005). This layer formation may be a principal factor in minimizing leakage by filling the gap along the interface and by interacting with dentin. It can also be considered a hybridized layer, since it is an intercrossed chemically bonded layer of collagen and MTA (Torabinejad *et al.* 1993). The layer formed resembles hydroxyapatite in structure and composition when examined by X-ray diffraction analysis (Sarkar *et al.* 2005; Bozeman *et al.* 2006). The combination of the resulting mineralized interstitial layer and the sustained, elevated pH for protracted periods (12.5 after curing) may therefore provide potent bacteriostatic and bactericidal properties, allowing improved entombment and killing of surviving microorganisms (Torabinejad *et al.* 1995a; Camilleri *et al.* 2005).

Fracture resistance

Teeth root filled with MTA have been reported to exhibit greater resistance to fracture than untreated controls (Bortoluzzi *et al.* 2007; Hatibović-Kofman *et al.* 2008). MTA may provide enhanced resistance to fracture and also contribute to strengthening of tooth structure. This characteristic of MTA has been shown *in vivo* after storage of extracted teeth for a period of one year (Topcuoğlu *et al.* 2012). The fracture resistance in MTA-treated teeth may be attributable in part to the presence of metalloproteinase-2, which has the capacity to inhibit collagen destruction (Tjaderhane 2009; Parirokh & Torabinejad 2010).

Chemomechanical instrumentation of the root canal significantly weakens dentin, making teeth more vulnerable to fracture when using conventional filling materials (Sim *et al.* 2001; Grigoratos *et al.* 2001; Topcuoğlu *et al.* 2012). In particular, calcium hydroxide used to disinfect root canals over extended periods can weaken immature teeth and considerably reduce fracture resistance (Andreasen *et al.* 2002). MTA has been shown to increase fracture resistance over time, findings that have been confirmed for MTA and other proprietary calcium silicate-based cements (Tuna *et al.* 2011). This feature of MTA obturation can positively influence the retention and long-term outcome for the involved tooth.

Sealing ability and setting expansion

In order to properly seal a canal and prevent bacterial penetration, the material should be dimensionally stable, adhering and adapting precisely to the dentin wall (Storm *et al.* 2008). The sealing capacity of MTA has been shown to be superior to that of other filling materials currently used (Torabinejad *et al.* 1993, 1995b; Wu *et al.* 1998; Roberts *et al.* 2008). It also resists leakage at a higher rate when placed in a moist environment (Torabinejad *et al.* 1995c; Gondim *et al.* 2003; Chogle *et al.* 2007). It has been postulated that this favorable characteristic may be at least in part due to the inherent property of both GMTA, and to a lesser degree WMTA, to expand during setting (Storm *et al.* 2008; Okiji & Yoshiba 2009; Hawley *et al.* 2010). The interaction of calcium ions and phosphate ions in the medium that facilitate the formation of apatite crystals at the MTA-dentin interface may contribute to this linear expansion (Sarkar *et al.* 2005; Tay *et al.* 2007; Okiji & Yoshiba 2009).

A study comparing white and GMTA as apical barriers showed GMTA to produce the superior seal (Matt *et al.* 2004). When challenged using human saliva it appears that GMTA is superior and that both are preferable to vertically condensed GP and sealer (Al-Hezaimi *et al.* 2005). Storm *et al.* (2008) showed that the linear expansion in water at 24 hours was 1.02% for GMTA and 0.08% for WMTA. When hydrated with Hank's balanced salt solution, the expansion was 0.68% for GMTA and 0.11% for WMTA. There is some speculation that the linear expansion of MTA when used as an obturation material may contribute to the propagation of undetected root infractions (De Bruyne & De Moor 2008). Although the seal achieved with GMTA may be superior, when infractions are suspected or detected, WMTA may be the preferable material.

APPLICATIONS/USES

Conventional obturation

Using MTA as the filling material in uncomplicated root canals is an acceptable treatment option for conventional obturation, patients with holistic treatment concerns and cases with extensive pathosis. Teeth with external inflammatory or internal root resorption, open apices or patients seeking "alternative" filling materials may be prime candidates for MTA obturation during initial treatment. Although some clinicians may argue that MTA limits or precludes retreatment options, surgical intervention can be initiated if healing is unfavorable. The advantages of MTA when selected in initial treatment can provide remarkable outcomes without the need for surgical root-resection and related post-treatment morbidity (Kvist & Reit 2000) (see Fig. 8.1).

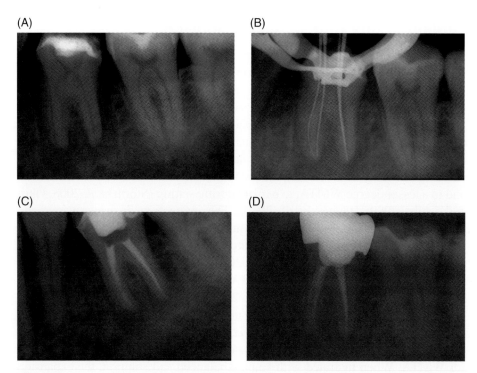

Fig. 8.1 (A) Forty-one year-old male patient with mandibular left first molar exhibiting extensive periradicular pathosis. The patient was concerned about gutta-percha and elected MTA obturation "alternative" treatment. (B) Radiographic working length confirmation. (C) MTA obturation of all three canals to the level of the pulpal floor. (D) Nine-year 8 month radiographic recall. Tooth restored with zinc phosphate cement core and full gold crown. Note absence of periradicular pathosis.

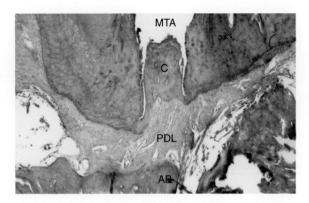

Fig. 8.2 Histological section of a dog tooth obturated with MTA at 180 days. Note biological closure of the main canal by new cementum (C), MTA plug, intact periodontal ligament (PDL), alveolar bone (AB) and absence of inflammatory cells. Hematoxylin and eosin, original magnification 100×. Courtesy of Dr. Roberto Holland, São Paulo, Brazil.

Inflammatory apical root resorption is a common complication of long-standing periapical disease (Kaffe *et al.* 1984; Laux *et al.* 2000; Vier & Figueiredo 2004). Root apices of teeth with necrotic pulps often exhibit moderate to severe foraminal and periforaminal resorption, depending on the duration of disease. Studies have identified internal apical resorption in teeth with periapical lesions in 74.7 to 81% of cases (Laux *et al.* 2000; Vier & Figueiredo 2002). This feature can impede healing when GP-based core materials are used, as they may not provide an adequate seal and do not promote repair. Moreover, these regions may also be vulnerable to biofilm formation from Gram-positive facultative anaerobes that can prevent periapical healing when GP is the filling material (Takemura *et al.* 2004; Noguchi *et al.* 2005). Inter-radicular biofilms are present in the majority of cases with large periapical lesions (Siqueira & Lopes 2001; Nair *et al.* 2005; Lin *et al.* 2008; Ricucci & Siqueira 2010), and they may be present in initial and refractory endodontic disease. Obturation using MTA may have an advantage in these challenging cases (Yildirim & Gencoglu 2010). Research in dog models has shown that teeth obturated with MTA feature cementum in the main canal, and in some instances the accessory canals (Holland *et al.* 1999b) (see Fig. 8.2).

If teeth present with radiographic evidence of apical root resorption, MTA should be considered as the ideal filling material. Furthermore, when uncontrolled hemorrhage is present after cleaning and shaping, a 3–5 mm apical plug of MTA is the preferred option (Matt *et al.* 2004; Al-Khatani *et al.* 2005; Pace *et al.* 2008). MTA can seal internal resorptive defects and counteract the possible effects of pathogenic biofilms and bacteria harbored in dentinal tubules (Matt *et al.* 2004; Ricucci & Siqueira 2010). The procedure is best executed using hand instrumentation with either pluggers or hand files, as extrusion of material is possible (see Fig. 8.3).

(A)
(B)

(C)

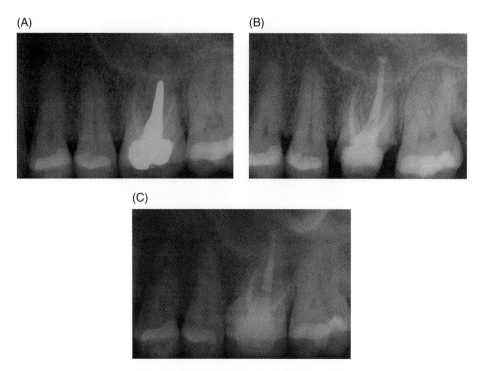

Fig. 8.3 (A) Radiograph of a symptomatic maxillary left first molar in a 38-year-old female featuring a large cast post and core and apical radiolucency with gutta-percha obturation and resorption at the palatal root. (B) Post-operative radiograph of MTA obturation of all canals, 5 mm apical fill at apex of palatal root. Canal was then backfilled with thermoplastic gutta-percha and a bonded core constructed. (C) Two-year 6 month review showing restoration with ceramic crown and complete periapical healing around palatal apex.

Retreatment

Retreatment of failed root canal treatments can be challenging when the original filling materials have sustained a long exposure to oral fluids. Bacteria in refractory or contaminated cases typically involve colonization of dentinal tubules by *E. faecalis*, *C. albicans*, and a host of Gram-positive bacteria, including *Proprionibacterium*, *Actinomyces*, *Streptococcus* and *Peptostreptococcus* species (Pinheiro *et al.* 2003; Siqueira & Rocas 2004; Williams *et al.* 2006). During long incubation periods, these micoorganisms have been known to advance and colonize dentinal tubules as far as 400 to 500 μm from the pulp–dentin interface (Orstavik & Haapasalo 1990; Peters *et al.* 2001; Love & Jenkinson 2002; Waltimo *et al.* 2003; Siqueira & Sen 2004). This characteristic can prevent their elimination even when long-term calcium hydroxide intracanal medication is used (Stuart *et al.* 2006). The eradication of these microbes is extremely difficult, even with the latest irrigants and technologies (Stuart *et al.* 2006). MTA

(A)

(B)

(C)

(D)

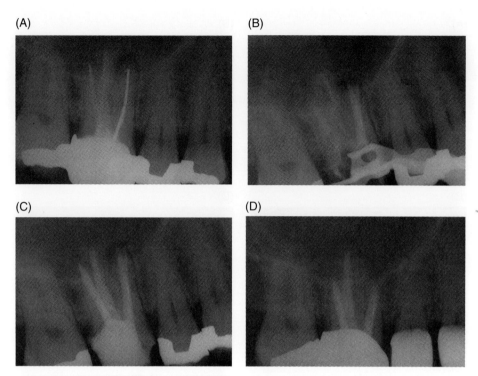

Fig. 8.4 (A) Forty-two year-old patient presented with his maxillary right first molar exhibiting ongoing symptoms and pathosis. Preoperative radiograph shows silver point obturation of mesiobuccal root associated with periapical pathosis and separated instrument at the apex of the distobuccal root. (B) Initial obturation of the MB root after silver point removal showing two portals of exit. (C) Complete obturation of three canals with MTA and placement of bonded core after MTA curing. (D) Eight-year recall showing absence of periapical pathosis. Patient was asymptomatic and the molar firm and in complete function.

obturation may impede the survival of these deeply imbedded microorganisms that might withstand conventional treatment (see Fig. 8.4).

A major problem with long-standing infections in previously treated teeth is the extent of bacterial invasion into the isthmuses, cul-de-sacs, accessory canals, and other anatomical ramifications (Nair *et al.* 2005; Ricucci & Siqueira 2010). These areas that were either not cleaned or are recolonized pose a challenge when using GP or resin-modified obturation materials due to their neutral pH and limited anti-microbial effect. Even if cleaning and shaping are completed with high regard for microscopic examination, ultrasonication and advanced irrigation systems using appropriate solutions, the elimination of these colonies may still not be adequate to avoid surgical indications. Long-standing colonization can also lead to biofilm formation within the canal system, which extends beyond the canal at the apex (Tronstad *et al.* 1990; Abou Rass & Bogen 1998; Sunde *et al.* 2000; Noguchi *et al.* 2005). These survival properties of polymicrobial colonies can prevent periradicular

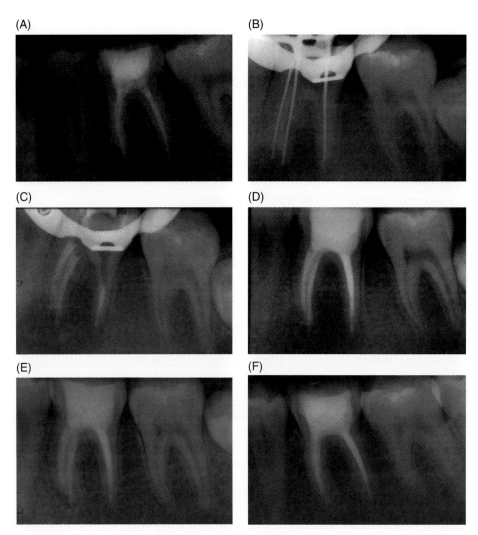

Fig. 8.5 (A) Periapical radiograph of a previously treated mandibular left first molar in a 12-year-old male patient with acute apical abscess and submandibular space infection. (B) Working length radiograph. (C) Initial MTA obturation with 5 mm apical plug to distal canal. (D) Radiograph of distal canal obturated with thermoplastic gutta-percha and sealer backfill. Bonded composite restoration is present. (E) Three-year 3 month radiographic review. (F) Nine-year 4 month radiographic recall without permanent cuspal coverage restoration. The molar exhibited normal probing and mobility.

healing and may necessitate surgery to allow resolution of periapical disease when conventional filling materials are used. Healing seen with MTA retreatment can produce improved outcomes and appears to minimize the need for surgical intervention typically seen in some GP retreatments (see Fig. 8.5).

Obturation prior to surgery

Obturation of teeth with MTA prior to surgical intervention allows clinicians to approach cases where anatomical access may be more than challenging. In particular, the mesial and distal roots of mandibular second and third molars and the palatal roots of maxillary premolars and molars may be considered. In other cases obturation of the distolingual root of mandibular first and second molars prior to surgery can simplifiy management of the resected root. After MTA has cured, resection does not affect seal integrity and encourages complete healing after removal of infected tissues (Andelin *et al.* 2002; Lamb *et al.* 2003). This surgical technique also allows a more conservative osteotomy site as the remaining root may not require enhanced access for the introduction of micromirrors, ultrasonic tips and materials. Nevertheless, the presence of GP remaining against the canal wall after resection mandates retrofill placement. A root-end filling material should also be considered if plastic or metal GP carriers are present.

Gutta-percha remaining at the canal interface poses a dilemma since tenacious Gram-positive bacteria and fungi show an ability to survive between GP/sealer and dentin (Friedman 2008). This aspect of MTA retreatment and surgical execution is an important consideration since previous treatments can present with transportation, pulpal remnants, voids, sealer absence, accessory canals, untreated isthmuses, separated instruments and biofilms, all of which can delay or prevent healing. Placement of a root-end filling material after root resection of canals filled with MTA should be considered when radiographs or microscopic examination raise concern (see Figs 8.6 and 8.7).

Large and long-standing lesions (over 5 mm) can show extensive bone loss leading some clinicians to condemn these treatment failures to extraction and implant placement (Greenstein *et al.* 2008). MTA obturation in retreatment combined with surgery can now provide patients an opportunity to retain teeth that have been compromised by advanced and extensive pathosis (see Fig. 8.8).

Obturation with perforation repair

Perforations are iatrogenic or pathologic communications between the root canal and the periodontium. MTA has been shown to be the preferred material in managing this complication (Main *et al.* 2004; Pace *et al.* 2008). Repair using MTA involves the identification of the involved area and application of the cement in a thickness that provides an adequate seal to promote repair and healing. This procedure can be performed nonsurgically or surgically using a dental operating microscope (DOM). However, perforations do not always occur on

(A)
(B)
(C)
(D)

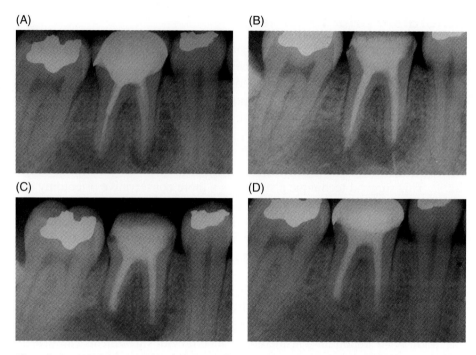

Fig. 8.6 (A) Radiograph of previously treated symptomatic mandibular right first molar with extensive apical pathosis and submandibular space infection in a 26-year old female. (B) Postoperative radiograph after disassembly, gutta-percha removal, MTA obturation and bonded core placement. Note extruded gutta-percha after retreatment. (C) Surgical root resection with removal of extruded gutta-percha and inflammatory tissue. Microscopic examination after resection revealed remaining gutta-percha located in distal canal wall interface and MTA retrofill was placed. (D) One year 6-month recall radiograph shows new full coverage restoration and complete remineralization of the previous osteotomy site.

the pulpal floor or accessible areas that allow for simple repair and further visits follow, often with GP and sealer obturations. The possibility of dislodging the MTA when placing the second obturation material is a strong argument for obturation of the entire canal with MTA when the perforation site is below the canal orifice.

There is no documented advantage to repairing a radicular perforation followed by GP and sealer obturation. The most logical sequence involves obturating the entire canal, unless a post space is to be prepared which may complicate treatment options. Obturation of the entire canal in resorption and perforation cases can be more predictable owing to MTA thickness and overall cement stability (Tsai *et al.* 2006). If the canal is treatment planned for post

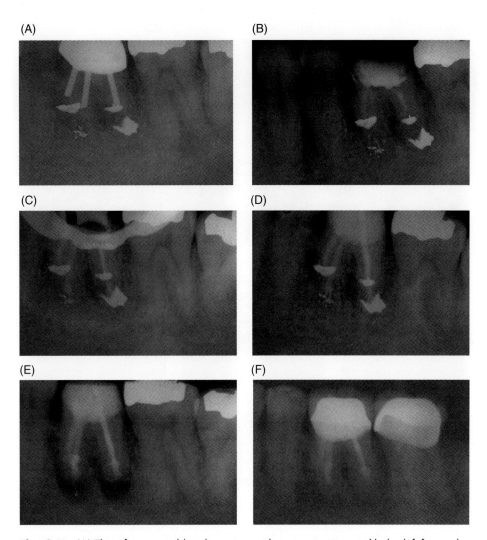

Fig. 8.7 (A) Thirty-four year-old male patient with symptomatic mandibular left first molar with three metal posts. Previously treated surgically with amalgam retrofills and treatment planned for extraction and an implant. (B) Calcium hydroxide dressing after crown and post disassembly. (C) All canals obturated with MTA. (D) Post and core constructed after MTA curing. (E) Postoperative radiograph after second surgery, removal of amalgam retrofills and MTA root-end restorations. (F) Eight-year 5 month recall showing remineralization of osteotomy site. The patient was symptom-free.

placement, then the MTA repair must be customized to accommodate the indicated restorative requirements. Clinicians should consider the simplicity of using only one material to fill the entire canal to the orifice when these defects are present (see Fig. 8.9).

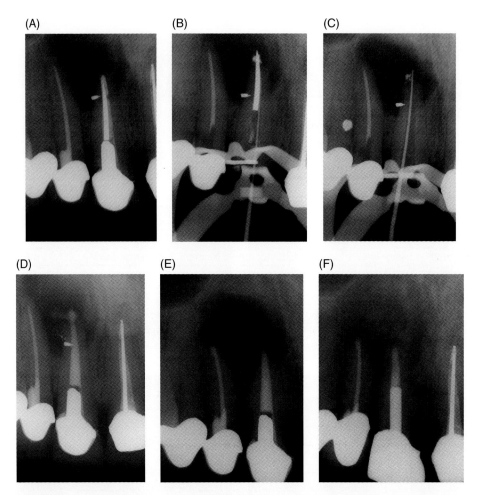

Fig. 8.8 (A) Preoperative radiograph of failed silver point treatment. Sinus tract formation and a large periapical lesion associated with the maxillary right central incisor extending to the right lateral incisor. (B) Attempted bypass of silver point during orthograde retreatment. (C) Radiograph after silver point removal and extrusion of canal materials. (D) MTA obturation prior to provisional cementation of the disassembled cast post and core. (E) Root resection of both the central and lateral incisors and removal of extruded material and silver point debris. (F) Four-year 6 month radiographic recall showing normal periapical structures and alveolar bone. Courtesy of Dr. Laureen M. Roh, Los Angeles, California.

Apexification using MTA obturation

The induction of root-end closure by MTA is a predictable and desired goal for treating nonvital, infected immature permanent teeth (Shabahang & Torabinejad 2000; Giuliani *et al.* 2002; Witherspoon *et al.* 2008; Pace *et al.* 2008; Bogen & Chandler 2008; Nayar *et al.* 2009; Güneş *et al.* 2012). If regenerative endodontic

(A)

(B)

(C)

(D)

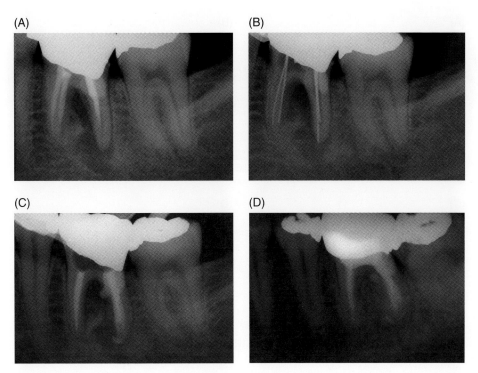

Fig. 8.9 (A) Preoperative radiograph of a failed gutta-percha obturation on the left first mandibular molar in a 67-year-old patient. Note presence of furcation bone loss. (B) Working length radiograph; apical resorption at distal apex. (C) Initial obturation of all canals with gray MTA revealing extrusion of material through perforating resorptive defect at furcation. (D) Eighteen month recall showing complete osseous repair of furca and periapical area.

procedures are not elected (see Chapter 6), then the formation of a root-end plug using MTA can provide an option that encourages root maturation. MTA stimulates cementogenesis and odontogenesis, allowing the cells of the apical papilla to complete root formation and apical closure (Huang *et al.* 2008). This process is completed by the cells of the apical papilla that differentiate into cementoblasts and odontoblasts (see Fig. 8.10).

The obturation technique in teeth with open apices is completed after proper cleaning and shaping to the working length. Length is usually determined by estimation using pretreatment images and confirmed using a large master apical file. The aim during careful instrumentation is to clean the canal walls to the limit of the apical extension, protecting and preserving the tissue beyond the root apex. Tissues beyond or at the apex will act as a natural barrier or diaphragm during the obturation process. Apical obturation must be completed using gentle force and with extreme tactile care. The obturation should ideally be positioned 1 mm short or level with the apical rim or collar (see Chapter 5).

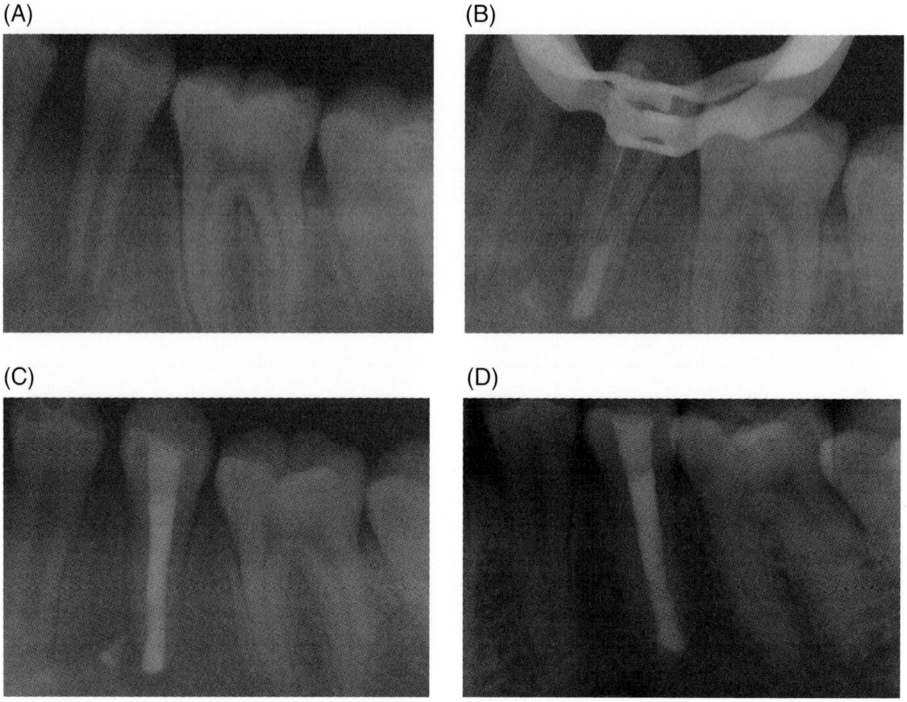

(A)

(B)

(C)

(D)

Fig. 8.10 (A) A 10 year-old patient with a symptomatic mandibular left second premolar with dens evaginatus and open apex with extensive periapical disease. (B) Obturation of apical foramen with 5.0 mm gray MTA apical plug. (C) Final obturation with thermoplastic gutta-percha and a bonded restoration. (D) Nine-year radiographic review. Note mature apex formation.

Compaction can be completed with a master apical file (MAF) one or two sizes smaller, endodontic pluggers, a Glick instrument, a large GP master cone, or the back end of a coarse paper point. Ultrasonic tips can be used, but care must be given to use the device at a low setting to avoid forcing an excess of MTA beyond the apex. Although MTA extrusion routinely occurs, it should not adversely affect the outcome (Tahan *et al.* 2010) (see MTA Compaction Techniques). When the apical plug is completed, it should ideally be 4–5 mm in length (Matt *et al.* 2004). After radiographic verification of adequate density and position, the coronal cement can be condensed with a large plugger and dried with a sterile paper point while using the DOM. A flowable resin-modified glass ionomer (RMGI) cement or compomer can be placed over the MTA and the remainder of the canal filled later with thermoplastic or laterally compacted GP and sealer to or near the cemento-enamel junction. Alternately, a bonded core build-up or other reinforcing technique may be used to permanently seal the canal system (Desai & Chandler 2009a).

Obturation for dental anomalies

An important feature of MTA obturation is its ability to address disease related to internal root resorption and a variety of anatomical variants. These include dens invaginatus, dens evaginatus, gemination, fusion, and C– shaped canal systems (Bogen & Kuttler 2009). The advantages of MTA in these cases are substantial and the indications multifactorial. Due to the small particle size of MTA, and particularly WMTA, the material can access and fill partially or completely anatomical spaces that can include fissures, fins, cul-de-sacs, and isthmuses. When dens invaginatus (dens in dente) is encountered, MTA obturation can neutralize microorganisms in one compartment while allowing another region of pulp to remain vital (see Fig. 8.11).

Teeth with C– shaped canal anatomy are also excellent candidates for MTA as the filling material (Tsai *et al.* 2006). This morphology presents a challenge and failed cases are often planned for retrograde treatment to resolve refractory disease. MTA obturation as a retreatment option is a viable alternative to surgery. Healing rates for MTA retreated C– shaped molars are consistently superior to the majority of GP obturated teeth (see Fig. 8.12).

The most commonly seen crown anomaly leading to endodontic problems in the developing dentition is dens evaginatus (de Lima *et al.* 2007; Alani & Bishop 2009). Patients of Mongoloid origin show a higher prevalence, and are diagnosed with infected pulp spaces, typically in premolars of both arches (Cho 2005; Rao *et al.* 2010). Clinically, there is an enamel extension or small talon cusp on the occlusal surface and a small portal of entrance can be seen under magnification. The extensions may break away or be subject to extreme wear leading to pulp exposure, acute apical abscesses, open apices and large periapical radiolucencies. Regenerative endodontic procedures or MTA obturation with an apical plug and thermoplastic obturation with a composite coronal restoration provides treatment that allows apical closure, root maturation and healing of periapical disease.

OBTURATION TECHNIQUES

Techniques for compaction of MTA are multiple and include the Lawaty technique, conventional compaction with stainless steel files and endo pluggers, and also using engine driven nickel-titanium (NiTi) files in reverse as augers. (Video). Obturating the entire canal system when possible creates simplicity for the operator and allows a greater volume of MTA in the canal against any defect site and therefore a better seal. (Video).

(A)   (B)   (C)

(D)   (E)   (F)

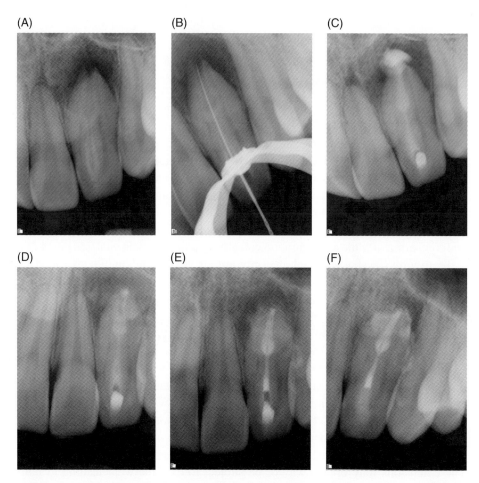

Fig. 8.11   (A) Radiograph of 16-year-old patient with left maxillary lateral incisor exhibiting a dens invaginatus anatomical anomaly. (B) Working length radiograph. (C) Canal filled with calcium hydroxide paste. (D) Recall radiograph after two months. (E) Radiograph showing MTA obturation of the central canal with access cavity provisionally restored. (F) Four-year recall shows periapical healing. Tooth was asymtomatic and responded normally to cold testing. Courtesy of Dr. Adrian Silberman, Murrieta, California.

Standard compaction technique*
(*Bogen & Kutler 2008)

Canal obturation with MTA requires the same preparation and irrigation normally executed for GP placement with or without smear layer removal (Yildirim *et al.* 2008). The retention of the smear layer does not appear to affect the interstitial layer formation of MTA and its presence may improve the seal over time

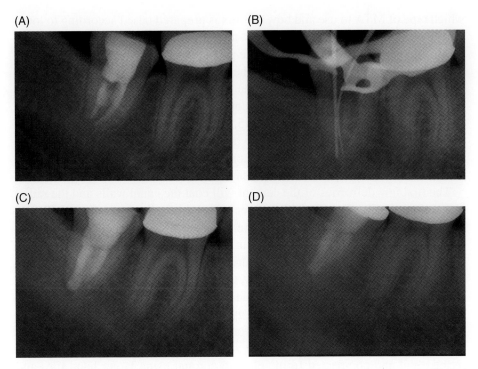

Fig. 8.12 (A) Twenty-eight-year-old patient with C– shaped second molar root filled 4 months previously with gutta-percha. Patient had ongoing pain and was unable to place occlusal force on the tooth; note small periapical radiolucency. (B) Radiograph of files in distal root after cleaning and shaping. (C) Completed MTA obturation with bonded composite core. (D) Two-year review. Patient was asymptomatic with tooth firm and functioning normally.

(Hatibović-Kofman *et al.* 2008; Tuna *et al.* 2011). The smear layer may act as a "coupling agent" that enhances MTA bonding to root canal dentin, similar to the hybrid layer formation when self-etching primer and bonding systems are used in restorative dentistry. Since the data are inconclusive regarding smear layer removal, clinicians may choose to leave the smear layer in selected cases and fill canals with MTA without apparently compromising outcome (Yildirim *et al.* 2010).

In initial or retreatment nonsurgical root canal preparation of teeth with closed apices, the master apical file (MAF) should be a minimum of size 25; however, a size 35 or 40 MAF is more desirable. White MTA has better handling characteristics and compactibility, attributed to smaller particle sizes compared to its counterpart, but GMTA appears to have superior sealing properties *in vitro* (Al-Hezaimi *et al.* 2006b). MTA can also be mixed with 0.12% chlorhexidine rather than sterile water or anesthetic solution, which may increase its antibacterial properties (Stowe *et al.* 2004; Holt *et al.* 2007). Clinicians should judge which type of MTA to use and how the mix is prepared based according to tooth location, esthetics, surgical indications, and difficulty of placement.

After the canals are dried with sterile paper points, the mixed MTA is placed in the canal with a carrier gun and pushed apically with an endodontic plugger, size 1/3, 5/7, 9/11, or a Glick instrument. A stainless steel K-file, one or two sizes smaller than the MAF is used to compact the apical 3–5 mm of wet MTA. If the last MAF file size used was a 35, then a size 25 or 30 K file is used to advance the wet MTA apically to the working length. The pilot tip of the MAF can be cut off with a high speed diamond bur to create a flat end to facilitate compaction after the apical plug has been formed.

The first few deliveries of the cement will coat the canal walls and the radial lands of the K-file. The file is then directed off the walls circumferentially and pushed with light to moderate pressure until resistance is encountered. If the tooth apex is closed, firmer pressure can be applied. Hand pluggers can also be used to complete the compaction, but they may be challenging to use in curved canals. As the MTA condenses apically, the working length will shorten, and an endodontic plugger (size 1/3 or 5/7) can now be applied to the top of the compacted apical material. Ultrasonic energy via the plugger can further compress the material using a low-range setting for the unit. A radiograph is then taken to check for voids and confirm acceptable density. Fresh MTA can then be placed in the canal and compacted from apical to coronal using larger hand files and pluggers, or the canal backfilled with thermoplastic GP and sealer.

If the radiograph reveals that the obturation density is inadequate, the existing (wet) MTA can be recompacted using a smaller K-file (i.e., size 20) until an acceptable result is attained. If voids are still present, the MTA can be rinsed out with sterile water or anesthetic solution using a 27 or 30 gauge needle under high pressure. If this is unsuccessful an ultrasonically activated 30 or 35 K-file can used. If these procedures are unsuccessful, then the remaining canal can be filled with MTA and the tooth monitored for healing and surgical indications. In cases where MTA is packed to the canal orifice and over the pulpal floor, a brief spray from a two-way syringe will remove any residual material from the access cavity walls or pulp floor.

If the decision is made to backfill the canal with GP or a resin-based material after placing a MTA plug, the canal can be irrigated with sterile water using a side-venting needle. After rinsing the canal it is dried with paper points and the MTA packed flat with the end of an appropriately sized plugger. A carefully directed force will prevent the extrusion of large amounts of MTA if the root apex is immature or open due to apical root resorption (Felippe *et al.* 2005; Tahan *et al.* 2010).

With large open apices, the MTA can be pushed down using the back end of an extra coarse paper point, GP point, Glick instrument, or large plugger. Endodontic pluggers can be used with ultrasonic energy on lower settings, but caution is advised, as large amounts of MTA may extrude when open apices are present. Although extruded MTA should not affect the outcome, the esthetics of placement may be an issue when attempting to achieve an ideal radiographic result. If extensive hemorrhage is present with open apices, perforating resorptive defects, or large long-standing perforation sites, the MTA must be placed in larger amounts and more rapidly delivered using a larger carrier (e.g., amalgam carrier) or brought to the canal in bulk as a less moist mixture. Excess moisture or blood is then removed from the top of the MTA with dry cotton pellets, with or without calcium hydroxide powder pressed over the entire volume of the material. This can also be achieved with the back end of an extra coarse paper point pressed continually against the mixture until seepage is controlled and stabilized. If the region has uncontrollable hemorrhaging that cannot be stabilized, then calcium hydroxide placement and provisionalization is recommended.

Lawaty technique*
(*Bogen & Kutler 2008)

The technique for cleaning and shaping the canal in preparation for MTA obturation requires the same mechanochemical preparation for conventional GP obturation. The canal may be prepared more conservatively, avoiding .06–.08 taper preparations and preserving more of the natural architecture and canal walls. The small particle size of WMTA facilitates its travel apically along a glide path with an apical diameter as small as a #20 K-file (GMTA requires a minimum MAF approximating a #25–30 K-file.) The use of a .04 taper ProFile (used in graded sizes from #15 to #35) will produce the desired glide path. Canals are irrigated throughout the preparation with 6.0% sodium hypochlorite before being rinsed with sterile water. Removal of smear layer can be implemented with ethylenediaminetetra-acetic acid (EDTA), BioPure™MTAD, or QMix™, but the outcome should be unaffected if the layer remains (Yildirim *et al.* 2008). The canals are dried with appropriately sized paper points.

Mixing the desired amount of white or gray MTA is carried out in a glass Dappen dish, using a syringe of sterile water or anesthetic solution and a Glick instrument. The quantity of MTA to be mixed should be sufficient to fill the pulpal floor in the access cavity over the prepared dry canal orifices. Excess moisture may be removed by gently swabbing the side of the Dappen dish with a cotton tip applicator. The Glick instrument is used to transfer the mixed MTA from the dish to the chamber.

The mixed MTA should be similar to wet sand and if it begins to dry out in the dish or access chamber, its consistency may be restored with sterile water or anesthetic solution. MTA in the chamber acts as a reservoir during the compaction process, and is replenished as needed. A series of K-files are used to transfer the prepared MTA to the terminus of the canal. The first file will be one size smaller than the MAF and the last will most often be size #60. In canals with abrupt curvature or dilaceration, Flexo-files may be a superior choice.

An apex locator is attached to the initial K-file to aid in the location of the canal terminus, reducing the chance of MTA extrusion. This file is moved circumferentially and passively along the canal glide path, with a gentle apical pumping motion, using the coronal section of the canal as a funnel. As the MTA flows from the access reservoir to the terminus, the apex locator will signal less frequently, and the practitioner will feel resistance and observe binding of the MTA to the file, as the apical plug is formed. When this resistance dissipates, the

(A) (B)

(C) (D)

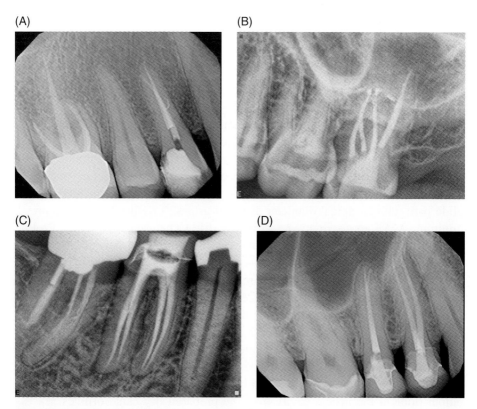

Fig. 8.13 (A) Digital radiograph of maxillary right first premolar with provisional restoration after MTA obturation of two canals. Note the inclusion of mid-root lateral canal with MTA fill. (B) Maxillary left second molar with bonded core and MTA obturation showing four canals. (C) Radiograph showing mandibular right first molar with acrylic provisional and four-canalled MTA obturation. (D) One year postoperative radiograph review of MTA fills of maxillary right first and second premolars.

file will be more passively manipulated once again, and a reduction in the depth of the canal glide path will become evident. Once apical resistance is lost, the next file in the sequence may be used. This pattern is repeated, concluding at size 60. In order to prevent voids, it is important not to omit any instrument in the sequence. Periapical radiographs are taken during the procedure to confirm the density of compaction.

The coronal portion of the canal may also be obturated with MTA; however, in appropriate cases, the coronal portion may be back-filled with GP or a post space created. If MTA is chosen for the coronal fill, Schilder pluggers may be employed, using a light, passive stroking technique, without putting undue pressure on the lateral canal walls, progressing from size 8.0 to larger sizes, if

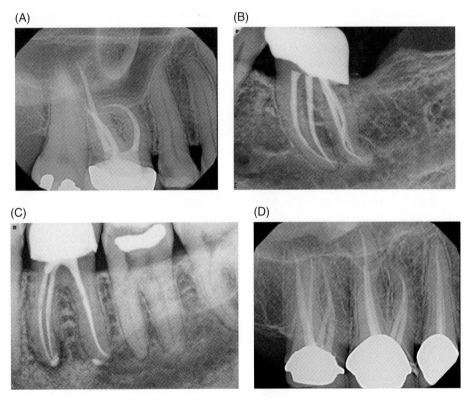

(A)   (B)   (C)   (D)

Fig. 8.14 (A) Digital 10-year recall radiograph of maxillary right first molar with full coverage restoration after MTA obturation. Note curvature of mesiobuccal root. (B) Radiograph of mandibular left first molar with four canals obturated. (C) Three-month recall radiograph of mandibular left first molar MTA obturation. Note presence of several lateral canals and minor MTA extrusion. (D) Postoperative 4-year recall radiograph of two maxillary right molars and a second premolar obturated with vertically compacted MTA.

necessary. Unless restorative considerations dictate otherwise, the remaining MTA in the access cavity may be compacted onto the pulpal floor, with a moist cotton pellet being placed. Once set the material helps to seal accessory canals on the pulp floor and may strengthen the dentin in the furcation area. Final restoration with a bonded core can be completed after setting of the material. Alternatively, all of the MTA may be rinsed/aired away using a two-way air/water syringe. The MTA canal filled orifices can be covered with a flowable composite after which a bonded composite core is placed to seal the pulpal floor and access chamber (See Figs 8.13 and 8.14).

Auger technique

The compaction of MTA can also be implemented using rotary instrumentation. The process involves using conventional .04 and .06 taper NiTi rotary files in the reverse mode. The technique is relatively new and demands modifications to allow proper filling of the apical 3–5 mm. This delivery method requires the same cleaning and shaping procedures as conventional therapies, but employs several different adaptations to secure consistent results. Since the preparation does not involve achieving a resistance form as required for warm vertical compaction, the mid-root and cervical canal preparations can be more conservatively executed to conserve radicular structure using .04 tapered files.

In teeth with relatively straight roots and closed apices entire canals can be obturated with the auger technique from apex to pulpal floor (see Fig. 8.15). MTA may better adapt to this technique when it is not too dry, and slightly wetter mixes allow easier delivery to the apical area. The technique can be completed with a 0.04 taper file one or two sizes smaller than the MAF. After delivery of the MTA with a carrier gun to the designated canal, the cement is pushed in with a plugger and the rotary instrument taken to the apical limit using a combined circumferential and pecking action. After the initial 4 to 5 mm is compacted, a paper point can be used to dry the mix if too wet. The compaction can be checked at this stage for location and density. At mid-root, a larger rotary file can be used, applying the same motion to complete the mid-root and cervical area.

A primary consideration with this technique is the apical 2–3 mm that can be difficult to obturate due to the mechanical properties of the files and the consistency of the MTA. This can be a challenge in teeth with abrupt apical curvature or open apices due to inflammatory root resorption or the presence of an immature apex. In cases with abrupt apical curvature, it is recommended that the apical 2–3 mm be packed to the extent of the designated working length using a precurved stainless steel K-file one size smaller than the MAF. When the apical part of the obturation is secure and a radiograph confirms its density and location, the remaining canal can be filled using the auger technique with the

(A)   (B)

(C)   (D)

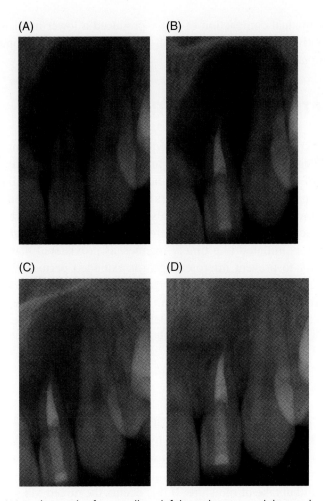

Fig. 8.15 (A) Radiograph of a maxillary left lateral incisor exhibiting dens invaginatus anatomy with a large periapical lesion in 12-year-old male patient. The patient presented with a sinus tract and profound swelling of the buccal vestibule. (B) Post-treatment radiograph after MTA obturation using the auger technique and sealing with a bonded composite core. (C) Postoperative 3 month radiographic review. (D) One-year radiographic recall showing remineralization of the previous periapical pathosis. The patient was asymptomatic with normal function of the tooth.

appropriate NiTi files. Clinical situations where this technique may be contraindicated include severe anatomical challenges or uncontrolled hemorrhaging.

This technique, although relatively new, is potentially safer than ultrasonic placement as less energy is involved. While ultrasonication in a few investigations shows greater density of fill, the chance of overfilling open apices or resorption defects is greater. Moreover, a recent study using microcomputed tomography revealed that manual compaction of MTA produced a lower incidence of voids and significantly denser root fillings than those attained by ultrasonic activation (El-Ma'aita *et al.* 2012).

RESTORATIVE CONSIDERATIONS

In cases where post placement may be required, backfilling the canals with thermoplastic GP or resin-based materials can be considered. This may include the distal canals of mandibular molars, palatal canals of maxillary molars, the long and straight canals of maxillary premolars and canals of anterior teeth. Placement of easily removable obturation materials can be completed after 4–5 mm of MTA is compacted in the apical area. Care should be taken to ensure that restorative treatment is initiated in a timely manner, as provisional materials do not have the ability to prevent microleakage for extended periods (Uranga *et al.* 1999; Balto 2002; Naoum & Chandler 2002; Weston *et al.* 2008). MTA may take considerable time to place in certain teeth and results will depend on case requirements and operator experience. Delivery techniques also require patience and practice and are subject to a learning curve.

DRAWBACKS

A frequently overlooked disadvantage of MTA application is the hygroscopic properties of the material. Since it has a hydrophilic nature, the material will set if precautions are not observed during storage. If the operator intends to use the unused portion of an opened pack, the material must be sealed in an airtight canister to avoid uptake of moisture. If this occurs the mixed MTA appears normal but does not harden. This has led many to believe that the material does not set properly and it is rejected in favor of other materials (Table 8.2).

Setting characteristics have been a hindrance to treatment delivery since most patients and operators want procedures completed in a timely manner. Several

Table 8.2 MTA disadvantages when used in obturation.

Slow setting time
Difficulty in removal during retreatment
May not set in presence of high pH
Discoloration of dentin
Hygroscopic characteristic may increase risk of premature setting
Setting expansion may propagate pre-existing root infractions

methods have been proposed to accelerate the set of MTA and include adding calcium chloride or removing calcium sulfate (Bortoluzzi *et al*. 2009). Recent investigations using different technologies may provide improvements to resolve this problem (M. Torabinejad, personal communication). Drawbacks with fast setting calcium-silicate cements include the possible weakening of interstitial layer formation, lower initial pH and sustained alkalinity for the eradication of microorganisms.

Discoloration of teeth filled with MTA can be an esthetic shortcoming. White MTA still produces some darkening of dentin (Karabucak *et al*. 2005). A technique has been proposed which uses hydrophilic resins to seal the inner chamber prior to MTA obturation and appears to show good results (Akbari *et al*. 2012). Also, MTA may not set properly when used in an acidic environment, compromising the compressive strength, surface hardness and resistance to dislodgement (Watts *et al*. 2007; Namazikhah *et al*. 2008; Hashem *et al*. 2012). If unset material is detected it should be replaced. The cement may be structurally stronger when allowed to harden for longer periods (e.g., 1 week) before placing permanent restorations (Kayahan *et al*. 2009).

Another clinical consideration is the linear expansion of MTA during setting. Teeth diagnosed for retreatment may contain pre-existing undetected radicular infractions from previous post placement, amalgam cores or heavy occlusal loads (Fuss *et al*. 2001; De Bruyne & De Moor 2008). This is particularly important when GMTA is used (Matt *et al*. 2004; Storm *et al*. 2008). In general, MTA obturation must be considered a permanent procedure in teeth with curved roots. Removal of the material can be completed with ultrasonics in straight canals, but removal in curved canals is extremely challenging beyond the curvature (Boutsiokis *et al*. 2008). Teeth which fail to demonstrate periradicular healing after MTA obturation in initial and retreatment cases must be considered for surgical treatment.

SEALERS

Sealer cements are primarily used in combination with a core root filling material such as gutta-percha, for the purpose of obliterating irregularities between the root canal wall and the core material.

Sealers generally:

- lute the core to the canal;
- act as a lubricant;
- have an antimicrobial effect;
- migrate into accessory canals, resorptive defects and other spaces not penetrated by the core material.

The requirements of an ideal sealer are that it be nonirritating, insoluble in tissue fluids, dimensionally stable, provide a hermetic seal, be radiopaque and bacteriostatic, adhere to the canal wall, be nonstaining, have adequate working time, and be easy to remove (Grossman *et al.* 1988).

No current sealer satisfies all these requirements, with many being toxic when newly applied (Spångberg & Langeland 1973) and absorbed when exposed to tissue fluid (Ørstavik 1983), so their volume must be kept to a minimum and entry into the periradicular tissues avoided.

Contemporary sealers may be divided into seven groups:

- zinc oxide–eugenols
- calcium hydroxides
- epoxy resins
- glass ionomers
- silicone-based
- monoblock sealer systems
- calcium silicate sealers.

Zinc oxide–eugenol sealers

Most are based on Grossman's formula (Grossman 1958). All are relatively weak, porous and cytotoxic. Modifications have allowed a variety of setting times and flow characteristics making the group probably the most popular sealers worldwide.

Calcium hydroxide sealers

Calcium hydroxide-based sealers have been developed in order to stimulate healing around the pulp stump and the formation of hard tissue apically (Desai & Chandler 2009b). Their seal is similar to that of zinc oxide-eugenol types (Jacobsen *et al.* 1987) but their solubility raises questions of long term integrity during exposure to tissue fluids (Tronstad *et al.* 1988).

Epoxy resin-based sealers

The first resin sealer, AH 26 (De Trey, Dentsply, Ballaigues, Switzerland), consists of an epoxy resin base which sets slowly when mixed with an activator. It has good sealing, adhesive and antimicrobial properties. The release of formaldehyde explains its strong antibacterial effect (Heling & Chandler 1996). AH 26 has largely been superseded by AH Plus which offers less cytotoxicity, a thinner film thickness and lower solubility.

Glass ionomer sealers

The ability of glass ionomers to adhere to dentin led to research investigations as a potential sealer soon after its introduction as a restorative material (Pitt Ford 1979). It was many years before a manufactured product for endodontic use was formulated, and sealers of this type are no longer available.

Silicone-based sealers

RoekoSeal (Coltène/Whaledent, Altstätten, Switzerland) is a polydimethylsiloxane-based sealer, said to expand 0.2% on setting and to have high radiopacity. A variety of silicone formulations, some combined with gutta-percha particles, are available. A potential concern is extrusion of material beyond the apex (Zielinski *et al.* 2008) although its cytotoxicity is lower than some other sealers.

Monoblock sealer systems

Gutta-percha does not adhere to dentin, so low viscosity composite resins to seal root canals were investigated in the late 1970s (Tidmarsh 1978). The development of a polycaprolactone thermoplastic material with bioactive glass, bismuth and barium salts as fillers now provides an alternative core material to GP (Resilon, Pentron Corp, Wallingford, CT, USA). This may bond to a urethane dimethacrylate (UDMA) based sealer (e.g. Epiphany, Pentron Corp) to create a "monoblock" (Tay & Pashley 2007). With the smear layer removed, a primer is applied and the dual-cured sealer coated onto the dentin wall. Early claims regarding these systems have been questioned. Many factors are involved in their effectiveness, including the nature of the smear layer (if present), dentin permeability, sealer thickness and polymerization contraction. The stability of the polymers over time may also be a concern.

Calcium silicate-based sealers

The most recent innovations in sealers have come with the introduction of calcium silicate or MTA-based sealers. The materials have been characterized as biocompatible and promote the deposition of hydroxyapatite crystalline deposits from amorphous calcium-phosphate precursors along the surface of the root canal (Weller *et al.* 2008; Camilleri 2009; Salles *et al.* 2012). They are designed for use with a core material in cold lateral, warm vertical, or carrier-based techniques, but can be used separately without a core. These contemporary sealers include ProRoot Endo sealer (Maillefer, Ballaigues, Switzerland), MTA Fillapex and MTA Obtura (Angelus, Londria, Brazil), Endo-CPM-Sealer (EGEO S.R.L., Buenos Aires, Argentina), Endosequence BC sealer (Brasseler USA, Savannah, GA), and iRoot SP sealer (Innovative Bioceramix Inc, Vancouver, BC, Canada).

ProRoot Endo sealer includes a powder that contains tricalcium silicate, tricalcium aluminate, and dicalcium silicate, with calcium sulfate as a setting retardant. Bismuth oxide is the radiopacifier. The liquid is a viscous aqueous polyvinyl-pyrrolidone homopolymer (Weller *et al.* 2008). After storage in simulated body fluid, the sealer demonstrated the formation of spherical amorphous calcium-like phases and apatite-like phases in ex vivo specimens. Similarly, an experimental MTA sealer with a water-soluble polymer revealed sealer release of calcium ions in solution that encouraged the deposition of calcium phosphate crystals when in contact with distilled water or a physiological solution (Camilleri 2009; Massi *et al.* 2011; Camilleri *et al.* 2011).

iRoot SP sealer is another newly introduced calcium silicate-based sealer with desirable properties such as apatite formation. This mineralization phenomenon also occurs with Endosequence BC Sealer (Candeiro *et al.* 2012), Endo-CPM-Sealer (Gomes-Filho *et al.* 2009), and MTA Fillapex (Salles *et al.* 2012). Calcium silicate-based sealers are also typically characterized by high viscosity and small particle size that allows excellent adaptation to dentin and they have shown superior bond strengths at the middle and apical third of extracted teeth (Huffman *et al.* 2009; Ersahan & Avdin 2010; Sagsen *et al.* 2011). The favorable biocompatibility and physiochemical properties of calcium silicate/MTA based sealers may provide superior outcomes in conventional root canal obturation and their future development and implementation appears promising.

SUMMARY

MTA exhibits many desirable physiochemical properties when used as a root canal filling material and may promote improved healing rates for compromised teeth. The bioactive properties of MTA encourage osteoblast cell differentiation and bone deposition, stimulate cementum repair and promote periodontal ligament reformation. MTA as an obturation material offers superior characteristics that include the formation of an interstitial layer at the dentin interface, superior sealability and the provision of a sustained alkaline pH during the slow setting process. Moreover, the fine particle size penetrates dentinal tubules and may inhibit the growth of *E. faecalis*, *C. albicans*, and other opportunistic pathogens.

The unique features of this hydraulic calcium-silicate cement can provide an important advantage when treating refractory endodontic cases compromised by substandard orthograde and retrograde treatment, restorative microleakage, inflammatory root resorption, anatomical anomalies, and teeth that exhibit immature apices. The cement also provides a technique for conventional obturation or for cases where alternative filling materials are indicated. MTA at its present stage of development is not the ideal root canal filling material. However, when used alone or combined with surgical treatment, MTA obturation can provide an opportunity for improved healing rates in patients with challenging and complex endodontic conditions.

REFERENCES

Abedi, H.R., Ingle, J.I. (1995) Mineral Trioxide Aggregate: a review of a new cement. *Journal of the Californian Dental Association* **23**, 36–9.

Abou-Rass, M., Bogen, G. (1998) Microorganisms in closed periapical lesions. *International Endodontic Journal* **31**, 39–47.

Aggarwal, V., Singla, M. (2010) Management of inflammatory root resorption using MTA obturation - a four year follow up. *British Dental Journal* **208**, 287–9.

Akbari, M., Rouhani, A., Samiee S., *et al.* (2012) Effect of dentin bonding agent on the prevention of tooth discoloration produced by mineral trioxide aggregate. *International Journal of Dentistry* 2012:563203.

Alani, A., Bishop, K. (2009) The use of MTA in the modern management of teeth affected by dens invaginatus. *International Dental Journal* **59**, 343–8.

Al-Hezaimi, K., Naghshbandi, J., Oglesby, S., *et al.* (2005) Human saliva penetration of root canals obturated with two types of mineral trioxide aggregate. *Journal of Endodontics* **31**, 453–6.

Al-Hezaimi, K., Naghshbandi, J., Oglesby, S., *et al.* (2006a) Comparison of antifungal activity of white-colored and gray colored mineral trioxide aggregate (MTA) at similar concentrations against Candida albicans. *Journal of Endodontics* **32**, 365–7.

Al-Hezaimi, K., Al-Shalan, TA., Naghshbandi, J., *et al.* (2006b) Antibacterial effect of two mineral trioxide aggregate (MTA) preparations against *Enterococcus faecalis* and *Streptococcus sanguis* in vitro. *Journal of Endodontics* **32**, 1053–6.

Al-Kahtani, A., Shostad, S., Schifferle, R., *et al.* (2005) In-vitro evaluation of microleakage of an orthograde apical plug of mineral trioxide aggregate in permanent teeth with simulated immature apices. *Journal of Endodontics* **31**, 117–19.

Al-Nazhan, S., Al-Judai, A. (2003) Evaluation of antifungal activity of mineral trioxide aggregate. *Journal of Endodontics* **29**, 826–7.

Anantula, K., Ganta, A.K. (2011) Evaluation and comparison of sealing ability of three different obturation techniques - Lateral condensation, Obtura II, and GuttaFlow: An in vitro study. *Journal of Conservative Dentistry* **14**, 57–61.

Andelin, W.E., Browning, D.F., Hsu G.H., *et al.* (2002) Microleakage of resected MTA. *Journal of Endodontics* **28**, 573–4.

Andreasen, J.O., Farik, B., Munksgaard, E.C. (2002) Long-term calcium hydroxide as a root canal dressing may increase risk of root fracture. *Dental Traumatology* **18**, 134–137.

Ari, H., Belli, S., Gunes, B. (2010) Sealing ability of Hybrid Root SEAL (MetaSEAL) in conjunction with different obturation techniques. *Oral Surgery Oral Medicine Oral Pathology Oral Radiolology and Endodontics* **109**, e113–e116.

Asgary, S., Parirokh, M., Engbal, M.J., *et al.* (2006) A qualitative X-ray analysis of white and grey mineral trioxide aggregate using compositional imaging. *The Journal of Materials Science: Materials in Medicine* **17**, 187–91.

Balto, H. (2002) An assessment of microbial coronal leakage of temporary materials in endodontically treated teeth. *Journal of Endodontics* **28**, 762–4.

Bogen, G., Kuttler, S. (2009) Mineral trioxide aggregate obturation: a review and case series. *Journal of Endodontics* **35**, 777–90.

Bogen, G., Chandler N. (2008) Vital pulp therapy. In: *Ingle's Endodontics*, 6th edn (eds. Ingle, J.I., Bakland L.K., Baumgartner, J.C.). BC Decker Inc, Hamilton, Ontario, pp.1310–1329.

Bortoluzzi, E.A., Souza, E.M., Reis, J.M., *et al.* (2007) Fracture strength of bovine incisors after intra-radicular treatment with MTA in an experimental immature tooth model. *International Endodontic Journal* **40**, 684–91.

Bortoluzzi, E.A., Broon, N.J., Bramante, C.M., *et al.* (2009) The influence of calcium chloride on the setting time, solubility, disintegration, and pH of mineral trioxide aggregate and white Portland cement with a radiopacifier. *Journal of Endodontics* **35**, 550–4.

Boutsioukis, C., Noula, G., Lambrianidis, T. (2008) Ex vivo study of the efficiency of two techniques for the removal of mineral trioxide aggregate used as a root canal filling material. *Journal of Endodontics* **34**, 1239–42.

Bozeman, T.B., Lemon, R.R., Eleazer, P.D. (2006) Elemental analysis of crystal precipitate from gray and white MTA. *Journal of Endodontics* **32**, 425–8.

Branchs, D., Trope, M. (2004) Revascularization of immature permanent teeth with apical periodontitis: New treatment protocol? *Journal of Endodontics* **30**, 196–200.

Budig, C.G., Eleazer, P.D. (2008) In vitro comparison of the setting of dry ProRoot MTA by moisture absorbed through the root. *Journal of Endodontics* **34**, 712–14.

Camilleri, J. (2007) Hydration mechanisms of mineral trioxide aggregate. *International Endodontic Journal* **40**, 462–70.

Camilleri, J. (2008a) The chemical composition of mineral trioxide aggregate. *Journal of Conservative Dentistry* **11**, 141–3.

Camilleri, J. (2008b) Characterization of hydration products of mineral trioxide aggregate. *International Endodontic Journal* **41**, 408–17.

Camilleri, J. (2009) Evaluation of selected properties of mineral trioxide aggregate sealer cement. *Journal of Endodontics* **35**, 1412–17.

Camilleri, J., Montesin, F.E., Brady, K., *et al.* (2005) The constitution of mineral trioxide aggregate. *Dental Materials* **21**, 297–303.

Camilleri, J., Gandolfik, M.G., Siboni, F., *et al.* (2011) Dynamic sealing ability of MTA root canal sealer. *International Endodontic Journal* **44**, 9–20.

Candeiro, G.T., Correia, F.C., Duarte, M.A., *et al.* (2012) Evaluation of radiopacity, pH, release of calcium ions, and flow of a bioceramic root canal sealer. *Journal of Endodontics* **38**, 842–5.

Carrotte, P. (2004) Endodontics: Part 8. Filling the root canal system. *British Dental Journal* **197**, 667–72.

Cho, S.Y. (2005) Supernumerary premolars associated with dens evaginatus: report of 2 cases. *Journal of the Canadian Dental Association* **71**, 390–3.

Chogle, S., Mickel, A.K., Chan, D.M., *et al.* (2007) Intracanal assessment of mineral trioxide aggregate setting and sealing properties. *General Dentistry* **55**, 306–11.

Cotton, T.P., Schindler, W.G., Schwartz, S.A., *et al.* (2008) A retrospective study comparing clinical outcomes after obturation with Resilon/Epiphany or gutta-percha/Kerr sealer. *Journal of Endodontics* **34**,789–97.

Dammaschke, T., Gerth, H.U., Zuchner, H., *et al.* (2005) Chemical and physical surface and bulk material characterization of white ProRoot MTA and two Portland cements. *Dental Materials* **21**, 731–8.

D'Arcangelo, C., D'Amario, M. (2007) Use of MTA for orthograde obturation of nonvital teeth with open apices: report of two cases. *Oral Surgery Oral Medicine Oral Pathology Oral Radiology Endodontics* **104**, e98–e101.

De Bruyne, M.A., De Moor, R.J. (2008) Influence of cracks on leakage and obturation efficiency of root-end filling materials after ultrasonic preparation: an in vitro evaluation. *Quintessence International* **39**, 685–92.

de Leimburg, M.L., Angeretti, A., Ceruti P., *et al.* (2004) MTA obturation of pulpless teeth with open apices: bacterial leakage as detected by polymerase chain reaction assay. *Journal of Endodontics* **30**, 883–6.

de Lima, M.V., Bramante, C.M., Garcia, R.B., *et al.* (2007) Endodontic treatment of dens in dente associated with a chronic periapical lesion using an apical plug of mineral trioxide aggregate. *Quintessence International*, e124–e128.

Desai, S., Chandler, N. (2009a) The restoration of permanent immature anterior teeth, root filled using MTA: A review. *Journal of Dentistry* **37**, 652–7.

Desai, S., Chandler, N. (2009b) Calcium hydroxide-based root canal sealers: a review. *Journal of Endodontics* **35**, 475–80.

Dreger, L.A., Felippe, W.T., Reyes-Carmona, J.F., *et al.* (2012) Mineral trioxide aggregate and Portland cement promote biomineralization in vivo. *Journal of Endodontics* **38**, 324–9.

Duarte, M.A., Demarchi, A.C., Yamashita, J.C., *et al.* (2003) pH and calcium ion release of 2 root-end filling materials. *Oral Surgery Oral Medicine Oral Pathology Oral Radiolology and Endodontics* **95**, 345–7.

El-Ma'aita, A.M., Qualtrough, A.J., Watts, D.C. (2012) A micro-computed tomography evaluation of mineral trioxide aggregate root canal fillings. *Journal of Endodontics* **38**, 670–2.

Ersahan, S., Aydin, C. (2010) Dislocation resistance of iRoot SP, a calcium silicate-based sealer, from radicular dentine. *Journal of Endodontics* **36**, 2000–2.

Felippe, M.C., Felippe, W.T., Marques, M.M., *et al.* (2005). The effect of the renewal of calcium hydroxide paste on the apexification and periapical healing of teeth with incomplete root formation. *International Endodontic Journal*, 436–42.

Fridland, M., Rosado, R. (2005) MTA solubility: a long term study. *Journal of Endodontics*, 376–9.

Friedman, S. (2008) Expected outcomes in the prevention and treatment of apical periodontitis. In: *Essential Endodontology: Prevention and Treatment of Apical Periodontitis*, 2nd edn. (eds. Ørstavik, D., Pitt Ford, T.R.). Blackwell Science, Oxford, pp. 408–69.

Fuss, Z., Lustig, J., Katz, A., *et al.* (2001) An evaluation of endodontically treated vertical root fractured teeth: impact of operative procedures. *Journal of Endodontics* **27**, 46–8.

Garberoglio, R., Brännström, M. (1976) Scanning electron microscopic investigation of human dentinal tubules. *Archives of Oral Biology* **21**, 355–62.

Giuliani, V., Baccetti, T., Pace R., *et al.* (2002) The use of MTA in teeth with necrotic pulps and open apices. *Dental Traumatology* **18**, 217–21.

Glick, D.H., Frank, A.L. (1986) Removal of silver points and fractured posts by ultrasonics. *Journal of Prosthetic Dentistry* **55**, 212–15.

Gomes-Filho, J.E., Watanabe, S., Bernabé, P.F., *et al.* (2009) A mineral trioxide aggregate sealer stimulated mineralization. *Journal of Endodontics* **35**, 256–60.

Gondim, E. Jr., Zaia, A.A., Gomez, B.P.F.A., *et al.* (2003) Investigation of the marginal adaptation of root-end filling materials in root-end cavities prepared with ultrasonic tips. *International Endodontic Journal* **36**, 491–9.

Greenstein, G., Cavallaro, J., Tarnow, D. (2008) When to save or extract a tooth in the esthetic zone: a commentary. *Compendium of Continuing Education in Dentistry* **29**, 136–45.

Grigoratos, D., Knowles, J., Ng, Y.L., *et al.* (2001) Effect of exposing dentine to sodium hypochlorite and calcium hydroxide on its flexural strength and elastic modulus. *International Endodontic Journal* **34**, 113–19.

Grossman, L.I. (1958) An improved root canal cement. *Journal of the American Dental Association* **56**, 381– 5.

Grossman, L.I. (1982) *Endodontic Practice*, 10th edn. Lea and Febiger, Philadelphia, p. 279.

Grossman L.I., Oliet, S., del Rio C.E. (1988) *Endodontic Practice*, 11th edn. Lea and Febiger, Philadelphia, pp. 242–270.

Guess, G.M. (2008) An alternative to gutta-percha for root canal obturation. *Dentistry Today* **27**, 84, 86, 88.

Güneş, B., Aydinbelge, H.A. (2012) Mineral trioxide aggregate apical plug method for the treatment of nonvital immature permanent maxillary incisors: Three case reports. *Journal of Conservative Dentistry* **15**, 73–6.

Hammad, M., Qualtrough, A., Silikas, N. (2009) Evaluation of root canal obturation: a three-dimensional in vitro study. *Journal of Endodontics* **35**, 541–4.

Hashem, A.A., Wanees Amin, S.A. (2012) The effect of acidity on dislodgment resistance of mineral trioxide aggregate and BioAggregate in furcation perforations: an in vitro comparative study. *Journal of Endodontics* **38**, 245–9.

Hatibović-Kofman, S., Raimundo, L., Zheng, L., *et al.* (2008) Fracture resistance and histological findings of immature teeth treated with mineral trioxide aggregate. *Dental Traumatology* **24**, 272–6.

Hawley, M., Webb, T.D., Goodell, G.G. (2010) Effect of varying water-to-powder ratios on the setting expansion of white and gray mineral trioxide aggregate. *Journal of Endodontics* **36**, 1377–9.

Heling, I., Chandler, N.P. (1996) The antimicrobial effect within dentinal tubules of four root canal sealers. *Journal of Endodontics* **22**, 257–9.

Holland, R., DeSouza V, Nery MJ., *et al.* (1999a) Reaction of rat connective tissue to implanted dentin tubes filled with mineral trioxide aggregate or calcium hydroxide. *Journal of Endodontics* **35**, 703–5.

Holland, R., de Souza, V., Nery, M.J., *et al.* (1999b) Reaction of dogs' teeth to root filling with mineral trioxide aggregate or a glass ionomer sealer. *Journal of Endodontics* **25**, 728–30.

Holland, R., Filho, J.A.O., de Souza, V., *et al.* (2001) Mineral trioxide aggregate repair of lateral root perforations. *Journal of Endodontics* **27**, 281–4.

Holland, R., de Souza, V., Nery, MJ., *et al.* (2002) Calcium salts deposition in rat connective tissue after the implantation of calcium hydroxide-containing sealers. *Journal of Endodontics* **28**, 173–6.

Holt, D.M., Watts, J.D., Beeson, T.J., *et al.* (2007) The anti-microbial effect against *Enterococcus faecalis* and the compressive strength of two types of mineral trioxide aggregate mixed with sterile water or 2% chlorhexidine liquid. *Journal of Endodontics* **33**, 844–7.

Huang, G.T., Sonoyama, W., Liu, Y., *et al.* (2008) The hidden treasure in apical papilla: the potential role in pulp/dentin regeneration and bioroot engineering. *Journal of Endodontics* **34**, 645–51.

Huffman, B.P., Mai, S., Pinna, L., *et al.* (2009) Dislocation resistance of ProRoot Endo Sealer, a calcium silicate-based root canal sealer, from radicular dentine. *International Endodontic Journal* **42**, 34–46.

Jacobovitz, M., Vianna, M.E., Pandolfelli, V.C., *et al.* (2009) Root canal filling with cements based on mineral aggregates: an in vitro analysis of bacterial microleakage. *Oral Surgery Oral Medicine Oral Pathology Oral Radiolology and Endodontics* **108**, 140–144.

Jacobsen, E.L., BeGole, E.A., Vitkus, D.D., *et al.* (1987) An evaluation of two newly formulated calcium hydroxide cements: a leakage study. *Journal of Endodontics* **13**, 164–9.

Jacobson, H.L., Xia, T., Baumgartner, J.C., *et al.* (2002) Microbial leakage evaluation of the continuous wave of condensation. *Journal of Endodontics* **28**, 269–71.

Kaffe, I., Tamse, A., Littner, M.M., *et al.* (1984) A radiographic survey of apical root resorption in pulpless permanent teeth. *Oral Surgery Oral Medicine Oral Pathology* **58**, 109–12.

Karabucak, B., Li, D., Lim, J., *et al.* (2005) Vital pulp therapy with mineral trioxide aggregate. *Dental Traumatology* **21**, 240–3.

Kato, H., Nakagawa, K. (2010) FP core carrier technique: thermoplasticized gutta-percha root canal obturation technique using polypropylene core. *Bulletin of the Tokyo Dental College* **51**, 213–20.

Kayahan, M.B., Nekoofar, M.H., Kazandağ, M., *et al.* (2009) Effect of acid-etching procedure on selected physical properties of mineral trioxide aggregate. *International Endodontic Journal* **42**, 1004–14.

Khayat, A., Lee, S.J., Torabinejad, M. (1993) Human saliva penetration of coronally unsealed obturated root canals. *Journal of Endodontics* **19**, 458–61.

Koh, E.T., Ford, T.R., Kariyawasam, S.P., *et al.* (2001) Prophylactic treatment of dens evaginatus using mineral trioxide aggregate. *Journal of Endodontics* **27**, 540–2.

Komabayashi, T., Spångberg, L.S. (2008a) Comparative analysis of the particle size and shape of commercially available mineral trioxide aggregates and Portland cement: a study with a flow particle image analyzer. *Journal of Endodontics* **34**, 94–8.

Komabayashi, T., Spångberg, L.S. (2008b) Particle size and shape analysis of MTA finer fractions using Portland cement. *Journal of Endodontics* **34**, 709–11.

Kvist, T., Reit, C. (2000) Postoperative discomfort associated with surgical and nonsurgical endodontic retreatment. *Endodontics and Dental Traumatology* **16**, 71–4.

Lamb, E.L., Loushine, R.J., Weller, R., *et al.* (2003) Effect of root resection on the apical sealing ability of mineral trioxide aggregate. *Oral Surgery Oral Medicine Oral Pathology Oral Radiology Endodontics* **95**, 732–5.

Laux, M., Abbott, P.V., Pajarola, G., *et al.* (2000) Apical inflammatory root resorption: a correlative radiographic and histological assessment. *International Endodontic Journal* **33**, 483–93.

Lee, S.J., Monsef, M., Torabinejad, M. (1993) The sealing ability of a mineral trioxide aggregate for repair of lateral root perforations. *Journal of Endodontics* **19**, 541–4.

Lee, Y.L., Lee, B.S., Lin F.H., *et al.* (2004) Effects of physiological environments on the hydration behaviour of mineral trioxide aggregate. *Biomaterials* **25**, 787–93.

Lin, S., Platner, O., Metzger, Z., *et al.* (2008) Residual bacteria in root apices removed by a diagonal root-end resection: a histopathological evaluation. *International Endodontic Journal* **41**, 469–75.

Love, R.M., Jenkinson, H.F. (2002) Invasion of dentinal tubules by oral bacteria. *Critical Reviews in Oral Biology and Medicine* **13**, 171–83.

Madison, S., Wilcox, L.R. (1988) An evaluation of coronal microleakage in endodontically treated teeth. Part III. In vivo study. *Journal of Endodontics* **14**, 455–8.

Main, C., Mirzayan, N., Shabahang, S., *et al.* (2004) Repair of root perforations using mineral trioxide aggregate: a long-term study. *Journal of Endodontics* **30**, 80–3.

Malagnino, V.A., Rossi-Fedele, G., Passariello, P., *et al.* (2011) 'Simultaneous technique' and a hybrid Microseal/PacMac obturation. *Dental Update* **38**, 477–8, 481–2, 484.

Massi, S., Tanomaru-Filho, M., Silva, G.F., *et al.* (2011) pH, calcium ion release, and setting time of an experimental mineral trioxide aggregate-based root canal sealer. *Journal of Endodontics* **37**, 844–6.

Matt, G.D., Thorpe, J.R., Strother, J.M., *et al.* (2004) Comparative study of white and gray mineral trioxide aggregate (MTA) simulating a one- or two-step apical barrier technique. *Journal of Endodontics* **30**, 876–9.

McKissock, A.J., Mines, P., Sweet, M.B., *et al.* (2011) Ten-month in vitro leakage study of a single-cone obturation system. *US Army Medical Department Journal* Jan–Mar, 42–7.

Mohammadi, Z., Modaresi, J., Yazdizadeh, M. (2006) Evaluation of the antifungal effects of mineral trioxide aggregate materials. *Australian Endodontic Journal* **32**, 120–2.

Molander, A., Reit, C., Dahlen, G., *et al.* (1998) Microbiological status of root-filled teeth with apical periodontitis. *International Endodontic Journal* **31**, 1–7.

Namazikhah, M.S., Nekoofar, M.H., Sheykhrezae, M.S., *et al.* (2008) The effect of pH on surface hardness and microstructure of mineral trioxide aggregate. *International Endodontic Journal* **41**, 108–16.

Nair, P.N., Henry, S., Cano V., *et al.* (2005) Microbial status of apical root canal system of human mandibular first molars with primary apical periodontitis after "one-visit" endodontic treatment. *Oral Surgery Oral Medicine Oral Pathology Oral Radiology Endodontics* **99**, 231–52.

Naoum, H., Chandler, N.P. (2002) Temporization for endodontics. *International Endodontic Journal* **35**, 964–78.

Nayar, S., Bishop, K., Alani, A. (2009) A report on the clinical and radiographic outcomes of 38 cases of apexification with mineral trioxide aggregate. *European Journal of Prosthodontics and Restorative Dentistry* **17**, 150–6.

Noguchi, N., Noiri, Y., Narimatsu, M., *et al.* (2005) Identification and localization of extraradicular biofilm-forming bacteria associated with refractory endodontic pathogens. *Applied Environmental Microbiology* **71**, 8738–43.

Okiji, T., Yoshiba, K. (2009) Reparative dentinogenesis induced by mineral trioxide aggregate: A review from the biological and physicochemical points of view. *International Journal of Dentistry* 464280.

Ordinola-Zapata, R., Bramante, C.M., Bernardineli, N., *et al.* (2009) A preliminary study of the percentage of sealer penetration in roots obturated with the Thermafil and RealSeal-1 obturation techniques in mesial root canals of mandibular molars. *Oral Surgery Oral Medicine Oral Pathology Oral Radiology Endodontics* **108**, 961–8.

O'Sullivan, S.M., Hartwell, G.R. (2001) Obturation of a retained primary mandibular second molar using mineral trioxide aggregate: a case report. *Journal of Endodontics* **27**, 703–5.

Ørstavik, D. (1983) Weight loss of endodontic sealers, cements and pastes in water. *Scandinavian Journal of Dental Research* **91**, 316–19.

Ørstavik, D., Haapasalo, M. (1990) Disinfection by endodontic irrigants and dressings of experimentally infected dentinal tubules. *Endodontics and Dental Traumatology* **6**, 142–9.

Ozdemir, H.O., Oznelik, B., Karabucak, B., *et al.* (2008) Calcium ion diffusion from mineral trioxide aggregate through simulated root resorption defects. *Dental Traumatology* **24**, 70–3.

Pace, R., Giuliani, V., Pagavino, G. (2008) Mineral trioxide aggregate as repair material for furcal perforation: case series. *Journal of Endodontics* **34**, 1130–3.

Pameijer, C.H., Zmener, O. (2010) Resin materials for root canal obturation. *Dental Clinics of North America* **54**, 325–44.

Parirokh, M., Torabinejad, M. (2010) Mineral trioxide aggregate: A comprehensive literature review – Part 1: Chemical, physical, and antibacterial properties. *Journal of Endodontics* **36**, 16–27.

Pawińska, M., Kierklo, A., Tokajuk, G., *et al.* (2011) New endodontic obturation systems and their interfacial bond strength with intraradicular dentine – ex vivo studies. *Advances in Medical Science* **22**, 1–7.

Peciuliene, V., Reynaud, A.H., Balciuniene, I., *et al.* (2001) Isolation of yeasts and enteric bacteria in root-filled teeth with chronic apical periodontitis. *International Endodontic Journal* **34**, 429–34.

Peters, L.B., Wesselink, P.R., Buijs, JF., *et al.* (2001) Viable bacteria in root dentinal tubules of teeth with apical periodontitis. *Journal of Endodontics* **27**, 76–81.

Pinheiro, E.T., Gomes, B.P., Ferraz, C.C., *et al.* (2003) Evaluation of root canal microorganisms isolated from teeth with endodontic failure and their antimicrobial susceptibility. *Oral Microbiology and Immunology* **18**, 100–3.

Pitt Ford, T.R. (1979) The leakage of root fillings using glass ionomer cement and other materials. *British Dental Journal* **146**, 273–8.

Pitt Ford, T.R., Torabinejad. M., McKendry, D.J., *et al.* (1995) Use of mineral trioxide aggregate for repair of furcal perforations. *Oral Surgery Oral Medicine Oral Pathology Oral Radiology Endodontics* **79**, 756–63.

Rao, Y.G., Guo, L.Y., Tao, H.T. (2010) Multiple dens evaginatus of premolars and molars in Chinese dentition: a case report and literature review. *International Journal of Oral Science* **2**, 177–80.

Ray, H.A., Trope, M. (1995) Periapical status of endodontically treated teeth in relationship to the technical quality of the root filling and the coronal restoration. *International Endodontic Journal* **28**, 12–18.

Reyes-Carmona, J.F., Felippe, M.S., Felippe, W.T. (2009) Biomineralization ability and interaction of mineral trioxide aggregate and white Portland cement with dentin in a phosphate-containing fluid. *Journal of Endodontics* **35**, 731–6.

Ribeiro, C.S., Kuteken, F.A., Hirata Júnior, R., *et al.* (2006) Comparative evaluation of antimicrobial action of MTA, calcium hydroxide and Portland cement. *Journal of Applied Oral Science* **14**, 330–3.

Ricucci, D., Siqueira, J.F. Jr. (2010) Biofilms and apical periodontitis: study of prevalence and association with clinical and histopathologic findings. *Journal of Endodontics* **36**, 1277–88.

Roberts, H.W., Toth, J.M., Berzins, D.W., *et al.* (2008) Mineral Trioxide Aggregate use in endodontic treatment: A review of the literature. *Dental Materials* **24**, 149–64.

Roig, M., Espona, J., Mercadé, M., *et al.* (2011) Horizontal root fracture treated with MTA, a case report with a 10-year follow-up. *Dental Traumatology* **27**, 460–3.

Salles, L.P., Gomes-Cornélio, A.L., Guimarães, F.C., *et al.* (2012) Mineral Trioxide Aggregate-based endodontic sealer stimulates hydroxyapatite nucleation in human osteoblast-like cell culture. *Journal of Endodontics* **38**, 971–6.

Sagsen, B., Ustün, Y., Demirbuga, S., *et al.* (2011) Push-out bond strength of two new calcium silicate-based endodontic sealers to root canal dentine. *International Endodontic Journal* **44**, 1088–91.

Santos, A.D., Moraes, J.C.S., Araújo, E.B., *et al.* (2005) Physico-chemical properties of MTA and a novel experimental cement. *International Endodontic Journal* **38**, 443–7.

Sarkar, N.K., Caicedo, R., Ritwik, P., *et al.* (2005) Physicochemical basis of the biologic properties of mineral trioxide aggregate. *Journal of Endodontics* **31**, 97–100.

Saunders, W.P., Saunders, E.M. (1994) Coronal leakage as a cause of failure in root canal therapy: a review. *Endodontics and Dental Traumatology* **10**, 105–8.

Savariz, A., González-Rodríguez, M.P., Ferrer-Luque, C.M. (2010) Long-term sealing ability of GuttaFlow versus AH Plus using different obturation techniques. *Medicina Oral Patología Oral y Cirugía Bucal* **15**, e936–e941.

Schlenker, M. (1880) Das füellen der wurzelkanäle mit Portland-cement nach Dr. Witte. *Deutsche Vierteljahrsschrift fuer Zahnheilkunde* **20**, 277–83 [in German].

Seltzer, S., Green, D.B., Weiner, N., *et al.* (2004) A scanning electron microscope examination of silver cones removed from endodontically treated teeth. *Journal of Endodontics* **30**, 463–74.

Sen, B.H., Piskin, B., Demirici, T. (1995) Observation of bacteria and fungi in infected root canals and dentinal tubules by SEM. *Endodontics and Dental Traumatology* **11**, 6–9.

Shabahang, S., Torabinejad, M. (2000) Treatment of teeth with open apices using mineral trioxide aggregate. *Practical Periodontics and Aesthetic Dentistry* **12**, 315–20.

Sim, T.P.C., Knowles, J.C., Ng Y-L., *et al.* (2001) Effect of sodium hypochlorite on mechanical properties of dentine and tooth surface strain. *International Endodontic Journal* **34**, 120–32.

Siqueira, J.F. Jr., Sen, B.H. (2004) Fungi in endodontic infections. *Oral Surgery Oral Medicine Oral Pathology Oral Radiology Endodontics* **97**, 632–41.

Siqueira, J.F. Jr., Lopes, H.P. (2001) Bacteria on the apical root surfaces of untreated teeth with periradicular lesions: a scanning electron microscopy study. *International Endodontic Journal* **34** 216–20.

Siqueira, J.F. Jr., Rocas, I.N. (2004) Polymerase chain reaction-based analysis of microorganisms associated with failed endodontic treatment. *Oral Surgery Oral Medicine Oral Pathology Oral Radiology Endodontics* **97**, 85–94.

Siqueira, J.F. Jr, Rôças, I.N., Favieri, A., *et al.* (2000) Bacterial leakage in coronally unsealed root canals obturated with 3 different techniques. *Oral Surgery Oral Medicine Oral Pathology Oral Radiology Endodontics* **90**, 647–50.

Spångberg, L., Langeland, K. (1973) Biologic effects of dental materials. 1. Toxicity of root canal filling materials on HeLa cells in vitro. *Oral Surgery, Oral Medicine, Oral Pathology* **35**, 402–14.

Storm, B., Eichmiller, F., Tordik, P., *et al.* (2008) Setting expansion of gray and white mineral trioxide aggregate and Portland cement. *Journal of Endodontics* **34**, 80–2.

Stowe, T.J., Sedgley, C.M., Stowe, B., *et al.* (2004) The effects of chlorhexidine gluconate (0.12%) on the antimicrobial properties of tooth-colored ProRoot mineral trioxide aggregate. *Journal of Endodontics* **30**, 429–31.

Stuart, C.H., Schwartz, S.A., Beeson, T.J., *et al.* (2006) Enterococcus faecalis: its role in root canal treatment failure and current concepts in retreatment. *Journal of Endodontics* **32**, 93–8.

Sunde, P.T., Tronstad, L., Eribe, E.R., *et al.* (2000) Assessment of periradicular microbiota by DNA-DNA hybridization. *Endodontics and Dental Traumatology* **16**, 191–6.

Sundqvist, G., Figdor, D. (1998) Endodontic treatment of apical periodontitis. In: *Essential Endodontology: Prevention and Treatment of Apical Periodontitis*, 1ˢᵗ edn (eds. Ørstavik, D., Pitt Ford, T.R.). Blackwell, Oxford, pp. 242–277.

Swanson, K., Madison, S. (1987) An evaluation of coronal microleakage in endodontically treated teeth. *Part I. Time periods. Journal of Endodontics* **13**, 56–9.

Tahan, E., Celik, D., Er, K., *et al.* (2010) Effect of unintentionally extruded mineral trioxide aggregate in treatment of tooth with periradicular lesion: a case report. *Journal of Endodontics* **36**, 760–3.

Tanomaru-Filho, M., Jorge, E.G., Guerreiro Tanomaru, J.M., *et al.* (2007) Radiopacity evaluation of new root canal filling materials by digitalization of images. *Journal of Endodontics* **33**, 249–51.

Takemura, N., Noiri, Y., Ehara, A., *et al.* (2004) Single species biofilm-forming ability of root canal isolates on gutta-percha points. *European Journal of Oral Science* **112**, 523–9.

Tay. F.R., Pashley, D.H. (2007) Monoblocks in root canals: a hypothetical or a tangible goal. *Journal of Endodontics* **33**, 391–8.

Tay, F.R., Pashley, D.H., Rueggerberg, F.A., *et al.* (2007) Calcium phosphate phase transformation produced by the interaction of the Portland cement component of white MTA with a phosphate-containing fluid. *Journal of Endodontics* **33**, 1347–51.

Taylor, H.F.N. (1997) *Cement Chemistry*, 2nd edn. Thomas Telford, London.

Tidmarsh, B.G. (1978) Acid-cleansed and resin-sealed root canals. *Journal of Endodontics* **4**, 117–21.

Tjaderhane, L. (2009) The role of matrix metalloproteinases and their inhibitors in root fracture resistance remains unknown. *Dental Traumatology* **25**, 142–3.

Topcuoğlu, H.S., Arsian, H., Keles, A., *et al.* (2012) Fracture resistance of roots filled with three different obturation techniques. *Medicina Oral Patología Oral y Cirugía Bucal*, **17**, e528–e532.

Torabinejad, M., Chivian, N. (1999) Clinical applications of mineral trioxide aggregate. *Journal of Endodontics* **25**, 197–205.

Torabinejad, M., Watson, T.F., Pitt Ford, T.R. (1993) The sealing ability of a mineral trioxide aggregate as a retrograde root filling material. *Journal of Endodontics* **19**, 591–5.

Torabinejad, M., Hong, C.U., McDonald, F., *et al.* (1995a) Physical and chemical properties of a new root-end filling material. *Journal of Endodontics* **21**, 349–53.

Torabinejad, M., Smith, P.W., Kettering, J.D., *et al.* (1995b) Comparative investigation of marginal adaptation of mineral trioxide aggregate and other commonly used root-end filling materials. *Journal of Endodontics* **21**, 295–9.

Torabinejad, M., Falah, R., Kettering, J.D., *et al.* (1995c) Comparative leakage of mineral trioxide aggregate as a root end filling material. *Journal of Endodontics* **21**, 109–21.

Tronstad, L., Barnett, F., Flax, M. (1988) Solubility and biocompatibility of calcium hydroxide-containing root canal sealers. *Endodontics and Dental Traumatology* **4**, 152–9.

Tronstad, L., Barnett, F., Cervone, F. (1990) Periapical bacterial plaque in teeth refractory to endodontic treatment. *Endodontics and Dental Traumatology* **6**, 73–7.

Tronstad, L., Asbjørnsen, K., Døving, L., *et al.* (2000) Influence of coronal restorations on the periapical health of endodontically treated teeth. *Endodontics and Dental Traumatology* **16**, 218–21.

Tsai, Y.L., Lan, W.H., Jeng, J.H. (2006) Treatment of pulp floor and stripping perforation by mineral trioxide aggregate. *Journal of the Formosan Medical Association* **105**, 522–6.

Tuna, E.B., Dinçol, M.E., Gençay, K., *et al.* (2011) Fracture resistance of immature teeth filled with BioAggregate, mineral trioxide aggregate and calcium hydroxide. *Dental Traumatology* **27**, 174–8.

Uranga, A., Blum, J.Y., Esber, S., *et al.* (1999) A comparative study of four coronal obturation materials in endodontic treatment. *Journal of Endodontics* **25**, 178–80.

Versiani, M..A., Sousa-Neto, M.D., Pécora, J.D. (2011) Pulp pathosis in inlayed teeth of the ancient Mayas: a microcomputed tomography study. *International Endodontic Journal* **44**, 1000–4.

Vier, F.V., Figueiredo, J.A. (2002) Prevalence of different periapical lesions associated with human teeth and their correlation with the presence and extension of apical external root resorption. *International Endodontic Journal* **35**, 710–19.

Vier, F.V., Figueiredo, J.A. (2004) Internal apical resorption and its correlation with the type of apical lesion. *International Endodontic Journal* **37**, 730–7.

Waltimo, T.M., Sen, B.H., Meurman, J.H., *et al.* (2003) Yeasts in apical periodontitis. *Critical Reviews in Oral Biology and Medicine* **14**, 128–37.

Watts, J.D., Holt, D.M., Beeson, T.J., *et al.* (2007) Effects of pH and mixing agents on the temporal setting of tooth-colored and gray mineral trioxide aggregate. *Journal of Endodontics* **33**, 970–3.

Weston, C.H., Barfield, R.D., Ruby, J.D., *et al.* (2008) Comparison of preparation design and material thickness on microbial leakage through Cavit using a tooth model system. *Oral Surgery Oral Medicine Oral Pathology Oral Radiology Endodontics* **105**, 530–5.

Weine, F.S. (1992) A preview of the canal-filling materials of the 21st century. *Compendium* **13**, 688, 690, 692.

Weller, R.N., Tay, K.C., Garrett, L.V., *et al.* (2008) Microscopic appearance and apical seal of root canals filled with gutta-percha and ProRoot Endo Sealer after immersion in a phosphate-containing fluid. *International Endodontic Journal* **41**, 977–86.

White, C. Jr., Bryant, N. (2002) Combined therapy of mineral trioxide aggregate and guided tissue regeneration in the treatment of external root resorption and an associated osseous defect. *Journal of Periodontology* **73**, 1517–21.

Williams, J.M., Trope, M., Caplan, D.J., *et al.* (2006) Detection and quantification of *E. faecalis* by real-time PCR (qPCR), reverse transcription-PCR (RT-PCR), and cultivation during endodontic treatment. *Journal of Endodontics* **32**, 715–21.

Williamson, A.E., Marker, K.L., Drake, D.R., *et al.* (2009) Resin-based versus gutta-percha-based root canal obturation: influence on bacterial leakage in an in vitro model system. *Oral Surgery Oral Medicine Oral Pathology Oral Radiology Endodontics* **108**, 292–6.

Witherspoon, D.E., Small, J.C., Regan, J.D., *et al.* (2008) Retrospective analysis of open apex teeth obturated with mineral trioxide aggregate. *Journal of Endodontics* **34**, 1171–6.

Witte, D. (1878) Das füellen der wurzelkanäle mit Portland-cement. *Deutsche Vierteljahrsschrift fuer Zahnheilkunde* **18**, 153–4 [in German].

Wu, M-K., Kontakiotis, E.G., Wesselink, P.R. (1998) Long-term seal provided by some root-end filling materials. *Journal of Endodontics* **24**, 557–60.

Yazdi, K.A., Bayat-Movahed, S., Aligholi, M., *et al.* (2009) Microleakage of human saliva in coronally unsealed obturated root canals in anaerobic conditions. *Journal of the Californian Dental Association* **37**, 33–7.

Yildirim, T., Gencoglu, N. (2010) Use of mineral trioxide aggregate in the treatment of large periapical lesions: reports of three cases. *European Journal of Dentistry* **4**, 468–74.

Yildirim, T., Oruçoğlu, H., Cobankara, F.K. (2008) Long-term evaluation of smear layer on the apical sealing of MTA. *Journal of Endodontics* **34**, 1537–40.

Yildirim, T., Er, K., Taşdemir, T., *et al.* (2010) Effect of smear layer and root-end cavity thickness on apical sealing ability of MTA as a root-end filling material: a bacterial leakage study. *Oral Surgery Oral Medicine Oral Pathology Oral Radiology Endodontics* **109**, e67–72.

Zhang, H., Pappen, F.G., Haapasalo, M. (2009) Dentin enhances the antibacterial effect of mineral trioxide aggregate and bioaggregate. *Journal of Endodontics* **35**, 221–4.

Zhu, Q., Haglund, R., Safavi, K.E., *et al.* (2000) Adhesion of human osteoblasts on root-end filling materials. *Journal of Endodontics* **26**, 404–6.

Zielinski, T.M., Baumgartner, J.C., Marshall, J.G. (2008) An evaluation of GuttaFlow and gutta-percha in the filling of lateral grooves and depressions. *Journal of Endodontics* **34**, 295–8.

9 Root-End Fillings Using MTA

Seung-Ho Baek[1] and Su-Jung Shin[2]

[1] School of Dentistry, Seoul National University, Korea
[2] College of Dentistry, Yonsei University, Gangnam Severance Hospital, Korea

Mineral Trioxide Aggregate: Properties and Clinical Applications, First Edition.
Edited by Mahmoud Torabinejad.
© 2014 John Wiley & Sons, Inc. Published 2014 by John Wiley & Sons, Inc.

INTRODUCTION OF ROOT-END FILLING MATERIALS

Purpose of root-end fillings

Surgical endodontic treatment is performed to resolve the inflammatory and/or procedural problems that cannot be treated by nonsurgical endodontic approaches.

The importance of placing a root-end filling for successful surgical endodontic treatment has been demonstrated in many clinical studies (Altonen & Mattila 1976; Lustmann *et al.* 1991; Rahbaran *et al.* 2001; Kim & Kratchman 2006). The major cause of periapical lesions that develop after nonsurgical endodontic treatment is apical leakage of bacteria and bacterial products from the contaminated canal space (Fig. 9.1). The removal of the infected periapical tissues by apical curettage without root-end filling does not eliminate the cause of Pathosis. The removal of the periapical lesion can only temporarily decrease the apparent symptoms and promote radiographic resolution of pathology. Periapical surgery entails not only the removal of the diseased periapical tissue and apex root, but also, resealing the root canal system.

There are some studies that have reported no significant differences in healing between teeth that were and were not root-end filled (Rapp *et al.* 1991; August 1996). Kim & Kratchman reported that the careful examination of these studies reveals many problems that are associated with their methodology and conclusions. First, the sample sizes are relatively small, leading to underpowered results. Second, the studies were conducted without microsurgical techniques and used amalgam as the root-end filling material. These old methods possessed inherent problems with steep angles of resection and the inconstancy of marginal adaptation of the root-end filling materials (Kim & Kratchman 2006). Therefore, the outcomes of the studies that are based on these conventional methods are less relevant for modern surgical endodontics.

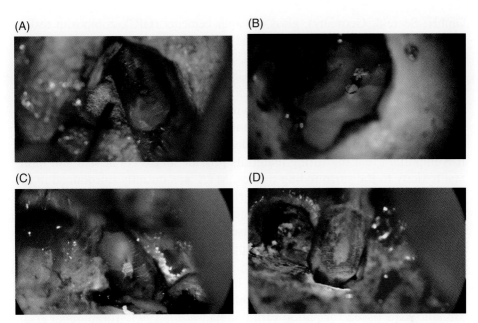

Fig. 9.1   Resected root surfaces that demonstrate apical leakage. (A,B) A 3-mm resected root surface, showing uncleaned areas in both canals. During apicoectomy, the unfilled canal space was examined with methylene blue staining. Although the curettage of apical granulation tissue and the removal of a root tip were performed, these bacterially contaminated surfaces can sustain periapical pathosis without proper retropreparation and root-end filling. (C,D) After a 3-mm root resection was completed, the resected surface was inspected under the microscope to investigate for isthmus presence, cracks or missed foramina. An unfilled canal space was observed, and MTA was applied into the retroprepared cavity.

The major cause of periapical lesions in many surgical cases may be due to leakage of bacteria and their toxins. Previous studies (Altonen and Mattila 1976; Lustman *et al.* 1991; Rahbaran *et al.* 2001) demonstrated the importance of root-end fillings in outcomes of apicoectomies by reporting that teeth with root-end fillings showed favorable results compared with those without root-end fillings. Therefore, sealing the root apex with a proper root-end filling material is crucial.

The purpose of the root-end filling is the hermetic sealing of the apex so that remaining bacteria or bacterial byproducts cannot enter or leave the canal.

HISTORY OF ROOT-END FILLING MATERIALS

A number of materials have been suggested as root-end filling materials including gutta-percha, amalgam, gold foil, zinc oxide eugenol (ZOE) cements, polycarboxylate cements, Cavit (3M ESPE, St. Paul, MN, USA), Diaket (ESPE

GmbH, Seefeld, Germany), glass ionomer cements (GIC), composite resins, Intermediate Restorative Material (IRM, Caulk/Dentsply, Milford, DE, USA), SuperEBA (Bosworth, Skokie, IL, USA), and mineral trioxide aggregate (ProRoot MTA; Dentsply, Tulsa, OK, USA).

The root-end filling material is placed to fill the root-end cavity, which is prepared with an ultrasonic tip following root end resection. With an understanding of this specific environment in which a root-end filling material is placed, several requirements for an ideal filling material can be established. It is important that the filling materials provide an excellent seal and minimal toxicity to the surrounding tissues. MTA was initially introduced in the early 1990s as a root-end filling material for use in periapical surgery. MTA was initially developed by Dr. Torabinejad and introduced in the early 1990s as a root-end filling materials for use in periapical surgery (Torabinejad *et al*. 1993). Since then, its clinical applications have broadened to perforation repair, pulp capping, pulpotomy, and apexification (Torabinejad and Chivian 1999). Its popularity might be derived from its excellent sealing ability, biocompatibility, and possible bioactive properties, which may promote hard tissue formation (Torabinejad *et al*. 1993; Torabinejad *et al*. 1994; Koh *et al*. 1998; Torabinejad *et al*. 1995a; Torabinejad *et al*.1997). For the past 20 years, there have been numerous studies that aimed to investigate MTA's physical, chemical, and biological properties, as well as its long-term clinical outcomes.

Amalgam

Amalgam has been used for over 100 years, and currently it is a widely used material in restorative procedures but rarely applied in apical retrofilling during apical surgery. In recent years, many have questioned the safety and integrity of amalgam in general and as a retrofilling material in particular, as it presents many disadvantages, including cytotoxicity, mercury toxicity, corrosion, delayed expansion, and amalgam tattoos embedded in soft and hard tissues (Fig. 9.2) (Dorn & Gartner 1990; Torabinejad *et al*. 1995a, 1997). The current use of amalgam as a root-end filling material is extremely limited (Chong & Pitt Ford 2005).

ZOE-based materials: IRM and SuperEBA

IRM and SuperEBA have been used extensively, as they are considered clinically superior to amalgam as root-end filling materials. Both IRM and SuperEBA are modified forms of ZOE cements. The physical properties of ZOE cements, such as weak compressive and, tensile strengths, a long setting time, and solubility in

(A) (B)

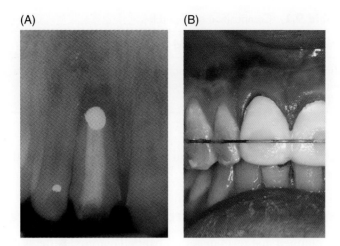

Fig. 9.2 An amalgam tattoo caused by an amalgam root-end filling. (A) A periapical radiograph demonstrated that an apicoectomy was performed on the maxillary right central incisor and a large root-end cavity was filled with amalgam. (B) An amalgam tattoo was broadly observed around the apical gingival area of the tooth. Source: Seung-Jong Lee, *Atlas of Endodontic Practice*, 3rd edition, Yenang Inc., p. 385, 2007. Source: Lee *et al*. 2007. Reproduced with permission of Dr. Seung-Jong Lee.

oral fluids, are improved in both IRM and SuperEBA. They exhibit similar and favorable properties, and they are clinically and histologically superior to amalgam (Baek *et al*. 2005; Baek *et al*.2010; Dorn & Gartner 1990).

IRM is composed of 80% zinc oxide powder, 20% polymethylethacrylate, and a 99% eugenol liquid. The sealing ability of IRM is better than that of amalgam, and it is not affected by the liquid/powder ratio (Crooks *et al*. 1994). The biologic response of IRM is similar to that observed with other ZOE-based materials. IRM appears to be well tolerated in the periapical tissues, but its use like super EBA does not result in regeneration of periapical tissues (Pitt Ford *et al*. 1994; Harrison & Johnson 1997).

SuperEBA was first suggested as a root-end filling material by Oynick & Oynick (1978). It is composed of 60% zinc oxide powder, 30% alumina, and 6% natural resin, and the liquid is 37.5% eugenol and 62.5% ortho-ethoxybenzoic acid (Table 9.1; Dorn & Gartner 1990; Pitt Ford *et al*. 1995a; Trope *et al*. 1996). SuperEBA was shown to be superior to amalgam in terms of sealing ability, apical tissue compatibility, and regeneration potential (Pitt Ford *et al*. 1995a; Torabinejad *et al*. 1995c). Rubinstein & Kim reported that the healing success after root-end surgery was 96.4% after one year when SuperEBA was used as a root-end filling material in conjunction with microsurgical techniques (Rubinstein & Kim 1999).

Table 9.1 Composition of SuperEBA.

Powder		Liquid	
Zinc oxide	60%	Eugenol	37.5%
Alumina	34%	Ortho-ethoxy benzoic acid	62.5%
Natural resin	6%		

Until MTA was developed, IRM and SuperEBA cements were the materials of choice for root-end fillings.

Resin-based materials: Retroplast and Geristore

Early studies claimed that resin materials exerted cytotoxic effects on periodontal ligament cells (Tai & Chang 2000; Huang *et al.* 2002). However, Rud and associates introduced Retroplast (Retroplast Trading, Dybersovej, Denmark] into endodontic surgery with favorable long-term outcomes (Rud *et al.* 1991, 1996; Yazdi *et al.* 2007). This material is placed on the concave root resected surface rather than being packed into a class I cavity. Retroplast has been mainly used in Europe. Similarly, Geristore (Den-Mat, Santa Maria, CA, USA) is a hybrid ionomer composite, and it has been used as a root-end filling material, especially in North America (Al-Sabek *et al.* 2005; Al-Sa'eed *et al.* 2008).

Al-Sabek and associates reported that human gingival fibroblasts attached and survived when in contact with Geristore, demonstrating less toxicity than IRM and Ketac-Fil (Al-Sabek *et al.* 2005). An *in vitro* study reported that extracts of both Geristore and Retroplast increased cell proliferation (Al-Sa'eed *et al.* 2008). However, conflicting results have been reported (Haglund *et al.* 2003; Tawil *et al.* 2009). In a study by Haglund and associates, Retroplast demonstrated decreased cell viability (Haglund *et al.* 2003). Compared with IRM and MTA, Geristore showed the least favorable histological results, even though there were no obvious radiographic differences between the materials (Tawil *et al.* 2009).

The major drawback of these resin-type materials is moisture sensitivity, especially to blood, during periapical surgery. Depending on the cavity design and hemorrhage control, the ideal conditions for bonding cannot be obtained in most surgical sites. Some researchers also have claimed handling difficulties with Geristore (Tawil *et al.* 2009).

Mineral trioxide aggregate (MTA)

MTA was introduced into surgical endodontic treatment as a root-end filling material by Torabinejad and associates in 1993 (Torabinejad *et al.* 1993). It was shown to have excellent sealing ability (Torabinejad *et al.* 1994, 1995e, f;

Bates *et al.* 1996), an antimicrobial effect (Torabinejad *et al.* 1995d), and it promoted osteoblast activity (Torabinejad *et al.* 1995c; Koh *et al.* 1998). MTA was also less cytotoxic than amalgam, IRM, or SuperEBA (Torabinejad *et al.* 1995f; Keiser *et al.* 2000). The results of studies in dogs and monkeys showed that MTA caused significantly less inflammation than amalgam (Torabinejad *et al.* 1995a, 1997) when used as a root end filling. MTA also exhibited the most favorable periapical tissue response, as cementum was shown to regenerate in direct contact with the MTA (Torabinejad *et al.* 1997; Rubinstein & Kim 1999; Baek *et al.* 2005, 2010).

Gray vs. White MTA

MTA was originally formulated as a gray powder, but white MTA was later developed to overcome tooth discoloration by the gray formula (Dammaschke *et al.* 2005). However, recent studies have demonstrated that white MTA also induces the discoloration (Felman & Parashos 2013; Camilleri 2014). When the sealing ability of the gray and white MTA was compared, there was no significant difference (Shahi *et al.* 2007).

There have been controversies among studies that examined whether there were any differences in biocompatibility between the gray and white MTA. Holland and associates evaluated the reaction of rat subcutaneous connective tissue to the implantation of dentin tubes filled with white MTA (Holland *et al.* 2002). They showed similar results to those reported for gray MTA, which indicated that white and gray MTA have similar mechanisms of action. On the other hand, a cell culture study by Perez and associates showed that osteoblasts behave differently on white MTA, suggesting that this might be due to the surface morphology of the materials (Perez *et al.* 2003). Most studies reported no significant difference in the biocompatibility between the two variants (Camilleri *et al.* 2004; Ribeiro *et al.* 2005; Shahi *et al.* 2006).

New types of MTA-like cements

Other types of MTA-like materials have been developed and marketed, including MTA angelus (Angelus, Londrina, PR, Brazil), MTA bio (Angelus, Londrina, PR, Brazil), CPM (Egeo, Buenos Aires, Argentina), Endosequence Root Repair Material (RRM) (Brasseler USA, Savannah, GA, USA), OrthoMTA (bioMTA, Seoul, South Korea), and Endocem MTA (Maruchi, Seoul, South Korea). Recent studies have compared these materials with ProRoot MTA. However, one of the major drawbacks of these relatively new products is the lack of clinical data to advocate long term successful outcomes.

REQUIREMENTS OF IDEAL ROOT-END FILLING MATERIALS

The ideal root-end filling material should be easy to manipulate, radiopaque, dimensionally stable, bactericidal or bacteriostatic, nonresorbable, and unaffected by the presence of moisture (Gartner & Dorn 1992). It should also adhere to the prepared cavity walls, seal the root canal system, promote healing, and it should be nontoxic and well-tolerated by periapical tissues (Table 9.2). Many studies have examined the sealing ability and biocompatability of retrograde filling materials, but none of these root-end filling materials, including MTA, fully satisfy these requirements (Aqrabawi 2000).

Advantages and disadvantages of MTA as a root-end filling material

Advantages of MTA

According to numerous previous studies (Torabinejad *et al.* 1995a, c, f, 1997; Trope *et al.* 1996; Baek *et al.* 2005, 2010; Chong & Pitt Ford 2005), MTA is superior or equivalent to other materials in terms of biocompatibility, sealing ability, and bactericidal properties. From a biological perspective MTA has a great advantage over other available materials. In addition to its excellent biocompatibility, MTA comes close to being an ideal filling material, as it has the capacity to promote bone, dentin, and cementum regeneration (Baek *et al.* 2005; Pitt Ford *et al.* 1995b). These outstanding features will be discussed later in this chapter.

Most dental filling materials exhibit the best results when they set in a dry environment or when moisture is properly controlled. MTA consists of hydrophilic powder and sets under wet conditions, except in environments with

Table 9.2 Requirements of the ideal root-end filling material (Gartner & Dorn 1992).

Easy to manipulate (proper working time)
Radiopaque
Long-term dimensional stability
Nonresorbable
Unaffected by moisture
Adhere to the dentin wall
Biocompatible
Bactericidal or bacteriostatic
Seal the root canal system (sealability)
Well-tolerated by periapical tissues (biocompatibility)
Ability to regenerate periapical tissues (bioactive)
Inexpensive

excessive bleeding or water contact. This property (insensitivity to the presence of moisture) is advantageous in most surgical conditions because it is almost impossible to obtain a completely dry environment, despite efforts to control hemorrhage with pressure and cotton pellets.

Disadvantages of MTA

MTA is known to be difficult to place into the prepared root-end cavities. In addition to these handling difficulties, freshly mixed MTA can be washed out whenever there is a significant communication between the oral cavity and MTA, limiting its periodontal applications. In situations without obvious communications, the blood flow in the surgical site will cause a certain amount of cement loss (Formosa *et al.* 2012).

MTA does not directly bond or adhere to bony or dental structure. The setting time of MTA is approximately 3–4 hours (Torabinejad *et al.* 1995b), which is considered to be a disadvantage in many clinical situations. The long setting time may evoke an increased solubility, exhibiting a detrimental effect on sealing ability. During apicoectomy, MTA might be exposed to an acidic environment, and the sealing ability of MTA under acidic conditions is controversial. Roy and associates reported that acidic environments did not hinder the sealing ability of MTA (Roy *et al.* 2001). On the other hand, the more extensive porosity of MTA was observed when it set in direct contact with acid (Namazikhah *et al.* 2008), and more leakage was observed in MTA when stored in low-pH solution (Saghiri *et al.* 2008).

To circumvent these problems, additives such as methylcellulose, calcium chloride, and dibasic sodium phosphate were employed to shorten the original setting time of MTA (Ber *et al.* 2007; Bortoluzzi *et al.* 2008; Huang *et al.* 2008). The mixing of MTA powder with different liquids may possibly alter other properties of the material. Adding calcium chloride solution might lower the final compressive strength relative to that of a mixture with sterile water (Kogan *et al.* 2006).

Another issue is its high cost, as many researchers and clinicians find that MTA is an expensive material (Casas *et al.* 2005; Mooney & North 2008).

The advantages and disadvantages of MTA are summarized in Table 9.3.

Table 9.3 Advantages and disadvantages of mineral trioxide aggregate (MTA).

Advantages	Disadvantages
Low cytotoxicity	Difficult to manipulate
Excellent biocompatibility	Long setting time
Hydrophilic	Cost
Radiopaque	
Sealing ability	
Bioactive	

MTA AS A ROOT-END FILLING MATERIAL

Cytotoxicity and biocompatibility

The most critical properties of root-end filling materials that come into contact with periapical and periodontal tissue are their cytotoxicity and biocompatibility. The biocompatibility of MTA is important to create an environment conducive to healing and bone fill.

Cytotoxicity of root-end filling materials has been evaluated by various methods, such as cell viability assays for mitochondrial dehydrogenase activity, an agar overlay method, and the evaluation of cell attachment and morphology. The cytotoxicity and biocompatibility of MTA were tested in *in vitro* cell culture studies, and the results showed the satisfactory attachment of osteoblasts and periodontal cells on MTA. In numerous previous studies, MTA has shown less or equivalent cytotoxicity compared with other root-end filling materials including amalgam, ZOE, IRM, composite resin and GIC. (Zhu *et al.* 2000; Balto 2004; Yoshimine *et al.* 2007; Bodrumlu 2008).

The cytotoxic effect on nerves and neural cells has also been measured to evaluate whether a root-end filling material inhibits nerve integrity or regeneration. When neurotoxicity was tested with several root-end filling materials, amalgam, SuperEBA, and Diaket induced neural cell death, while MTA did not (Asrari & Lobner 2003).

Most early studies were performed with a premixed MTA. It was suspected that freshly mixed MTA might create a detrimental environment for cells because it has a high pH during setting (Balto 2004). An inhibition zone was often observed in cell cultures that were grown in contact with fresh MTA. However, this cell-free zone seems to be transient (Fig. 9.3A, B). When fresh MTA was inserted *in vivo*, no evidence of a cell-free zone was reported (Pitt Ford *et al.* 1996; Apaydin *et al.* 2004). When the cytotoxicity of MTA, amalgam, and SuperEBA were measured, fresh MTA showed the least degree of toxicity compared with the other materials. The initial toxicity of MTA before setting may not create a detrimental environment when it is applied into a root-end cavity (Lustmann *et al.* 1991).

Biocompatibility is the ability of a material to enact its specific role with a favorable host response (Willians 1986). Several *in vivo* animal studies have reported that MTA is a biocompatible material with no adverse effect on the dental tissues (Chong & Pitt Ford 2005; Torabinejad *et al.* 1995c; Baek *et al.* 2005). When MTA was implanted into the bone of animal models, no inflammation was observed, and direct bone deposition was often found around the materials (Saidon *et al.* 2003). The mean distances from the newly regenerated bone to three different types of retrograde filling materials were measured

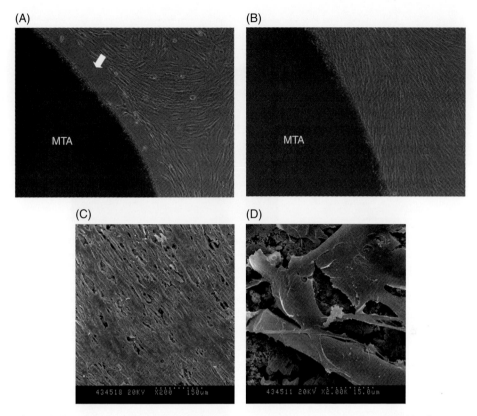

Fig. 9.3 Phase microscopy and scanning electron microscopy (SEM) showing human periodontal ligament (PDL) cells grown on freshly prepared white MTA for 48 (A) and 72 (B–D) hours. (A) The white arrow indicates the cell-free zone between the margin of the MTA and the cells. (B) No inhibition zone between MTA and cells was observed in 72-hour samples. (C) Cells were attached and healthy when they were plated on MTA (×200). (D) Cells on MTA were photographed at a high magnification (×2000).

four months after apical surgery. The distance from MTA to the newly formed bone was similar to the normal average periodontal ligament thickness in dogs, and this average distance was smaller than that of the Super EBA and amalgam groups (Fig. 9.4) (Baek *et al.* 2010). These findings suggest that MTA can create a favorable environment for bone and periodontal ligament (PDL) regeneration.

Histologically, little or no inflammation was detected when MTA was used as a root-end filling material in dogs and monkeys. Torabinejad and associates showed that MTA was covered with a cementum layer when used as a root-end filling material in dogs (Torabinejad *et al.* 1995a) and monkeys (Torabinejad

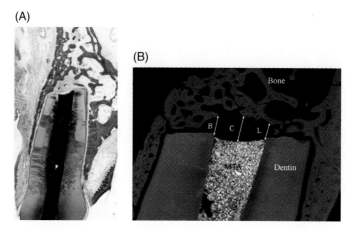

Fig. 9.4 Microradiographs of the MTA filling illustrated the distances between a root-end filling and the regenerated bone. This specimen was fabricated 4 months after apicoectomy in dogs. (B) is an enlargement of the area shown in (A). These figures showed the distance from MTA to the regenerated bone(mean: 0.397mm) was similar to normal average periodontal thickness in dogs and the distance in amalgam group was significantly higher than that in MTA group. Source: Baek *et al.* 2010. Reproduced with permission of Elsevier.

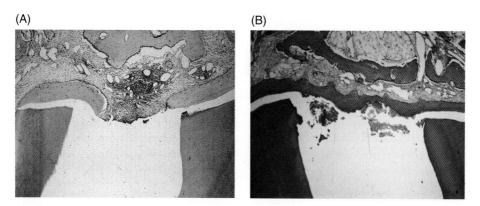

Fig. 9.5 (A) On top of the amalgam retrograde filling, no direct cementum deposition was noticed. (B) On the other hand, new cementum grew over the resected root-end dentin as well as on the MTA root-end filling. Source: Torabinejad *et al.* 1997. Reproduced with permission of Elsevier.

et al. 1997) (Fig. 9.5). In their study, cementum was present on the surface of MTA in all the samples. Baek and associates investigated the tissue responses when amalgam, SuperEBA, and MTA were used as root-end filling materials, and they showed persistent low levels of inflammation and a favorable periapical tissue response, with new cementum formation over the MTA (Huang *et al.* 2002, Baek *et al.* 2005). The regenerated cementum on the MTA might be important for the regeneration of periodontal tissue (Fig. 9.6) (Lindskog *et al.* 1983).

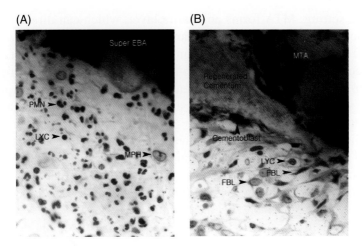

Fig. 9.6 (A,B) Inflammatory cell infiltration on SuperEBA (A) and MTA (B) specimens (Giemsa staining, ×800) in dogs. (a) Around the SuperEBA retrofilling, polymorphonuclear leukocytes (PMNs), lymphocytes (LYC), plasma cells, and macrophages (MPH) were observed. (B) MTA specimens exhibited the deposition of fibroblasts (FBL) and minor inflammatory cells. Source: Baek *et al.* 2005. Reproduced with permission of Elsevier.

MTA appears to be the most biocompatible root-end filling material and is considered the first choice of material for root-end filling.

Bioactivity

Several histological studies have found that thick cementum was deposited on the surfaces of MTA root-end fillings, confirming MTA's biocompatibility and bioactivity. (Torabinejad *et al.* 1995a, 1997; Baek *et al.* 2005). Pitt Ford and associates reported the continuous formation around excess MTA when it was used to repair a perforation (Pitt Ford *et al.* 1995b). A material is considered to be bioactive when it results in positive host responses, such as hard tissue induction properties (Pitt Ford *et al.* 1995b). Several studies have shown that MTA has the capacity to promote hard tissue formation (Torabinejad *et al.* 1995a, c, 1997; Koh *et al.* 1998; Baek *et al.* 2005, 2010).

MTA is reported to stimulate cytokine release, which controls inflammatory responses and hard tissue formation (Koh *et al.* 1997). MTA increases the levels of interleukin IL-6, IL-8, and osteocalcin expression. Osteocalcin is a bone-specific marker, which supports the role of MTA in osteogenic cell proliferation. However, IL-6 stimulates osteoclast formation and recruitment. Based on this data it appears that, MTA may actually promote bone turnover by increasing osteoclastic and osteoblastic activity.

During setting, MTA forms an apatite layer, which can directly bond to living bone and dental tissue (Sarkar *et al.* 2005; Bozeman *et al.* 2006; Gandolfi *et al.* 2010). The formation of apatite may enhance sealability and osteoblast growth (Gandolfi *et al.* 2010; Camilleri & Pitt Ford 2006). MTA promotes osteoblast attachment and increases Runx2 expression, which is critical for osteoblast differentiation (Perinpanayagam & Al-Rabeah 2009).

In addition, MTA preferentially induces the alkaline phosphatase activity of PDL and gingival fibroblasts, which can promote osseous repair (Bonson *et al.* 2004). The mechanisms for the stimulatory effect of MTA on PDL cell proliferation are unknown. However, given that calcium ions are a major component of MTA, it is quite plausible that the calcium ions released from MTA play an important role in cell proliferation. More recently, it was demonstrated that MTA stimulates human pulp cell proliferation (Takita *et al.* 2006). In this study, it was hypothesized that one of the main causes of MTA-induced cell proliferation is the continuous release of calcium ions from MTA. Other than cell proliferation, the functional competency of a cell is achieved through differentiation, and the process of cell differentiation is characterized by the expression of tissue-specific genes. Bonson and associates showed that MTA increases the expression of alkaline phosphatase, osteonectin, and osteopontin genes in PDL fibroblasts. This suggests that MTA induces bone formation by stimulating osteogenic cell differentiation (Bonson *et al.* 2004).

On the other hand, it has been claimed that MTA is osteoconductive rather than osteoinductive, based on the finding that a subcutaneous implant of MTA elicited severe initial reactions with coagulation necrosis and dystrophic calcification, which later subsided, and osteogenesis occurred in intraosseous MTA implants (Moretton *et al.* 2000).

The exact mechanism has not yet been proven; however, MTA seems to be a bioactive material that can enhance the healing process.

Sealability

The sealing ability of a retrograde filling material is critical because the remaining intracanal irritants (in most cases, microorganisms) can cause refractory pathosis and the possible need for further surgical endodontics. A large number of investigations on bacterial leakage were performed using the current root-end filling materials. The majority of these studies showed that MTA is more resistant to bacterial leakage than amalgam (Torabinejad *et al.* 1995e; Fischer *et al.* 1998). The results from leakage tests that compared MTA and SuperEBA are controversial. In some studies, there was no significant difference between the two root-end filling materials (Scheerer *et al.* 2001; Mangin *et al.* 2003). However, others have shown that the sealability of MTA is superior to that of SuperEBA (Torabinejad *et al.* 1995e; Fischer *et al.* 1998; Wu *et al.* 1998; Gondim *et al.* 2005).

The excellent sealing ability of MTA cannot be guaranteed in an acidic environment. Teeth stored in low pH after being retrofilled with MTA showed a lower resistance to leakage than teeth stored in high pH (Saghiri *et al.* 2008).

The thickness of the retrograde filling material affects the sealability of MTA. Because MTA leaks when it is applied at lower thicknesses, a 4-mm thickness is recommended (Valois & Costa 2004).

More recently, studies have focused on the formation of the hydoxyapatite layer of MTA during setting. This layer is expected to create a biologic seal between MTA and the dentin interface (Sarkar *et al.* 2005; Bozeman *et al.* 2006; Gandolfi *et al.* 2010; Reyes Carmona *et al.* 2009).

Antibacterial effect

A root-end filling is often placed in an environment in which infection or irritants remain.

Based on a large number of previous studies, MTA has antibacterial effects against many species of microbes (Torabinejad *et al.* 1995d; Yasuda *et al.* 2008; Estrela *et al.* 2011). When several available root-end filling materials, including amalgam, IRM, Superbond C&B, MTA, Geristore, Dyract, and composite resin, were tested for bacterial leakage, IRM and MTA were generally more potent inhibitors of bacterial growth (Eldeniz *et al.* 2006). However, some conflicts exist in other studies indicating that MTA does not show any anti microbial activity (Miyagak *et al.* 2006; Yasuda *et al.* 2008).

CLINICAL APPLICATIONS OF MTA

Retropreparation and root-end filling

Cavity preparation for MTA root-end filling

The purpose of a root-end preparation is to clean and create a space for a root-end filling material. One of the most significant recent improvements in endodontic surgery was the introduction of ultrasonic tips by Dr. Carr for root-end preparation in the early 1990s. These replaced the use of conventional air-turbine handpieces with burs. Many ultrasonic tips for root-end preparation are available in various shapes, sizes, and designs: CT series tips (SybronEndo, CA, USA), KiS ultrasonic tips (Obtura-Spartan, Fenton, MO, USA), ProUltra Surgical tips (ProUltra, Dentsply Tulsa Dental, Tulsa, OK, USA), and B&L JET tips (B&L Biotech USA, PA, USA). The cavity preparation for MTA root-end fillings is the same as for other root-end filling materials. Under a microscope, root-end preparation with ultrasonic tips can make a class I preparation to a depth of 3 mm along the long axis of the root.

Mixing procedure

The powder/liquid ratio of MTA is three parts powder to one part sterile aqueous solution (Fig. 9.7). After 30 s of mixing, the mixture should exhibit a wet sand consistency.

Methods for placement of MTA

MTA is difficult to deliver to a small cavity for root-end filling because its physical properties differ from those of other root-end filling materials.

For delivery of the MTA, most clinicians use a syringe-type carrier or MTA pellet forming block.

Carrier- and syringe-type devices

Carrier- and syringe-type devices are most often used for the delivery of MTA, and they include: the Retro Amalgam filling carrier (Moyco Union Broach, York, PA, USA), the Messing Root Canal Gun (R. Chige, Inc., Boca Raton, FL, USA), Dovgan MTA Carriers (Quality Aspirators, Duncanville, TX, USA), the MTA Carrier (G. Hartzell & Sons, Concord, CA, USA), MAP System (PD, Vevey, Switzerland), and the C-R Syringe (Centrix Inc., Shelton, CT, USA).

The tips of carriers are placed on the mixture of MTA and lightly tapped to insert a small amount of material into the tip. With this method, the amount of MTA powder used can be minimized, and the precise placement of MTA is possible. However, these carrier- and syringe-type devices also have several limitations. When the root-end preparation is small, the carrier-type devices can be difficult to use. Sometimes, syringe tips may not reach the anatomically complex regions. If a large amount of MTA is delivered to the root-end cavity, especially when the tip of the delivery device is large, an excess of MTA is deposited into the bone cavity and over the root surface (Fig. 8.8). It is important to clean the carries immediately after use to prevent clogging of the syringe. (Video).

Lee MTA pellet forming block

Lee first introduced an MTA block, which was made by cutting a groove into a 0.5 inch × 0.5 inch × 2 inch plastic block (Tap Plastics, San Rafael, CA, USA) using a #169 fissure bur. The formation and delivery of an MTA pellet with an MTA block can overcome the difficulties presented by carrier- and syringe-type devices.

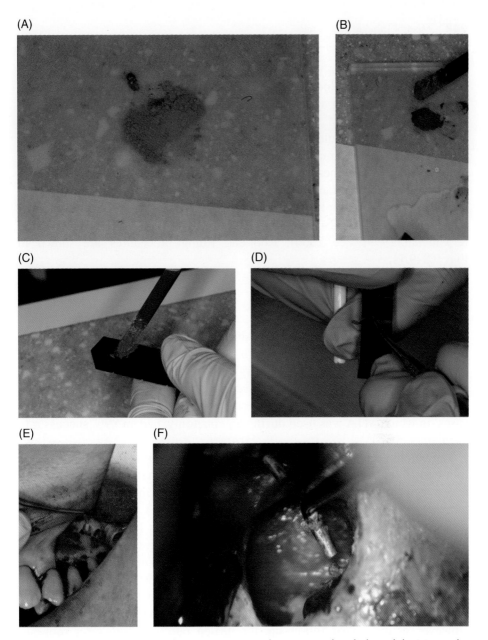

Fig. 9.7 MTA mixing procedure. (A) MTA powder on a sterilized glass slab. (B) Powder is mixed with sterilized water using a cement spatula. This mixture should have a wet sand consistency. (C) A small amount of the MTA mixture is placed into the groove of the Lee MTA pellet forming flock (G. Hartzell & Sons, Concord, CA, USA). (D) After wiping the filling surface of MTA block with sterile gauze, the MTA pellet is scooped out using the Lee Carver (G. Hartzell & Sons). (E) This scooped pellet is delivered to a cavity formed after retropreparation. (F) The MTA pellet is condensed using a microplugger. Depending on the size of the retroprepared cavity, this procedure can be repeated as needed until MTA fills the cavity. (Courtesy of Dr. Jung Lim at UCLA.)

The MTA, mixed to a wet sand consistency, is immediately placed into the grooves of the MTA block using a cement spatula, and the excess material MTA application using a Lee MTA pellet forming block is demonstrated in Figure 9.7.

The MTA pellets should be placed into the root end preparation as quickly as possible because the small pellets will quickly dehydrate. When the MTA mixture is dry, it becomes crumbly and unmanageable. Using several grooves on each of the four surfaces of the plastic block will help maintain rapidity in the placement of multiple pellets of MTA. Covering the plastic block with moistened gauze will also help prevent desiccation of the MTA (Torabinejad & Chivian 1999; Lee 2000). Root-end filling procedures are shown in Figs 9.8–9.11.

Clinical outcomes

MTA is often the material of choice during apical surgeries and intentional replantations due to its biocompatibility and positive clinical outcomes (Rubinstein & Torabinejad 2004). Surgical cases that used MTA retrofillings have shown excellent results when combined with modern microscopic endodontic surgical procedures. A prospective case series study of 276 cases, in which MTA was used during apicoectomy, had an 89% success rate (Saunders 2008).

The outcomes and success rates of apicoectomies with the various types of root-end filling materials have been investigated in many studies. Although the success rate for MTA was higher (84% after 12 months, 92% after 24 months) than that of IRM (76% and 87%, respectively), there was no significant difference in success between the two materials (Chong *et al.* 2003). These findings were consistent with those of other studies that compared MTA and IRM (Lindeboom *et al.* 2005; Tawil *et al.* 2009). When the success rate in the MTA retrofilling group was compared with that of SuperEBA, one prospective study claimed that no difference existed between the two materials (95.6% success in MTA versus 93.1% in SuperEBA) (Song *et al.* 2012). However, at the 5-year follow-up, the healed rate was higher for root-end fillings with MTA (86%) than with SuperEBA (67%) (von Arx *et al.* 2012). MTA showed favorable results regardless of tooth type, which contrasts with Retroplast's variable healing rates that depend on the tooth type (von Arx *et al.* 2010). Based on the currently available studies, MTA appears to be the material of choice for root-end fillings. Outcomes from two case studies are shown in Figs 9.12 and 9.13.

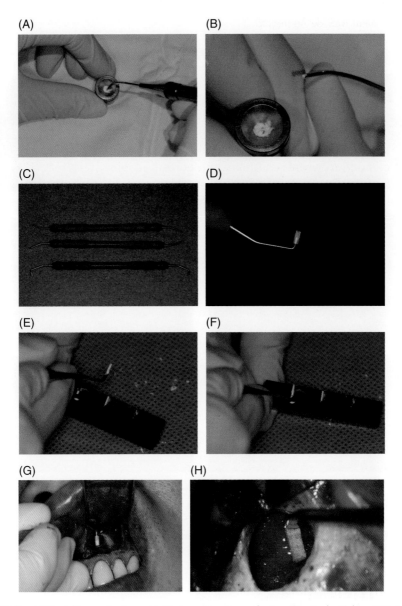

Fig. 9.8 MTA delivery devices. (A,B) A syringe-type device (Dentsply, Tulsa, OK, USA). MTA powder is placed into the mixing pot and mixed with sterile liquid or water. With light tapping, a small amount of MTA is placed into the tip of the syringe. By pushing the finger holder, the inserted MTA is extracted through the tip. (C,D) Surgical carriers of MTA (Dentsply, Tulsa, OK, USA). The Teflon sleeve is inserted into the tip of carrier, which is configured with the proper angle to reach the surgical site. The MTA mixture is placed into the sleeve by tapping the carrier (Courtesy of Dr. Dong-Ryul Shin at Luden Dental Clinic.) (E,F). The Lee MTA pellet forming blocks seen in this image (G. Hartzell & Sons, Concord, CA, USA). A small amount of MTA mixture is placed into a groove of the block. A special carrier is used to scoop a pellet of MTA. (G) MTA application using surgical carriers of MTA delivery system. (H) MTA application using Lee MTA Pellet forming block and Lee carver (G. Hartzell & Sons). (Courtesy of Dr. Dong-Ryul Shin.)

(A)   (B)

(C)   (D)

(E)   (F)

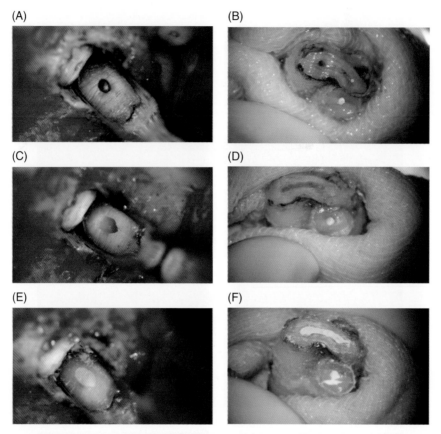

Fig. 9.9 Root-end filling procedure during apical surgery (A,C,E) and intentional replantation (B,D,F). (A,B) Resected root ends (C,D) 3-mm deep root end cavity preparations (E,F). Root end cavities filled with MTA and observed under the microscope. (Courtesy of Dr. Minju Song at Yonsei University.)

CONCLUSION

Various types of materials have been used in root-end fillings. Based on the numerous studies to date, MTA appears to have clear advantages over the other materials. The literature regarding the effects of moisture on MTA speaks to the increased porosity of the material when in contact with acidic solution and therefore does not accurately reflect this conclusion regarding MTA and the effects of moisture on the material. MTA has also been recognized as a bioactive material, although the specific mechanism is not yet fully understood. Over the last two decades, extensive studies on MTA have demonstrated

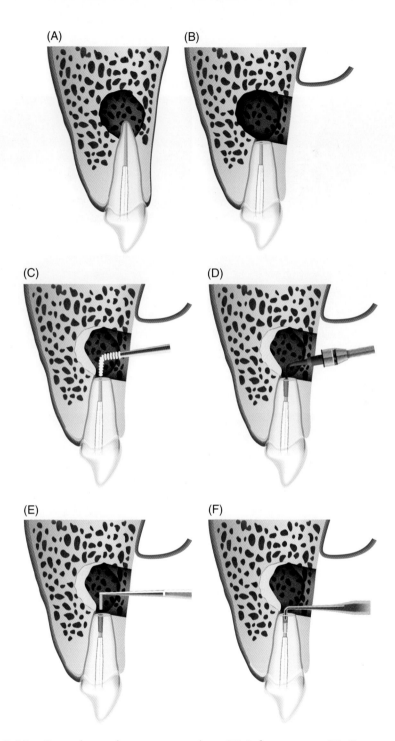

Fig. 9.10 General apical surgery procedure. (A) Before surgery. (B) Osteotomy and root resection. (C) Retropreparation using an ultrasonic tip. (D) Cavity dry using a proper air syringe. (E) MTA application. (F) MTA condensation.

(A)

(B)

(C)

(D)

(E)

(F)

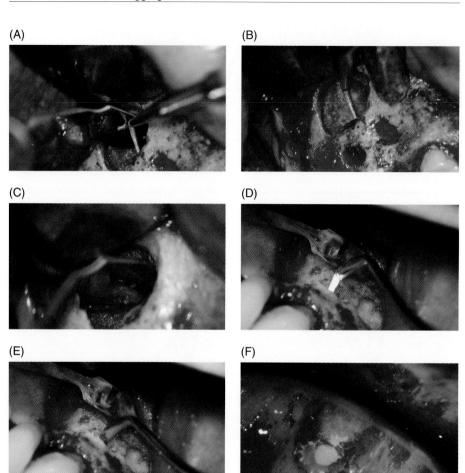

Fig. 9.11 Apical Microsurgery procedure. (A) An ultrasonic tip is positioned in the direction of the long axis of the root. (B) Old gutta-percha and apical root canal dentin is removed using an ultrasonic tip until the depth of cavity is 3 mm. (C) A surgical micromirror is used to inspect the retropreparation. (D,E) The MTA pellet is applied into the cavity. (F) Excess MTA is removed using a cotton pellet or an endodontic spoon excavator. A clean root surface filled with MTA is observed under the microscope.

that it is a promising material. As a root-end filling material, the most common complaint is the difficulty in placing the material into a retroprepared cavity. This handling problem can be overcome by utilizing some devices and instruments that are especially designed for this purpose.

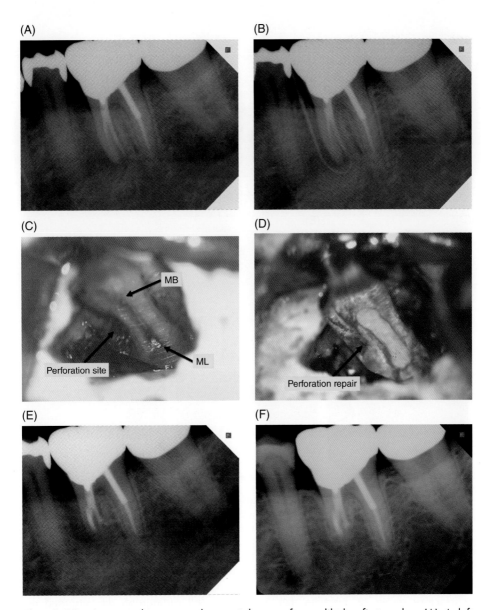

Fig. 9.12 A surgical case on the mesial root of mandibular first molar. (A) A left mandibular first molar was mobile, with a probing depth of 6 mm in the mesiobuccal and mesiolingual pockets. Preoperative radiographs showed previous root canal therapy on the first molar with periapical radiolucency on the mesial root. (B) A gutta-percha cone was inserted into a sinus tract until it reached the apex of the mesial root. (C) Inspection of the resected mesial root surface showed that the mesiobuccal canal was completely missed during cleaning and shaping, which caused the apical leakage and perforation. (D) Retropreparation, including the mesiobuccal and mesiolingual canals and their isthmuses, was performed, and MTA was applied as a root-end filling material. (E) Postoperative radiographs showed that the resected mesial root was retrofilled with MTA. (F) Four-year recall X-ray demonstrated the complete healing of previous apical pathosis. The patient was asymptomatic and the mobility of the tooth was decreased. (Courtesy of Dr. Euiseong Kim at Yonsei University.)

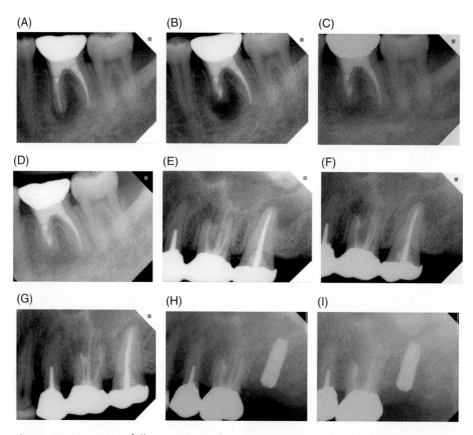

Fig. 9.13 Long-term follow-up surgical cases using MTA as a root-end filling material. (A) The pre-operative radiograph of a mandibular first molar showed the presence of a previous root canal therapy on the first molar with periapical radiolucency on the mesial root. This radiograph was taken after the retreatment. The mesiobuccal canal was not negotiated due to severe calcification. A periapical surgery was planned because the patient was symptomatic. (B) Postoperative radiographs showed that the resected mesial root was retrofilled with MTA. (C) A 3-year recall radiograph shows satisfactory results at this time. (D) A 5-year recall radiograph demonstrated the complete healing of the lesion. (E) Preoperative radiograph of a left maxillary first molar. Root canal therapy was previously performed by a general dentist and recurrent apical swelling was reported. (F) Postoperative radiograph. A missed mesiolingual canal was detected during apicoectomy. (G) A postoperative radiograph with different angles showed mesioligual canal and isthmus was also filling with MTA. (H,I) A 5-year recall X-rays demonstrated the complete healing of the previous apical lesion. (Courtesy of Dr. Euiseong Kim at Yonsei University.)

REFERENCES

Al-Sabek, F., Shostad, S., Kirkwood, K.L. (2005) Preferential attachment of human gingival fibroblasts to the resin ionomer Geristore. *Journal of Endodontics* **31**(3), 205–8.

Al-Sa'eed, O.R., Al-Hiyasat, A.S., Darmani, H. (2008) The effects of six root-end filling materials and their leachable components on cell viability. *Journal of Endodontics* **34**(11), 1410–4.

Altonen, M., Mattila, K. (1976) Follow-up study of apicoectomized molars. *International Journal of Oral Surgery* **5**(1), 33–40.

Apaydin, E.S., Shabahang, S., Torabinejad, M. (2004) Hard-tissue healing after application of fresh or set MTA as root-end-filling material. *Journal of Endodontics* **30**(1), 21–4.

Aqrabawi, J. (2000) Sealing ability of amalgam, super EBA cement, and MTA when used as retrograde filling materials. *British Dental Journal* **188**(5), 266–8.

Asrari, M., Lobner, D. (2003) In vitro neurotoxic evaluation of root-end-filling materials. *Journal of Endodontics* **29**(11), 743–6.

August, D.S. (1996) Long-term postsrugical results on teeth with periapical radiolucencies. *Journal of Endodontics* **22**, 380–3.

Baek, S.H., Plenk, H., Jr., Kim, S. (2005) Periapical tissue responses and cementum regeneration with amalgam, SuperEBA, and MTA as root-end filling materials. *Journal of Endodontics* **31**(6), 444–9.

Baek, S.H., Lee, W.C., Setzer, F.C., *et al.* (2010) Periapical bone regeneration after endodontic microsurgery with three different root-end filling materials: amalgam, SuperEBA, and mineral trioxide aggregate. *Journal of Endodontics* **36**(8), 1323–5.

Balto, H.A. (2004) Attachment and morphological behavior of human periodontal ligament fibroblasts to mineral trioxide aggregate: a scanning electron microscope study. *Journal of Endodontics* **30**(1), 25–9.

Bates, C.F., Carnes, D.L., del Rio, C.E. (1996) Longitudinal sealing ability of mineral trioxide aggregate as a root-end filling material. *Journal of Endodontics* **22**(11), 575–8.

Ber, B.S., Hatton, J.F., Stewart, G.P. (2007) Chemical modification of proroot mta to improve handling characteristics and decrease setting time. *Journal of Endodontics* **33**(10), 1231–4.

Bodrumlu, E. (2008) Biocompatibility of retrograde root filling materials: a review. *Australian Endodontics Journal* **34**(1), 30–5.

Bonson, S., Jeansonne, B.G., Lallier, T.E. (2004) Root-end filling materials alter fibroblast differentiation. *Journal of Dental Research* **83**(5), 408–13.

Bortoluzzi, E.A., Broon, N.J., Bramante, C.M., *et al.* (2006) Sealing ability of MTA and radiopaque Portland cement with or without calcium chloride for root-end filling. *Journal of Endodontics* **32**(9), 897–900.

Bozeman, T.B., Lemon, R.R., Eleazer, P.D. (2006) Elemental analysis of crystal precipitate from gray and white MTA. *Journal of Endodontics* **32**(5), 425–8.

British Standards Institute (2007) Terminology for the bio-nano inferface. PAS 132. http://shop.bsigroup.com/forms/Nano/PAS-132/

Camilleri, J. (2014) Color stability of white mineral trioxide aggregate in contact with hypochlorite solution. *Journal of Endodontics* **40**(3), 436–40.

Camilleri, J., Pitt Ford, T.R. (2006) Mineral trioxide aggregate: a review of the constituents and biological properties of the material. *International Endodontics Journal* **39**(10), 747–54.

Camilleri, J., Montesin, F.E., Papaioannou, S., *et al.* (2004) Biocompatibility of two commercial forms of mineral trioxide aggregate. *International Endodontics Journal* **37**(10), 699–704.

Casas, M.J., Kenny, D.J., Judd, P.L., *et al.* (2005) Do we still need formocresol in pediatric dentistry? *Journal of the Canadian Dental Association* **71**(10), 749–51.

Chong, B., Pitt Ford, T. (2005) Root-end filling materials: rationale and tissue response. *Endodontics Topics* **11**(1), 114–30.

Chong, B.S., Pitt Ford, T.R., Hudson, M.B. (2003) A prospective clinical study of Mineral Trioxide Aggregate and IRM when used as root-end filling materials in endodontic surgery. *International Endodontics Journal* **36**(8), 520–6.

Crooks, W.G., Anderson, R.W., Powell, B.J., *et al.* (1994) Longitudinal evaluation of the seal of IRM root end fillings. *Journal of Endodontics* **20**(5), 250–2.

Dammaschke, T., Gerth, H.U., Zuchner, H., *et al.* (2005) Chemical and physical surface and bulk material characterization of white ProRoot MTA and two Portland cements. *Dental Materials* **21**(8), 731–8.

Dorn, S.O., Gartner, A.H. (1990) Retrograde filling materials: a retrospective success-failure study of amalgam, EBA, and IRM. *Journal of Endodontics* **16**(8), 391–3.

Eldeniz, A.U., Hadimli, H.H., Ataoglu, H., *et al.* (2006) Antibacterial effect of selected root-end filling materials. *Journal of Endodontics* **32**(4), 345–9.

Estrela, C., Bammann, L.L., Estrela, C.R., *et al.* (2011) Antimicrobial and chemical study of MTA, Portland cement, calcium hydroxide paste, Sealapex and Dycal. *Brazilian Dental Journal* **1**, 3–9.

Felman, D., Parashos. P. (2013) Coronal tooth discoloration and white mineral trioxide aggregate. *Journal of Endodontics* **39**(4), 484–7.

Fischer, E.J., Arens, D.E., Miller, C.H. (1998) Bacterial leakage of mineral trioxide aggregate as compared with zinc-free amalgam, intermediate restorative material, and Super-EBA as a root-end filling material. *Journal of Endodontics* **24**(3), 176–9.

Formosa, L.M., Mallia, B., Camilleri, J. (2012) A quantitative method for determining the antiwashout characteristics of cement-based dental materials including mineral trioxide aggregate. *International Endodontics Journal* **46**(2), 179–86.

Gartner, A.H., Dorn, S.O. (1992) Advances in endodontic surgery. *Dent Clin North Am* **36**(2), 357–78.

Gandolfi, M.G., Taddei, P., Tinti, A., *et al.* (2010) Apatite-forming ability (bioactivity) of ProRoot MTA. *International Endodontics Journal* **43**(10), 917–29.

Gondim, E., Jr., Kim, S., de Souza-Filho, F.J. (2005) An investigation of microleakage from root-end fillings in ultrasonic retrograde cavities with or without finishing: a quantitative analysis. *Oral Surgery, Oral Medicine, Oral Pathology, Oral Radiology and Endodontics* **99**(6), 755–60.

Haglund, R., He, J., Jarvis, J., *et al.* (2003) Effects of root-end filling materials on fibroblasts and macrophages in vitro. *Oral Surgery, Oral Medicine, Oral Pathology, Oral Radiology and Endodontics* **95**(6), 739–45.

Harrison, J.W., Johnson, S.A. (1997) Excisional wound healing following the use of IRM as a root-end filling material. *Journal of Endodontics* **23**(1), 19–27.

Holland, R., Souza, V., Nery, M.J., *et al.* (2002) Reaction of rat connective tissue to implanted dentin tubes filled with a white mineral trioxide aggregate. *Brazilian Dental Journal* **13**(1), 23–6.

Huang, F.M., Tai, K.W., Chou, M.Y., *et al.* (2002) Cytotoxicity of resin-, zinc oxide-eugenol-, and calcium hydroxide-based root canal sealers on human periodontal ligament cells and permanent V79 cells. *International Endodontics Journal* **35**(2), 153–8.

Huang, T.H., Shie, M.Y., Kao, C.T., *et al.* (2008) The effect of setting accelerator on properties of mineral trioxide aggregate. *Journal of Endodontics* **34**(5), 590–3.

Lee, E.S. (2000) A new mineral trioxide aggregate root-end filling technique. *Journal of Endodontics* **26**(12), 764–5.

Lindeboom, J.A., Frenken, J.W., Kroon, F.H., *et al.* (2005) A comparative prospective randomized clinical study of MTA and IRM as root-end filling materials in single-rooted teeth in endodontic surgery. *Oral Surgery, Oral Medicine, Oral Pathology, Oral Radiology and Endodontics* **100**(4), 495–500.

Lindskog, S., Blomlof, L., Hammarstrom, L. (1983) Repair of periodontal tissues in vivo and in vitro. *Journal of Clinical Periodontology* **10**(2), 188–205.

Lustmann, J., Friedman, S., Shaharabany, V. (1991) Relation of pre- and intraoperative factors to prognosis of posterior apical surgery. *Journal of Endodontics* **17**(5), 239–41.

Keiser, K., Johnson, C.C., Tipton, D.A. (2000) Cytotoxicity of mineral trioxide aggregate using human periodontal ligament fibroblasts. *Journal of Endodontics* **26**(5), 288–91.

Kim, S., Kratchman, S. (2006) Modern endodontic surgery concepts and practice: a review. *Journal of Endodontics* **32**(7), 601–23.

Kogan, P., He, J., Glickman, G.N., *et al.* (2006) The effects of various additives on setting properties of MTA. *Journal of Endodontics* **32**(6), 569–72.

Koh, E.T., Torabinejad, M., Pitt Ford, T.R., *et al.* (1997) Mineral trioxide aggregate stimulates a biological response in human osteoblasts. *Journal of Biomedical Materials Research* **37**(3), 432–9.

Koh, E.T., McDonald, F., Pitt Ford, T.R., *et al.* (1998) Cellular response to Mineral Trioxide Aggregate. *Journal of Endodontics* **24**(8), 543–7.

Mangin, C., Yesilsoy, C., Nissan, R., *et al.* (2003) The comparative sealing ability of hydroxyapatite cement, mineral trioxide aggregate, and super ethoxybenzoic acid as root-end filling materials. *Journal of Endodontics* **29**(4), 261–4.

Miyagak, D.C., de Carvalho, E.M., Robazza, C.R., *et al.* (2006) In vitro evaluation of the antimicrobial activity of endodontic sealers. *Brazilian Oral Research* **20**(4), 303–6.

Mooney, G.C., North, S. (2008) The current opinions and use of MTA for apical barrier formation of non-vital immature permanent incisors by consultants in paediatric dentistry in the UK. *Dental Traumatology* **24**(1), 65–9.

Moretton, T.R., Brown, C.E., Jr., Legan, J.J., *et al.* (2000) Tissue reactions after subcutaneous and intraosseous implantation of mineral trioxide aggregate and ethoxybenzoic acid cement. *Journal of Biomedical Materials Research* **52**(3), 528–33.

Namazikhah, M.S., Nekoofar, M.H., Sheykhrezae, M.S., *et al.* (2008) The effect of pH on surface hardness and microstructure of mineral trioxide aggregate. *International Endodontics Journal* **41**(2), 108–16.

Oynick, J., Oynick, T. (1978) A study of a new material for retrograde fillings. *Journal of Endodontics* **4**(7), 203–6.

Perez, A.L., Spears, R., Gutmann, J.L., *et al.* (2003) Osteoblasts and MG-63 osteosarcoma cells behave differently when in contact with ProRoot MTA and White MTA. *International Endodontics Journal* **36**(8), 564–70.

Perinpanayagam, H., Al-Rabeah, E. (2009) Osteoblasts interact with MTA surfaces and express Runx2. *Oral Surgery, Oral Medicine, Oral Pathology, Oral Radiology and Endodontics* **107**(4), 590–6.

Pitt Ford, T.R., Andreasen, J.O., Dorn, S.O., *et al.* (1994) Effect of IRM root end fillings on healing after replantation. *Journal of Endodontics* **20**(8), 381–5.

Pitt Ford, T.R., Andreasen, J.O., Dorn, S.O., *et al.* (1995a) Effect of super-EBA as a root end filling on healing after replantation. *Journal of Endodontics* **21**(1), 13–5.

Pitt Ford, T.R., Torabinejad, M., McKendry, D.J., *et al.* (1995b) Use of mineral trioxide aggregate for repair of furcal perforations. *Oral Surgery, Oral Medicine, Oral Pathology, Oral Radiology and Endodontics* **79**(6), 756–63.

Pitt Ford, T.R., Torabinejad, M., Abedi, H.R., *et al.* (1996) Using mineral trioxide aggregate as a pulp-capping material. *Journal of the American Dental Association* **127**(10), 1491–4.

Rahbaran, S., Gilthorpe, M.S., Harrison, S.D., *et al.* (2001) Comparison of clinical outcome of periapical surgery in endodontic and oral surgery units of a teaching dental hospital: a retrospective study. *Oral Surgery, Oral Medicine, Oral Pathology, Oral Radiology and Endodontics* **91**(6), 700–9.

Rapp, E.L., Brown, C.E., Jr, Newton, C.W. (1991) An analysis of success and failure of apicoectomies. *Journal of Endodontics* **17**, 508–12

Reyes-Carmona, J.F., Felippe, M.S., Felippe, W.T. (2009) Biomineralization ability and interaction of mineral trioxide aggregate and white portland cement with dentin in a phosphate-containing fluid. *Journal of Endodontics* **35**(5), 731–6.

Ribeiro, D.A., Matsumoto, M.A., Duarte, M.A., *et al.* (2005) In vitro biocompatibility tests of two commercial types of mineral trioxide aggregate. *Brazilian Oral Research* **19**(3), 183–7.

Roy, C.O., Jeansonne, B.G., Gerrets, T.F. (2001) Effect of an acid environment on leakage of root-end filling materials. *Journal of Endodontics* **27**(1), 7–8.

Rubinstein, R.A., Kim, S. (1999) Short-term observation of the results of endodontic surgery with the use of a surgical operation microscope and Super-EBA as root-end filling material. *Journal of Endodontics* **25**(1), 43–8.

Rubinstein, R., Torabinejad, M. (2004) Contemporary endodontic surgery. *Journal of the California Dental Association* **32**(6), 485–92.

Rud, J., Munksgaard, E.C., Andreasen, J.O., *et al.* (1991) Retrograde root filling with composite and a dentin-bonding agent. 1. *Endodontics and Dental Traumatology* **7**(3), 118–25.

Rud, J., Rud, V., Munksgaard, E.C. (1996) Long-term evaluation of retrograde root filling with dentin-bonded resin composite. *Journal of Endodontics* **22**(2), 90–3.

Saghiri, M.A., Lotfi, M., Saghiri, A.M., *et al.* (2008) Effect of pH on sealing ability of white mineral trioxide aggregate as a root-end filling material. *Journal of Endodontics* **34**(10), 1226–9.

Saidon, J., He, J., Zhu, Q., *et al.* (2003) Cell and tissue reactions to mineral trioxide aggregate and Portland cement. *Oral Surgery, Oral Medicine, Oral Pathology, Oral Radiology and Endodontics* **95**(4), 483–9.

Sarkar, N.K., Caicedo, R., Ritwik, P., *et al.* (2005) Physicochemical basis of the biologic properties of mineral trioxide aggregate. *Journal of Endodontics* **31**(2), 97–100.

Saunders, W.P. (2008) A prospective clinical study of periradicular surgery using mineral trioxide aggregate as a root-end filling. *Journal of Endodontics* **34**(6), 660–5.

Scheerer, S.Q., Steiman, H.R., Cohen, J. (2001) A comparative evaluation of three root-end filling materials: an in vitro leakage study using *Prevotella nigrescens*. *Journal of Endodontics* **27**(1), 40–2.

Shahi, S., Rahimi, S., Lotfi, M., *et al.* (2006) A comparative study of the biocompatibility of three root-end filling materials in rat connective tissue. *Journal of Endodontics* **32**(8), 776–80.

Shahi, S., Rahimi, S., Yavari, H.R., *et al.* (2007) Sealing ability of white and gray mineral trioxide aggregate mixed with distilled water and 0.12% chlorhexidine gluconate when used as root-end filling materials. *Journal of Endodontics* **33**(12), 1429–32.

Song, M., Chung, W., Lee, S.J., *et al*. (2012) Long-term outcome of the cases classified as successes based on short-term follow-up in endodontic microsurgery. *Journal of Endodontics* **38**(9), 1192–6.

Tai, K.W., Chang, Y.C. (2000) Cytotoxicity evaluation of perforation repair materials on humanperiodontal ligament cells in vitro. *Journal of Endodontics* **26**(7), 395–7.

Takita, T., Hayashi, M., Takeich,i O., *et al*. (2006) Effect of mineral trioxide aggregate on proliferation of cultured human dental pulp cells. *International Endodontics Journal* **39**(5), 415–22.

Tawil, P.Z., Trope, M., Curran, A.E., *et al*. (2009) Periapical microsurgery: an in vivo evaluation of endodontic root-end filling materials. *Journal of Endodonticsontics* **35**(3), 357–62.

Torabinejad, M., Chivian, N. (1999) Clinical applications of mineral trioxide aggregate. *Journal of Endodontics* **25**(3), 197–205.

Torabinejad, M., Watson, T.F., Pitt Ford, T.R. (1993) Sealing ability of a mineral trioxide aggregate when used as a root end filling material. *Journal of Endodontics* **19**(12), 591–5.

Torabinejad, M., Higa, R.K., McKendry, D.J., *et al*. (1994) Dye leakage of four root end filling materials: effects of blood contamination. *Journal of Endodontics* **20**(4), 159–63.

Torabinejad, M., Hong, C.U., Lee, S.J, Monsef, M., *et al*. (1995a) Investigation of mineral trioxide aggregate for root-end filling in dogs. *Journal of Endodontics* **21**(12), 603–8.

Torabinejad, M., Hong, C.U., McDonald, F., *et al*. (1995b) Physical and chemical properties of a new root-end filling material. *Journal of Endodontics* **21**(7), 349–53.

Torabinejad, M., Hong, C.U., Pitt Ford, T.R., *et al*. (1995c) Tissue reaction to implanted super EBA and mineral trioxide aggregate in the mandible of guinea pigs: a preliminary report. *Journal of Endodontics* **21**(11), 569–71.

Torabinejad, M., Hong, C.U., Pitt Ford, T.R., *et al*. (1995d) Antibacterial effects of some root end filling materials. *Journal of Endodontics* **21**(8), 403–6.

Torabinejad, M., Rastegar, A.F., Kettering, J.D., *et al*. (1995e) Bacterial leakage of mineral trioxide aggregate as a root-end filling material. *Journal of Endodontics* **21**(3), 109–12.

Torabinejad, M., Smith, P.W., Kettering, J.D., *et al*. (1995f) Comparative investigation of marginal adaptation of mineral trioxide aggregate and other commonly used root-end filling materials. *Journal of Endodontics* **21**(6), 295–9.

Torabinejad, M., Pitt Ford, T.R., McKendry, D.J., *et al*. (1997) Histologic assessment of mineral trioxide aggregate as a root-end filling in monkeys. *Journal of Endodontics* **23**(4), 225–8.

Trope, M., Lost, C., Schmitz, H.J., *et al*. (1996) Healing of apical periodontitis in dogs after apicoectomy and retrofilling with various filling materials. *Oral Surgery, Oral Medicine, Oral Pathology, Oral Radiology and Endodontics* **81**(2), 221–8.

Valois, C.R., Costa, E.D., Jr. (2004) Influence of the thickness of mineral trioxide aggregate on sealing ability of root-end fillings in vitro. *Oral Surgery, Oral Medicine, Oral Pathology, Oral Radiology and Endodontics* **97**(1), 108–11.

von Arx, T., Hanni, S., Jensen, S.S. (2010) Clinical results with two different methods of root-end preparation and filling in apical surgery: mineral trioxide aggregate and adhesive resin composite. *Journal of Endodontics* **36**(7), 1122–9.

von Arx, T., Jensen, S.S., Hanni, S., *et al*. (2012) Five-year longitudinal assessment of the prognosis of apical microsurgery. *Journal of Endodontics* **38**(5), 570–9.

Willians, D.F. (1986) Definitions in biomaterials. Proceedings of a Consensus Conference of the European Society for Biomaterials. England co. 4. Elsevier, New York.

Wu, M.K., Kontakiotis, E.G., Wesselink, P.R. (1998) Long-term seal provided by some root-end filling materials. *Journal of Endodontics* **24**(8), 557–60.

Yasuda, Y., Kamaguchi, A., Saito, T. (2008) In vitro evaluation of the antimicrobial activity of a new resin based endodontic sealer against endodontic pathogens. *Journal of Oral Science* **50**(3), 309–13.

Yazdi, P.M., Schou, S., Jensen, S.S., *et al.* (2007) Dentine-bonded resin composite (Retroplast) for root-end filling: a prospective clinical and radiographic study with a mean follow-up period of 8 years. *International Endodontics Journal* **40**(7), 493–503.

Yoshimine, Y., Ono, M., Akamine, A. (2007) In vitro comparison of the biocompatibility of mineral trioxide aggregate, 4META/MMA-TBB resin, and intermediate restorative material as root-end-filling materials. *Journal of Endodontics* **33**(9), 1066–9.

Zhu, Q., Haglund, R., Safavi, K.E., *et al.* (2000) Adhesion of human osteoblasts on root-end filling materials. *Journal of Endodontics* **26**(7), 404–6.

10   Calcium Silicate–Based Cements

Masoud Parirokh[1] and Mahmoud Torabinejad[2]

[1]Department of Endodontics, Kerman University of Medical Sciences
School of Dentistry, Iran
[2]Department of Endodontics, Loma Linda University School
of Dentistry, USA

Mineral Trioxide Aggregate: Properties and Clinical Applications, First Edition.
Edited by Mahmoud Torabinejad.
© 2014 John Wiley & Sons, Inc. Published 2014 by John Wiley & Sons, Inc.

INTRODUCTION

Calcium silicate-based cements {mineral trioxide aggregate (MTA) lookalike materials} are cements or root canal sealers that have been made based on a composition of calcium and silicate. Due to promising results obtained by MTA and its excellent sealing ability, biocompatibility, and clinical applications for pulp capping in primary and permanent teeth, root-end filling, perforation repair, and apical plug for teeth with open apices, researchers have been encouraged to investigate materials with similar favorable properties while being less expensive as well as fewer of the current drawbacks of the original MTA (Parirokh & Torabinejad 2010a, b; Torabinejad & Parirokh 2010). Since 75% of MTA is composed of Portland cement (PC) (Parirokh & Torabinejad 2010a), some investigators introduced their novel formulations as PC-based materials. These investigators claimed that their new materials had a similar composition to MTA with some modifications that may improve some of the properties such as handling characteristics, lower setting time, prevention of tooth discoloration, and higher radiopacity. In this chapter, several materials, mostly composed of calcium and silicate (main components of PC) that are commercially available, are discussed. In addition, several new formulations of experimental calcium silicate-based cements are briefly introduced.

PORTLAND CEMENT (PC)

High cost has been claimed to be one of the major drawbacks for MTA (Parirokh & Torabinejad 2010b). Since PC is an inexpensive material and is chemically similar to MTA, some researchers have suggested PC as an acceptable substitute material for MTA.

Chemical composition

Except for the bismuth oxide component, PC and MTA have a similar main composition of tricalcium and dicalcium silicate, which during hydration, produce calcium silicate hydrate gel and calcium hydroxide (CH). However, MTA showed lack of potassium, and less calcium dialuminate, and calcium sulfate unhydrated compared to type I PC (Parirokh & Torabinejad 2010a).

Despite the similarity, several differences are reported between the materials in terms of setting expansion, chemical composition, surface chemical composition, porosity, compressive strength, radiopacity, calcium ion release, and particle size. Several investigators have tried to add various amounts of bismuth oxide (as radiopacifiers) to PC. However, an increase in porosity, solubility, and degradation of the material were observed with increasing amounts of bismuth oxide. Moreover, because of the presence of more flaws in the composition of bismuth oxide and PC, the mixture showed a higher amount of cracks in the set material (Parirokh & Torabinejad 2010a).

Despite similarities in the composition of white and gray ProRoot MTA to white and gray PC (Asgary et al. 2009b; Parirokh & Torabinejad 2010a), both types of ProRoot MTA showed significantly lower levels of arsenic compared to white and gray PC. In addition, gray PC showed significantly higher lead concentrations than gray and white ProRoot MTA and white PC. Also the amounts of chromium, copper, manganese, and zinc in gray PC were significantly higher compared to white PC and gray and white ProRoot MTA (Chang et al. 2010). The amount of trace elements released from PC in both physiologic solution (Hank's balanced solution: HBSS) and acidic environment was higher than that in several calcium silicate-based materials such as BioAggregate (BA), Biodentine (BD), tricalcium silicate, and Angelus MTA (AMTA). PC had higher concentrations of chromium, lead, and arsenic compared to AMTA (Camilleri *et al.* 2012). Despite having no significant difference in amounts of arsenic in their composition, white PC and AMTA released higher amounts of arsenic than ProRoot MTA when the samples were either placed in water or synthetic body fluid. Gray PC not only has significantly higher levels of lead, arsenic, and chromium in its material composition compared to AMTA and ProRoot MTA, but it also releases significantly higher amounts of these elements in water or synthetic body fluid (Schembri *et al.* 2010). The amounts of arsenic in all types of white PC are not the same. One investigation showed that despite the presence of 4.7 ± 0.36 ppm type III arsenic in white PC from one manufacturer (Irajazinho; Votorantim Cimentos, Rio Branco, SP, Brazil), another manufacture's white PC (Juntalider; Brasilatex Ltda, Diadema, SP, Brazil) had lower detectable levels of type III arsenic in its composition (De-Deus *et al.* 2009a).

Physical properties

It has been suggested that the presence of iron and manganese in MTA may be the cause of tooth discoloration after treatment (Asgary *et al.* 2005; Dammaschke *et al.* 2005; Parirokh & Torabinejad 2010b). Recently however, the discoloration potential of MTA has been attributed to the presence of bismuth in the material's composition (Krastl *et al.* 2013; Vallés *et al.* 2013). An investigation showed that PC had significantly lower discoloration potential compared to gray ProRoot MTA, while no significant difference was measured against white ProRoot MTA. The contamination of white ProRoot MTA and PC with blood resulted in the cements' discoloration with no significant difference between the tested materials (Lenherr *et al.* 2012).

There are some controversies regarding the solubility of PC. Early investigations reported a high solubility of PC compared to MTA (Parirokh & Torabinejad 2010a). One investigation reported that AMTA had higher solubility than modified PC (75% PC + 20% bismuth oxide + 5% calcium sulfate) (Vivan *et al.* 2010). According to ISO 6876/2001, white ProRoot MTA showed significantly higher solubility compared to white PC. When the white PC and white ProRoot MTA was stored in either water or HBSS, the latter material showed significantly higher liquid uptake. Both white PC and white ProRoot MTA showed expansion in contact with HBSS. White PC released calcium, aluminum, and silicon in higher amounts in HBSS compared to the water (Camilleri 2011). Washout resistance of PC was higher when the material was stored in both distilled water and HBSS compared to AMTA (Formosa *et al.* 2013).

Several criteria have been introduced for evaluating a material's bioactivity such as: releasing calcium ions, electroconductivity, production of CH, formation of an interfacial layer between the cement and dentinal wall, and formation of apatite crystals over the material's surface in a synthetic tissue fluid environment

(Parirokh *et al.* 2007; Asgary *et al.* 2009a; Parirokh *et al.* 2009; Parirokh & Torabinejad 2010a, 2010b). PC showed an alkaline pH and the production of port-landite (CH) after hydration (Camilleri 2008; Gonçalves *et al.* 2010; Massi *et al.* 2011; Formosa *et al.* 2012). However, a long-term investigation showed that for-mation of CH throughout a one-year period after setting in PC was significantly lower compared to ProRoot MTA. Maturation of structure and hydration mecha-nism is not obvious in PC compared to ProRoot MTA throughout the one-year period of time (Chedella & Berzins 2010). This suggests that MTA is more bioac-tive than PC (Formosa *et al.* 2012).

The particle size of white PC is significantly larger than white ProRoot MTA (Asgary *et al.* 2011b) and, after hydration, the crystalline particles in white MTA were smaller than those present in white PC (Asgary *et al.* 2004).

White and gray PC did not fulfill the requirement of ANSI/ADA specification 57 for radiopacity (Borges *et al.* 2011). According to ANSI/ADA specification number 57/2000 and ISO 6876/2001, each root canal sealing material should have radiopacity equal to 3 mm aluminum, which is enough for MTA, but PC did not exhibit this amount of radiopacity. Several investigations have been performed to evaluate the effect of adding different opacifiers to various properties of PC (Camilleri 2010; Camilleri *et al.* 2011b; Cutajar *et al.* 2011; Formosa *et al.* 2012).

Bioactivity of white PC has been confirmed by precipitation and formation of the interfacial layer between the cement and the root dentin in separate *in vitro* investigations (Parirokh & Torabinejad 2010a). PC showed bioactivity when placed in a synthetic body fluid such as HBSS (Formosa *et al.* 2012), Dulbecco's phosphate-buffered saline (Gandolfi *et al.* 2010), or phosphate-buffered saline (PBS) (Reyes-Carmona *et al.* 2010). Both white and gray PC showed calcium ion release (Gonçalves *et al.* 2010; Massi *et al.* 2011). The formation of apatite crystals took different amounts of time when various physiologic solutions were used (Gandolfi *et al.* 2010).

The push-out bond strength of PC was reported to be significantly lower than that of AMTA and ProRoot MTA following storage of the materials in PBS (Reyes-Carmona *et al.* 2010).

From the physical and chemical properties, the major differences between MTA and PC are the presence of bismuth oxide, lower levels of calcium alumi-nate and calcium sulfate, lower solubility, and smaller particle size of MTA compared to PC (Parirokh & Torabinejad 2010a).

Antibacterial activity

There are a few reports regarding the antibacterial activity of PC and MTA. Some investigators reported no antibacterial activity of PC and MTA against several bacterial species, whereas others showed that PC, like MTA, has antibacterial and antifungal properties against *Enterococcus faecalis, Micrococcus luteus,*

Staphylococcus aureus, Staphylococcus epidermidis, Psuedomonas aeruginosa, and *Candida albicans* (Parirokh & Torabinejad 2010a).

Sealing ability

White and gray ProRoot MTA showed similar dye penetration compared to white and gray PC when used as root-end filling materials (Rekab & Ayoubi 2010; Shahi *et al*. 2011). When used as perforation repair material, white PC showed significantly less protein leakage compared to white and gray ProRoot MTA (Shahi *et al*. 2009).

Biocompatibility

Cell culture studies

Investigations that compared PC and MTA reported different results regarding cell viability, proliferation, and migration. Several cell culture investigations revealed no significant differences between the tested PC and MTA (Parirokh & Torabinejad 2010a). Moreover, an investigation reported that white PC with 15% bismuth oxide (similar to white AMTA) showed no genotoxicity or cytotoxicity in murine fibroblast cell culture (Zeferino *et al*. 2010). In contrast, addition of bismuth oxide to PC powder at all ratios resulted in significantly lower cell viability compared to the control during early evaluation time (Parirokh & Torabinejad 2010a). PC did not affect cell viability or induce expression of osteonectin and dentin sialophosphoprotein mRNAs in human dental pulp cell culture (Min *et al*. 2007). Both ProRoot MTA- and PC-induced expression of collagen, fibronectin, and transforming growth factor (TGF) β1 in periodontal fibroblast cell culture (Fayazi *et al*. 2011). However, ProRoot MTA showed significantly higher cell proliferation and migration compared to PC in human bone marrow-derived mesenchymal stem cells (D'Antò *et al*. 2010). Varying results in cell culture investigations, despite the use of similar materials, might be because of the employment of various cell types, the choice of study duration, use of a fresh or cured material, frequency of changing the medium, the use of direct contact or extract of MTA, and the concentration of the material in the cell culture media (Torabinejad & Parirokh 2010).

Subcutaneous implantation

Subcutaneous implantation of dentin tubes filled with PC promotes mineralization between PC and the dentinal tube. However, PC showed significantly lower biomineralization compared to AMTA mainly after 30 and 60 days (Dreger *et al*. 2012). Another subcutaneous implantation study showed that both white and gray ProRoot MTA were more biocompatible compared to white and gray PC (Shahi *et al.* 2010). Subcutaneous implantation of PC showed a similar reaction to AMTA by inducing moderate inflammation at 7 days followed by a reduction in the number of inflammatory cells as well as signs of mineralization by presence of Von Kossa positive structures at longer time intervals (Viola *et al.* 2012).

In vivo investigations

Animal investigations reported no significant difference between white ProRoot MTA and white PC as pulp capping agents in terms of the calcified bridge thickness over the capping area. However, both materials were significantly superior compared to CH in that regard (Parirokh & Torabinejad 2010b; Al-Hezaimi *et al.* 2011a). Another investigation used a combination of Emdogain with either white PC or white ProRoot MTA as pulp capping agents. Results showed that there was no significant difference between reparative dentin thicknesses with either of the combinations (Al-Hezaimi *et al.* 2011b).

Clinical applications

A human investigation using AMTA and PC for pulpotomy in carious primary molars reported successful clinical and radiographic outcomes up to 24 months after treatment. However, more pulp canal obliteration was observed in the teeth that were treated with PC compared to the gray AMTA (Sakai *et al.* 2009).

Limitations

1 Separate investigations reported scarce results regarding the composition of PC (De-Deus *et al.* 2009a; Parirokh & Torabinejad 2010a). Since PC is manufactured widely around the world, it is difficult if not impossible to evaluate the purity of all manufacturers' compositions.
2 PC had higher concentrations of chromium, lead, and arsenic, is acid-soluble, and leaches out in HBSS compared to AMTA (Camilleri *et al.* 2012). In addition, PC contains higher concentrations of heavy metals such as copper, manganese, and strontium, which are known to be toxic, compared to white ProRoot MTA (Parirokh & Torabinejad 2010a). One of the major concerns about using PC is the amount of lead and arsenic in its composition that are released from the material into the surrounding tissues (Schembri *et al.* 2010). Because of some reports regarding the high solubility of some types

of PC and the release of toxic elements into the surrounding tissues, its long-term safety is questioned (Parirokh & Torabiejad 2010a). In addition, gray PC showed significantly higher lead concentrations than gray and white ProRoot MTA, as well as white PC. Moreover, the amount of cadmium, chromium, copper, manganese, and zinc in gray PC were significantly higher compared to white PC and gray and white ProRoot MTA. Finally, the amount of arsenic in gray and white PC is significantly higher than that in both white and gray ProRoot MTA (Chang *et al.* 2010).

3 Another concern for PC's higher solubility is the fact that the material might degrade after one of its clinical applications and therefore jeopardize the seal of the material (Borges *et al.* 2010; Parirokh & Torabinejad 2010a).

4 Lower compressive strength of some types of PC compared to white and gray MTA might be important for some of the clinical applications of MTA such as repairing perforations and pulp capping because these procedures need materials with sufficient compressive strength during mastication (Parirokh & Torabinejad 2010a).

5 Excessive setting expansion of a material, particularly as a root-end filling substance, might result in a cracked tooth, which is undesirable. The scarcity of results regarding setting expansion of PC is another concern for the use of the material as an MTA substitute for root-end filling (Parirokh & Torabinejad 2010a).

6 Carbonation of PC in inflamed tissue results in lower tensile strength and resiliency of the material, which might cause cracks and buckle under mastication force instead of deforming, particularly in some clinical applications of MTA such as perforation repair or pulp capping (Parirokh & Torabinejad 2010a).

7 MTA as a medical material is manufactured under intensive supervision to ensure its composition and to prevent contamination. The material is approved by the US Food and Drug Administration (FDA) for use in humans (Parirokh & Torabinejad 2010a).

8 PC produces a significantly lower amount of portlandite after setting, compared to white ProRoot MTA, up to 1 year after hydration, which may affect long-term efficacy of the material (Chedella & Berzins 2010).

9 Biomineralization by MTA-based materials is more effective than PC, which is crucial for a biomaterial (Dreger *et al.* 2012).

In conclusion, despite some similarity in chemical composition and physical properties between white and gray MTA with white and gray PC, there have been several limitations that prevent practitioners from using PC as a substitute for MTA.

ANGELUS MTA

Angelus MTA (MTA-Angelus, Angelus, Londrina, PR, Brazil) was developed in Brazil. Similar to ProRoot MTA (Asgary *et al.* 2005; Parirokh *et al.* 2005) the material is marketed in both forms of white and gray AMTA. Unfortunately, most articles do not mention the type of AMTA used; therefore, they are combined as AMTA in this chapter.

Chemical composition

AMTA is composed of 80% PC and 20% bismuth oxide. Compared to gray ProRoot MTA, gray AMTA contains a lower amount of bismuth oxide and magnesium phosphate, but a higher amount of calcium carbonate, calcium silicate, and barium zinc phosphate. Furthermore, AMTA contains less carbon, oxygen, and silica than gray ProRoot MTA, but more calcium. In addition, AMTA showed the presence of aluminum and the absence of iron, in contrast to gray ProRoot MTA, which exhibited the opposite. The amount of bismuth oxide in crystalline structures of gray ProRoot MTA is greater than that in gray AMTA. Based on present available data, AMTA has a different chemical composition compared to gray ProRoot MTA (Parirokh & Torabinejad 2010a). The amount of aluminum oxide in AMTA was reported to be more than twice as high that in white ProRoot MTA (Asgary *et al.* 2009b).

De-Deus and associates (2009a) have shown that both gray ProRoot MTA and gray AMTA had a below-the-limit amount of arsenic (<2 mg/kg-ISO 9917–1/2007) in their compositions, whereas the white ProRoot MTA (3.3±0.46 ppm) and white AMTA (6.5±0.56 ppm) had a higher than permitted amount of arsenic in their compositions. AMTA and white ProRoot MTA and white PC had similar amounts of metallic ions. The amount of acid-soluble level of arsenic in both white ProRoot MTA and AMTA is higher than the ISO 9917–1/2007 specification. AMTA released significantly less chromium compared to ProRoot MTA in synthetic body fluid. However, the amount of arsenic released in AMTA is significantly higher than that in white ProRoot MTA when the samples are either kept in water or synthetic body fluid (Schembri *et al.* 2010). Investigations (Monteiro Bramante *et al.* 2008; Parirokh & Torabinejad 2010a; Schembri *et al.* 2010; Camilleri *et al.* 2012) on arsenic and trace elements in the composition of MTA resulted in variations to ISO 9917–1/2007. The method of detecting acid-soluble elements in MTA was different in separate investigations and it may be the reason for reporting different amounts of arsenic and other trace elements in various types of MTA. Despite an acid-extractable arsenic level higher than ISO 9917–1/2007 (Schembri *et al.* 2010; Camilleri *et al.* 2012), Camilleri and associates (2012) concluded that AMTA is safe to be used in dentistry.

Physical properties

Some of the physical properties of AMTA, such as setting time and range of particles, are different from those of ProRoot MTA. However, there are similarities in pH and calcium ion release between these materials (Parirokh & Torabinejad 2010a).

Several discoloration reports regarding MTA have used either white or gray AMTA in their case reports, clinical trials, or *in vitro* investigations (Bortoluzzi *et al.* 2007; Moore *et al.* 2011; Ioannidis *et al.* 2013). Valles and associates (2013) attributed MTA discoloration to the formation of metallic bismuth under light irradiation. Discoloration potential of white and gray AMTA has been investigated (Ioannidis *et al.* 2013). Results showed that gray AMTA produced significantly greater discoloration compared to white AMTA. Gray AMTA's discoloration effect was observed after one month, whereas detectable discoloration in white AMTA samples was observed by human eyes after three months. Both types of AMTA reduced lightness, redness, and yellowness in human teeth. A recent *in vitro* investigation suggested that conditioning coronal dentinal tubules with dentin bonding agents prior to placing either gray or white AMTA as an orifice barrier inside the root canal may prevent future tooth discoloration (Akbari *et al.* 2012).

Both white and gray AMTA showed an alkaline pH following mixture. However, the latter material showed higher alkalinity up to 168 hours after mixing. The amount of calcium ions released in gray AMTA is higher than that in white AMTA up to 72 hours after mixing (de Vasconcelos *et al.* 2009). White AMTA showed an alkaline pH, lower calcium ion release, as well as lower initial and final setting time compared to PC (Massi *et al.* 2011; Hungaro Duarte *et al.* 2012). The AMTA solubility values meet the requirement of solubility described by ASNI/ADA specification 57/2000 (Borges *et al.* 2012). However, the material solubility did not fulfill the requirements that are determined by the International Standard Organization 6876/2001 (Parirokh & Torabinejad 2010a).

Microhardness of AMTA could be affected by the method of mixing. The best average of microhardness at 4 days following mixing was obtained for white and gray AMTA when both materials were mixed with ultrasonic vibration. However, at 28 days after mixing, white AMTA that triturated with amalgamator and gray AMTA that mixed with ultrasonic vibration obtained the best average of microhardness (Nekoofar *et al.* 2010). No temperature rise was observed up to 400 minutes following gray AMTA mixing. The porosity of the gray AMTA is reported to be about 28% and the size of pores was 2.5 μm. The compressive strength of gray AMTA was about 34 MPa after 15 days (Oliveira *et al.* 2010).

The resistance to displacement of AMTA was significantly higher than that of PC (Reyes-Carmona *et al.* 2010). In a long-term study, fracture resistance of teeth with immature roots that were filled with AMTA was significantly higher than that of teeth filled with CH after one year. However, no significant difference was found between gray AMTA and ProRoot MTA in that study (Tuna *et al.* 2011).

Fracture resistance of teeth with immature roots that were filled with gray AMTA was significantly greater than that of teeth filled with CH after 1 year. However, no significant difference was found between AMTA and white ProRoot MTA in the same period of time (Tuna *et al.* 2011).

According to the manufacturers' data sheets for AMTA, the absence of dehydrated calcium sulfate lowers the material setting time to 10 minutes. The setting time of AMTA (14.28 ± 0.49 min) is lower than white and gray ProRoot MTA (Parirokh & Torabinejad 2010a).

Results regarding radiopacity of various types of MTA showed that both types of gray and white AMTA have lower radiopacity than white and gray ProRoot MTA. Gray and white forms of AMTA had a higher number of dissimilar particles compared to white and gray ProRoot MTA (Parirokh & Torabinejad 2010a).

Antibacterial activity

AMTA showed some antibacterial and antifungal activities (Parirokh & Torabinejad 2010a). AMTA showed similar antifungal activity as ProRoot MTA. Despite no killing effect on C. *albicans* after one hour, both of the materials showed fungicidal activity at 24 hours and 48 hours (Kangarlou *et al.* 2012).

Sealing ability

AMTA showed reasonable sealing ability and marginal adaptation in several investigations (Torabinejad & Parirokh 2010).

Biocompatibility properties

Cell culture studies

White AMTA showed low or no genotoxicity and cytotoxicity in separate investigations on murine fibroblast cell culture, L929 mouse fibroblasts, fibroblasts (3T3), odontoblast-like cells, and human dermal fibroblast (Gomes-Filho *et al.* 2009c; Lessa *et al.* 2010; Zeferino *et al.* 2010; Damas *et al.* 2011; Hirschman *et al.* 2012; Silva *et al.* 2012). A cell culture study that used L929 mouse fibroblast cells showed that AMTA did not inhibit cell viability or induce interleukin (IL)-6 cytokine (with no significant difference compared to the control). However, AMTA significantly increased the release of IL-1β compared to the control (Gomes-Filho *et al.* 2009c). Comparing the effects of ProRoot MTA and AMTA on human periodontal fibroblasts, the former showed better biocompatibility

(Samara *et al.* 2011). AMTA showed gelatinolytic activity for matrix metallopro-
teinase-2 (Silva *et al.* 2012). Both white ProRoot MTA and AMTA showed similar human dermal fibroblast viability of greater than or equal to 91.8%. (Damas
et al. 2011).

Anti-inflammatory effects of gray AMTA have been confirmed by reducing
mRNA expression for CC5, IL-1α, and interferon-γ (Parirokh & Torabinejad
2010a). Immune cells produced greater amounts of TGF-β1, IL-1β, macrophage
inflammatory protein-2 (MIP-2), and Leukotriene-B4 in the presence of AMTA
(Torabinejad & Parirokh 2010).

Subcutaneous implantation

Separate investigations on AMTA subcutaneous implantation showed a moderate inflammatory reaction at seven days that was similar to the control at longer
time intervals (30 and 60 days) and subsided in terms of reduced intensity of
inflammatory cells. Mineralized structures were seen in close contact with the
implanted material at 30 days following the material implantation (Gomes-Filho
et al. 2009a, b, 2012; Viola *et al.* 2012). Biomineralization of AMTA was significantly higher than that of PC (Dreger *et al.* 2012).

Intraosseous implantation

AMTA produced a mild inflammatory reaction and dystrophic calcification fol-
lowing implantation of the material inside the socket of extracted teeth in rats.
In conclusion, AMTA was tolerated well by the rats' alveolar socket (Gomes-
Filho *et al.* 2010, 2011).

In vivo investigations

Animal investigations using AMTA as pulp capping and root-filling materials
reported successful outcomes (Parirokh & Torabinejad 2010b). Perforation repair
in rat maxillary molar teeth with AMTA resulted in a significant reduction in the
width of periodontal space and osteoclasts' number at 60 days (da Silva *et al.*
2011). A histologic investigation on dogs' teeth showed no significant difference
among AMTA, super EBA, and IRM as root-end filling material, although AMTA
was the most biocompatible material tested in terms of periapical tissue response
(Wälivaara *et al.* 2012). Another investigation on rats' avulsed teeth with extended
extraoral dry time conditions compared white AMTA and CH as root canal filling
materials. Results showed that despite no significant difference between CH and
white AMTA, the latter material induced more new bone deposition and less
inflammatory tissue reaction after 80 days (Marão *et al.* 2012).

Clinical applications

Several case reports illustrated successful use of AMTA for repairing resorptive defects, perforations, root-end filling materials, pulp capping, revitalization with triple antibiotics paste, and filling a root canal in a tooth with root fracture (Kvinnsland *et al.* 2010; Parirokh & Torabinejad 2010b; Yilmaz *et al.* 2010; dos Santos *et al.* 2011; Shetty & Xavier 2011; Lenzi & Trope 2012; Vier-Pelisser *et al.* 2012; Carvalho *et al.* 2013).

All human investigations that used AMTA as pulp capping agent in caries-free intact teeth showed favorable pulp response (Parirokh & Torabinejad 2010b; Zarrabi *et al.* 2010).

In a clinical and radiographic investigation on placing either white AMTA or white ProRoot MTA as an apical plug in 22 maxillary incisors, no significant difference was found between two groups up to an average of 23.4 months follow-up time. In this study, four out of five teeth that showed coronal discoloration following treatment were treated with AMTA (Moore *et al.* 2011).

In conclusion, despite promising reports of using AMTA through several case reports and case series, the limited amount of evidence-based investigations may be of concern to clinicians using the material for various clinical applications that have been tested for MTA.

BIOAGGREGATE (BA)

BioAggregate (BA) also referred to as DiaRoot (DiaDent) BioAggregate (Innovative Bioceramix, Vancouver, BC, Canada) (De-Deus *et al.* 2009b; Hashem & Wanees Amin 2012) is a material that was introduced for perforation repair, root-end filling, as well as pulp capping.

Chemical composition

The material is composed of fine nanoparticle size, aluminum-free powder that is mixed with deionized water to form a bioceramic paste. BA is composed of a powder (mixed with H_2O) consisting of SiO_2 (13.70%), P_2O_5 (3.92%), CaO (63.50%), and Ta_2O_5 (17%). The manufacturer adds tantalum oxide (Ta_2O_5) to the powder as radiopacifier (Camilleri *et al.* 2012). In addition, CH was detected in the set form of BA, similar to white ProRoot MTA (Park *et al.* 2010; Grech *et al.* 2013). BA has chromium in a similar amount to PC in material composition. In addition, BA has a higher amount of acid-extractable arsenic accepted by ISO 9917–1/2007 (2 mg/kg) and also shows an acceptable amount of lead in its composition. However, the material released negligible amount of trace elements (Camilleri *et al.* 2012).

Physical properties

BA has an alkaline pH after setting (Zhang *et al.* 2009a; Grech *et al.* 2013). BA and white ProRoot MTA showed bioactivity and precipitate apatite crystals when the materials are kept in PBS for up to two months (Shokouhinejad *et al.* 2012a; Grech *et al.* 2013). BA showed significantly less resistance to displacement compared to AMTA when the samples were kept in PBS. However, when the samples were exposed to an acidic environment for four days, BA's push-out bond strength had not been influenced, whereas AMTA's resistance to displacement significantly decreased. Surprisingly, if the exposed samples to acid kept in PBS for 30 days, the AMTA bond resorted and the samples showed significantly higher push-out bond strength compared to the BA samples in the same storage conditions (Hashem & Wanees Amin 2012). Fracture resistance of teeth with immature roots that were filled with BA was significantly greater than that of the teeth filled with CH after 1 year. However, no significant difference was found between AMTA, ProRoot MTA, and BA for the same period of time (Tuna *et al.* 2011).

Antibacterial activity

Both ProRoot MTA and BA killed *E. faecalis* with no significant difference between the materials. Interestingly, the set cement killed bacteria more quickly compared to the freshly mixed materials. Adding dentin powder to the BA cement increased its antibacterial activity (Zhang *et al.* 2009a).

Sealing ability

BA showed significantly lower dye leakage (El Sayed & Saeed 2012), whereas no significant glucose penetration was observed compared to white ProRoot MTA (Leal *et al.* 2011).

Biocompatibility

Cell culture studies

Results of a human periodontal ligament (PDL) fibroblast cell culture study reported that both ProRoot MTA and BA were able to differentiate the PDL cells as well as induce alkaline phosphates and collagen I gene expression (Yan *et al.* 2010). Another investigation on osteoblast cells reported that both materials were nontoxic. However, BA induced a significant increase in the expression of collagen type I, osteocalcin, and osteopontin genes compared to white ProRoot MTA on the second and third day of the study (Yuan *et al.* 2010). No significant difference regarding cell viability was reported between white

ProRoot MTA and BA when they were exposed to human mononuclear cell culture (derived from bone marrow) (De-Deus *et al.* 2009b).

In conclusion, BA is a material with fine particle size, bioactivity, certain antibacterial properties, and no reported toxicity. However, so far, all investigations on BA have been laboratory studies. One will need to see *in vivo* and evidence-based investigations to determine the material's efficacy in clinical applications.

BIODENTINE (BD)

Biodentine (Septodont, Saint-Maur-des-Fosse´s Cedex, France) is a powder/liquid material.

Chemical composition

The powder consists mainly of SiO_2 (16.90%), CaO (62.90%), ZrO_2 (5.47%), and the liquid is composed of Na (15.8%), Mg (5%), Cl (34.7), Ca (23.6%), and H_2O (20.9%) (Camilleri *et al.* 2012). The hydration of BD results in calcium silicate hydrate and CH that leach into the surrounding solution (Grech *et al.* in press). In one investigation, the amount of lead that leached into an acidic environment from BD was higher than that for AMTA, PC, BA, and tricalcium silicate. The amount of released arsenic from BD, however, was the same as that from BA and PC in the same environment. The amount of chromium released from BD in an acidic environment is lower than that from BA and PC. Despite the presence of high lead some investigators have concluded that BD is safe for use in dentistry (Camilleri *et al.* 2012).

Physical properties

Biodentine has an alkaline pH and is bioactive by releasing calcium ions when stored in HBSS (Grech *et al.* 2013). When BD is used as a root canal filling material, the amount of calcium and silicate uptake by the root dentin was significantly higher than that of the control and white ProRoot MTA specimens (Han & Okiji 2011). BD showed a significant adverse influence on flexural strength of dentin after two and three months of exposure (Sawyer *et al.* 2012). Prolonged contact of BD with dentin resulted in biodegradation of the collagen matrix (Leiendecker *et al.* 2012).

Biocompatibility and clinical applications

In an *in vitro* investigation, BD, white ProRoot MTA, and CH significantly elevated the secretion of TGFβ1 of the whole pulp following use as pulp capping agents. Moreover, an early form of reparative dentin was observed in the teeth capped with BD (Laurent *et al.* 2012).

Similar to those for BA, so far, all investigations on BD were conducted *in vitro*. More investigations, particularly *in vivo*, are needed to determine its effectiveness in clinical situations.

iROOT

iRoot (Innovative BioCeramix Inc., Vancouver, Canada) has been introduced in three forms: iRoot Sp, iRoot BP, and iRoot BP Plus. These forms have been introduced for use in root filling, root repair (iRoot BP and iRoot BP plus), and root canal sealer (iRoot Sp) materials (http://www.ibioceramix.com/iRootSP.html).

iRoot SP is an injectable, ready-to-use, insoluble, radiopaque white paste that needs moisture to initiate and complete its setting.

Chemical composition

iRoot SP is a calcium silicate aluminum-free-based root canal sealer that has a very similar composition to WMTA (http://www.ibioceramix.com/iRootSP. html). The root canal should not be completely free of moisture when iRoot Sp is used as a root canal sealer (Nagas *et al.* 2012).

Physical properties

The manufacturer has introduced the material as a root filling material that can be used with or without gutta-percha (Nagas *et al.* 2012). iRoot SP shows a significantly higher bond to dentin compared to MTA Fillapex and Epiphany (Sağsen *et al.* 2011; Nagas *et al.* 2012). The higher bond strength has been attributed to the smaller particle size, level of viscosity, and minimal shrinkage during setting period. The smaller particle size and high level of viscosity increase the flow of the material into the dentinal tubules, other anatomic structures of the root canal space, when gutta-percha is used as the root canal filling material (Shokouhinejad *et al.* 2013). In a study of three conditions of dry, wet, and slightly moist canal, the latter condition provided the highest bond strength between iRoot SP and the dentinal wall of the root canal space (Nagas *et al.* 2012). Placement of CH inside the root canal prior to using iRoot SP as a root canal sealer improves its bond strength to dentin (Amin *et al.* 2012). The results of another study have shown that using iRoot SP with gutta-percha improves resistance to fracture in simulated open apex teeth (Ulusoy *et al.* 2011). iRoot SP showed an alkaline pH up to 7 days after setting and was capable of killing *E. faecalis* in an antibacterial investigation (Zhang *et al.* 2009b).

iRoot BP is an injectable, ready-to-use white paste for root repair and root filling. The manufacturer claims that iRoot BP and iRoot BP Plus are insoluble, radiopaque, do not shrink during setting, and need moisture to set (http://www.ibioceramix.com/products.html). However, the results of a recent investigation showed that iRoot SP was very soluble and did not fulfill ANSI/ADA Specification 57/2000 requirement (Borges *et al.* 2012). The difference between iRoot BP and iRoot BP Plus is the consistency of the materials. iRoot BP is an injectable premixed paste while iRoot BP Plus is a premixed putty material (http://www.ibioceramix.com/products.html).

Biocompatibility

Results of a cell culture investigation on human osteoblast cells showed that iRoot BP Plus showed significantly lower viability compared to white ProRoot MTA (De-Deus *et al.* 2012). Another cell culture study on L929 cells showed fresh iRoot Sp had significantly higher toxicity compared to ProRoot MTA in a filter diffusion test, whereas the extracts of both materials were nontoxic (Zhang *et al.* 2010).

Recently, the manufacturer introduced iRoot FS as the next generation of root canal filling and repair materials with fast setting properties and the same characteristics of calcium silicate-based, aluminum-free materials that are insoluble, radiopaque, do not shrink during setting, and need moisture for setting (http://www.ibioceramix.com/products.html).

In conclusion, iRoot is a bioactive, alkaline material, high toxicity with certain antibacterial properties. However, so far, the material efficacy in clinical procedures has not been investigated.

CALCIUM ENRICHED MIXTURE (CEM) CEMENT

Calcium enriched mixture (CEM) cement (BioniqueDent, Tehran, Iran) is a powder/liquid material.

Chemical composition

CEM cement is composed of CaO (51.81%), SiO_2 (6.28%), Al_2O_3 (0.95%), MgO (0.23%), SO_3 (9.48%), P_2O_5 (8.52%), Na_2O (0.35%), Cl (0.18%), and H&C (22.2%) (Asgary *et al.* 2008c). It has been shown that lime is the major component of CEM cement. The concentrations of other constituents in CEM cement are different from those in ProRoot MTA, AMTA, and white and gray PC, except for some trace elements (Asgary *et al*. 2009b).

Physical properties

CEM cement and white ProRoot MTA have no significant difference in pH (10.61 versus 10.71), working times (4.5 min versus 5 min), or dimensional changes (0.075 versus 0.085 mm). However, there were significant differences between the materials' setting times, film thickness, and flow (Asgary *et al*. 2008c). CEM cement produces an alkaline pH and releases calcium in a similar manner to white ProRoot MTA (Asgary *et al*. 2008c; Amini Ghazvini *et al*. 2009). In addition, CEM cement releases significantly higher levels of phosphate compared to PC and white ProRoot MTA during the first hour after mixing (Amini Ghazvini *et al*. 2009). CEM cement radiopacity is reported to be 2.227 mm Al, which is lower than that of ProRoot MTA (5.009 mm Al) and AMTA (5.589 mm Al) (Torabzadeh *et al*. 2012). CEM cement's radiopacity did not fulfill the requirement of ANSI/ADA specification number 57/2000 and ISO 6876/2001 each for endodontic sealing materials (3 mm Al). The particle size of CEM cement is between 0.5 to 30 μm (Soheilipour *et al*. 2009). The percentage of the particle size between 0.5 and 2.5 μm diameter in CEM cement is significantly higher than that in white ProRoot MTA and white PC (Asgary *et al*. 2011b). The effect of using CH, ProRoot MTA, and CEM cement on flexural strength of bovine root dentin after 30 days showed that all tested materials significantly decreased flexural strength compared to the control. However, there was no significant difference among the tested materials in that regard (Sahebi *et al*. 2012). Shear bond strength of either CEM cement or ProRoot MTA to composite resin did not improve following acid etching. Therefore, the investigators encourage covering the bioactive materials used for vital pulp therapy such as CEM cement or MTA with resin modified glass ionomer before restoring the teeth with composite resin (Oskoee *et al*. 2011). Obturating the simulated open apex teeth with either white MTA or CEM cement significantly increases their resistance to fracture after six months. However, no significant difference was found between the materials tested (Milani *et al*. 2012). Push-out bond strength of CEM cement as root-end filling material was comparable with white ProRoot MTA. Both materials showed higher resistance to displacement when the root-end preparation was performed with ultrasonic technique rather than Er, Cr:YSGG laser (Shokouhinejad *et al*. 2012b).

Bioactivity of CEM cement was confirmed by the presence of crystals that had comparable composition to the standard hydroxyapatite over the material when the samples were placed in PBS for one week (Asgary *et al*. 2009a).

Antibacterial activities

Two separate antibacterial investigations evaluated the activity of CEM cement, gray and white ProRoot MTA, PC, and CH on *E. faecalis*, *P. areuginosa*, *Escherichia coli*, and *S. aureus*. Results showed that both CH and CEM cement had significantly higher antibacterial activity against the microorganisms used in these studies compared to white and gray ProRoot MTA and PC (Asgary *et al.* 2007; Asgary & Kamrani 2008). Both white ProRoot MTA and CEM cement showed similar fungicidal activity after 24 and 48 hours of incubation with *C. albicans* (Kangarlou *et al.* 2009).

Sealing ability

When used as a root-end filling material, CEM cement showed no significant difference with white ProRoot MTA and AMTA. However, all materials showed significantly lower dye leakage compared to IRM (Asgary *et al.* 2006a, 2008a). A fluid filtration study that stored CEM cement as a root-end filling material in different media reported that when the teeth were kept in PBS, the samples showed significantly less leakage compared to the ones that were stored in distilled water (Ghorbani *et al.* 2009). A bacterial penetration study showed no significant difference in bacterial leakage between white ProRoot MTA and CEM cement up to 70 days (Kazem *et al.* 2010). A dye leakage investigation on blood and saliva contamination compared to dry conditions when white ProRoot MTA and CEM cement were used as root-end filling materials showed no significant difference between the materials except for saliva contamination. As with saliva contamination, the CEM cement showed significantly lower dye leakage (Hasheminia *et al.* 2010). A fluid filtration investigation reported that using CH as a medicament prior to placement of CEM cement as an apical plug had no short- or long-term negative effect on the sealing ability of the material (Bidar *et al.* 2011).

Using MTA or CEM cement as an intra-orifice barrier showed significantly lower leakage compared to amalgam and composite resin in a polymicrobial leakage study (Yavari *et al.* 2012).

Biocompatibility

Cell culture studies

In an L929 mouse fibroblast cell culture study, both CEM cement and ProRoot MTA showed no significant difference in cell viability compared to the control (Ghoddusi *et al.* 2008). In another investigation on L929 mouse fibroblasts, MTA had significantly higher cell viability compared to CEM cement while both materials showed significantly less cytotoxicity compared to IRM (Mozayeni *et al.* 2012).

An *ex vivo* investigation on neural cells showed that both CEM cement and white ProRoot MTA have suppressive effects on neural cell excitability and neural cell firing frequency (Abbasipour *et al.* 2012). Another investigation evaluated cell morphology and adhesion of human gingival fibroblasts to CEM cement and white ProRoot MTA by scanning electron microscope (SEM) and reported no significant difference between the materials (Asgary *et al.* 2012).

Skin test and subcutaneous implantation

Skin test reactivity of CEM cement showed a significantly lower inflammatory reaction compared to white ProRoot MTA (Tabarsi *et al.* 2012). A subcutaneous implantation study reported that CEM cement induced no necrosis compared to white and gray ProRoot MTA. However, all tested materials induced calcific metamorphosis. Investigators concluded that all the materials tested were biocompatible at the end of the experiment (Parirokh *et al.* 2011).

Intraosseous implantation

An investigation on intraosseous implantation of CEM cement and ProRoot MTA resulted in no significant difference between the materials in terms of inflammation and new bone formation up to 8 weeks (Rahimi *et al.* 2012).

In vivo investigations

Three separate animal investigations showed that both ProRoot MTA and CEM cement were successfully used as pulp capping and pulpotomy agents with no significant difference between the materials. However, both of the materials were significantly better than Dycal for calcified bridge formation (Asgary *et al.* 2006b, 2008b; Tabarsi *et al.* 2010).

Another animal study compared CEM with ProRoot MTA as perforation repair materials and showed mild inflammation and formation of a hard tissue at the perforation site with no significant difference between the two materials after three months (Samiee *et al.* 2010).

In an animal investigation on dogs' teeth, both white ProRoot MTA and CEM cement were used as root-end filling materials. Results showed cementum deposition over both of the materials in the majority of the teeth with no significant difference (Asgary *et al.* 2010).

Clinical investigations

Several case reports illustrate successful outcomes of using CEM cement for furcation perforation repair, internal and external resorptive defects, vital pulp therapy in open apex teeth, clot covering during revitalization procedure of open apex teeth with necrotic pulps, and root-end filling for reimplanted or transplanted teeth (Asgary 2009, 2010, 2011; Nosrat & Asgary 2010a, b; Asgary *et al.* 2011a; Nosrat *et al.* 2011b; Asgary & Ahmadyar 2012; Asgary & Eghbal 2012).

A case series demonstrated successful use of CEM cement as an apical plug for 13 teeth with open apices and necrotic pulps up to an average of 14.5 months following treatment (Nosrat *et al.* 2011a).

In a human study that compared AMTA and CEM cement as pulp capping agents, the materials showed similar favorable responses in terms of calcified bridge formation eight weeks following the procedure (Zarrabi *et al.* 2010). Immunohistochemical staining for fibronectin and tenascin, two major glycoproteins involved in dentinogenesis, was confirmed in teeth capped with either AMTA or CEM cement with no significant difference between the materials (Zarrabi *et al.* 2011).

A randomized clinical trial on direct pulp capping of primary molar teeth compared CEM cement with ProRoot MTA. Clinical and radiographic success up to six months after pulp capping resulted in high success rates with no significant difference between the materials (Fallahinejad Ghajari *et al.* 2010). Similarly, another clinical trial that used CEM cement and white ProRoot MTA as pulpotomy agents in primary molar teeth reported high success rates with no significant difference in clinical and radiographic outcomes between the materials up to 24 months following the treatment (Malekafzali Ardekani *et al.* 2011). A case report illustrated successful pulp capping with CEM cement in a permanent molar tooth that had sensitivity to percussion and a small radiographic lesion (Nosrat *et al.* 2012). Another case report illustrated successful clinical and radiographic outcomes of a cariously exposed open apex molar tooth that received CEM cement as pulpotomy agent up to 12 months following the procedure (Nosrat & Asgary 2010b). A case series of cariously exposed permanent molars using CEM cement as a pulpotomy agent showed successful clinical and radiographic outcomes in 11 out of 12 teeth up to an average of 15.8 months following the treatment (Asgary & Ehsani 2009). Another investigation used CEM and white ProRoot MTA as pulpotomy agents for treating cariously exposed immature molar teeth. Radiographic and clinical outcomes up to 12 months following the treatment showed no significant difference between the materials (Nosrat *et al.* 2013).

A clinical trial compared pain relief after either one visit of root canal therapy or pulpotomy with CEM cement in teeth with irreversible pulpitis. Results showed that patients who received pulpotomy with CEM cement had significantly lower pain rates during the first week following the treatment (Asgary & Eghbal 2010). Another clinical trial compared pain rates as well as clinical and radiographic treatment outcomes following pulpotomy with CEM cement and white ProRoot MTA as pulpotomy agents in molar teeth with irreversible pulpitis. Results showed that not only there was no significant difference in the pain rates in the teeth, but there was also no significant difference in radiographic and clinical outcomes up to 12 months after the procedure (Asgary & Eghbal 2013). A multicenter clinical trial compared clinical and radiographic outcomes of the teeth that had irreversible pulpitis and received either pulpotomy with CEM cement or one visit of root canal therapy. Results showed that the teeth that received pulpotomy with CEM cement had significantly better radiographic outcomes compared to those that received one visit of root canal therapy (Asgary *et al.* 2013).

In conclusion, CEM cement is an alkaline material (after hydration) that has a fine particle size, is nontoxic, and is biocompatible with certain antibacterial properties. *In vivo* investigations on clinical applications are very encouraging. However, many of the human studies on CEM cement were only focused on vital pulp therapy. Except for vital pulp therapy, evidence for other clinical applications is limited to several case reports, and more research is recommended.

MTA FILLAPEX

MTA Fillapex (Angelus Industria de Produtos Odontologicos S/A, Londrina, Brazil) is a resin MTA-based root canal sealer that has nanosilicate particles (Nagas *et al.* 2012).

Chemical composition

MTA Fillapex is composed of natural resin, salicylate resin, diluting resin, bismuth trioxide, nanoparticulated silica, MTA, and pigments (Bin *et al.* 2012).

Physical properties

Results of a solubility test showed that MTA Fillapex did not fulfill the ANSI/ADA specification 57/2000 requirement. The material showed significantly higher solubility compared to AMTA and AH Plus. Calcium ion release was also detected during the solubility test of MTA Fillapex. After the solubility test, the surface showed morphologic changes with high amounts of calcium and carbon at the superficial layer of the material (Borges *et al.* 2012). MTA Fillapex has shown a lower to equal bond to dentin compared to Epiphany (Nagas *et al.* 2012). Despite an investigation reporting that there was no significant difference between the bond strength of MTA Fillapex to dentin compared to AH Plus (Assmann *et al.* 2012), two other investigations showed that both AH Plus and iRoot Sp had significantly higher bond strength to dentin compared to MTA Fillapex (Sağsen *et al.* 2011; Nagas *et al.* 2012). The resistance to dislodgment of MTA Fillapex was reported to be significantly lower than that of Endo-CPM sealer (Assmann *et al.* 2012). The material has an alkaline pH (pH value > 10) before and after setting (Morgental *et al.* 2011; Silva *et al.* 2013).

An investigation evaluated the resistance to fracture of the root canals that were obturated with gutta-percha and one of the following root canal sealers: MTA Fillapex, iRoot Sp, and AH Plus. Results showed that all root canal sealers significantly reinforced roots against fracture compared to the roots that were instrumented but not filled, although no significant difference was found among the sealers (Sağsen *et al.* 2012). In contrast, filling simulated open apex teeth with MTA Fillapex and gutta-percha showed significantly lower resistance to fracture compared to AH Plus and gutta-percha (Tanalp *et al.* 2012).

The root canal should not be completely free of moisture when MTA Fillapex and iRoot SP are used as root canal sealers (http://www.ibioceramix.com/products.html; Nagas *et al.* 2012). Placement of CH inside the root canal prior to using MTA Fillapex as a root canal sealer had no significant positive improvement on its bond strength to dentin. The bond strength of a root canal sealer is clinically important because it prevents the material from dislocating during tooth flexure and post space preparation. Therefore, if MTA Fillapex or iRoot SP are used as a root canal sealer in a single visit treatment, they would have similar bond strength to dentin in a matching-taper single cone obturation technique with gutta-percha, with lower bond strength to dentin compared to AH Plus (Amin *et al.* 2012). The flow of MTA Fillapex has been reported as 31.09 ± 0.67 mm, which is higher than the minimum 20 mm requirement for obtaining ISO 6876/2001 specification. The flow of MTA Fillapex is significantly higher than that of AH Plus. The radiopacity of MTA Fillapex is equal to 7.06 mm Al, which is higher than the ISO 6876/2001 requirement for root canal sealers (Silva *et al.* 2013).

Antibacterial activities

Freshly mixed MTA Fillapex has antibacterial activity against *E. faecalis* before setting. However, MTA Fillapex showed no antibacterial effect on *E. faecalis* after setting (Morgental *et al.* 2011).

Biocompatibility

Cell culture studies

MTA Fillapex is a bioactive material that increases alkaline phosphatase activity and deposits of calcium in human osteoblast-like cell culture. Results of cell culture investigations on MTA Fillapex were scarce. In an investigation, despite initial cytotoxicity, MTA Fillapex showed a less toxic effect on human osteo-blast-like cells seven days following exposure to the material. Both Epiphany SE and Endofill root canal sealer showed higher cytotoxicity compared to MTA Fillapex after setting (Salles *et al.* 2012). In contrast, three separate cell culture studies on Chinese hamster fibroblasts, primary human osteoblasts, and BALB/c 3 T3 cells reported high cytotoxicity and genotoxicity for MTA Fillapex through-out the experiments (Bin *et al.* 2012; Scelza *et al.* 2012; Silva *et al.* 2013). Results of a cell culture study based on ISO 10993–5 requirements for root canal sealers confirmed that MTA Fillapex had a cytotoxic effect on BALB/c 3 T3 cells up to 4 weeks following the procedure (Silva *et al.* 2013).

Subcutaneous implantation

A subcutaneous implantation study reported a severe inflammatory reaction to MTA Fillapex even at 90 days after implantation. In the study, despite a similar early high inflammatory reaction of MTA Fillapex and Grossman sealer, the latter material showed significantly lower tissue reaction 90 days after implantation, although both sealers remained toxic at this time interval (Zmener *et al.* 2012). Another subcutaneous implantation study reported that despite having MTA com-position, MTA Fillapex showed no superiority in terms of inflammatory reaction compared to AH Plus and Endofill root canal sealers. Among the materials tested, AH Plus showed a similar reaction to the control 60 days after implantation (Tavares *et al.* 2013). In contrast, a subcutaneous implantation reported a mild tis-sue reaction to MTA Fillapex 15 days after the procedure, similar to the reaction to AMTA. Moreover, the areas of mineralization were detected by Von Kossa staining in MTA Fillapex specimens (Gomes-Filho *et al.* 2012).

In conclusion, MTA Fillapex is a highly soluble, alkaline, bioactive root canal sealer while its biocompatibility is in question. In addition, no *in vivo* investigation has been conducted using MTA Fillapex to demonstrate the material's efficacy.

ENDO-CPM

Endo-CPM sealer (EGEO SRL, Buenos Aires, Argentina) is an MTA-based root canal sealer that was developed in Argentina in 2004 (Parirokh & Torabinejad 2010a).

Chemical composition

The composition of Endo-CPM Sealer after mixing is MTA in addition to calcium chloride, calcium carbonate, sodium citrate, propylene glycol alginate, and propylene glycol.

Physical properties

The addition of calcium carbonate to the material was for decreasing the pH after setting (Gomes-Filho *et al.* 2009c). Release of calcium ion from Endo-CPM was detected during two *in vitro* investigations (de Vasconcelos *et al.* 2009; Tanomaru-Filho *et al.* 2009). The sealer has an alkaline pH value (de Vasconcelos *et al.* 2009; Morgental *et al.* 2011) and significantly higher bond strength to dentin compared to MTA Fillapex and AH Plus (Assmann *et al.* 2012).

Antibacterial activity

Endo-CPM showed antibacterial activity similar to that of white ProRoot MTA and white AMTA (Parirokh & Torabinejad 2010a). End-CPM sealer has no antibacterial activity against *E. faecalis* (Morgental *et al.* 2011).

Sealing ability

The results of two dye leakage investigations using Endo-CPM and an epoxy resin sealer containing CH (MBPc) were in favor of the latter material, whereas no significant difference was observed in marginal adaptation evaluated by SEM of these two materials and AMTA when used as apical plugs in teeth with open apices (Orosco *et al.* 2008, 2010).

Biocompatibility

Cell culture studies

In a mouse fibroblast culture investigation, Endo-CPM sealer induced IL-6 release while it showed no inhibitory effect on cell viability (Gomes-Filho *et al.* 2009c).

Subcutaneous implantation

Two subcutaneous implantation investigations showed Endo-CPM, like MTA, producing an early mild to moderate reaction (Gomes-Filho *et al.* 2009a; Scarparo *et al.* 2010) followed by mineralization at 30 days (Gomes-Filho *et al.* 2009a).

In vivo investigations

In a rat investigation, both white AMTA and Endo-CPM sealer showed biocompatibility when used as perforation repair materials (da Silva *et al.* 2011).

In conclusion, Endo-CPM sealer is a bioactive alkaline material with some antibacterial activity. Despite encouraging laboratory and in *vivo* investigations, lack of human studies regarding the clinical applications of Endo-CPM is a major concern.

CIMENTO ENDODONTICO RAPIDO (CER)

CER is an abbreviation for *cimento endodontico rapido* (fast endodontic cement).

Chemical composition

The material's composition includes PC and a gel composed of water, barium sulfate, and an emulsifier (for improvement of handling properties) (Santos *et al.* 2005). The material is also known as MTA-exp (de Vasconcelos *et al.* 2009).

Physical properties

Santos and associates reported that calcium ion release and electrical conductivity from the material is significantly higher than those of AMTA 24 hours after mixing (Santos *et al.* 2005). Another investigation showed that in different study periods there was a significant difference in calcium ion release between CER and gray AMTA (at 24 hours in favor of gray AMTA, in contrast to no significant difference being found between the materials at 168 hours) (de Vasconcelos *et al.* 2009). The material changed the pH value of the storage solution in a similar way to AMTA (at first mildly acidic, alkaline after 24 hours, and neutral after 360 hours) (Santos *et al.* 2005). The setting time of the material is 7 min, which is significantly lower than that of AMTA. However, the material had no significant difference in thermal expansion compared to AMTA (Santos *et al.* 2008).

Biocompatibility

Subcutaneous implantation

Subcutaneous tissue reaction to CER was moderate at seven days, whereas it was similar to the control at longer time intervals (30 and 60 days), and Von Kossa positive structures (mineralized structures) were seen in close contact with the implanted materials (Gomes-Filho *et al.* 2009b).

In conclusion, it seems that more laboratory and *in vivo* investigation (as well as clinical investigations) are needed for further evaluation of the material.

ENDOSEQUENCE

EndoSequence (Brasseler, Savannah, GA, USA) has been introduced as EndoSequence Root Repair Material (RRM), EndoSequence Root Repair Putty (RRP) (Damas *et al.* 2011) and EndoSequence BC obturation system (EndoSequence BC Gutta-percha, EndoSequence BC sealer). It has been claimed that EndoSequence BC sealer and iRoot SP have had the same formula distributing with different manufacturers (Brasseler USA and Innovative BioCeramix Inc, respectively) (http://www.ibioceramix.com/iRootSP.html.).

EndoSequence RRM has been developed for pulp capping, perforation repair, apexification, root-end filling, and repair of root resorption.

Chemical composition

EndoSequence RRM is composed of zirconium oxide, calcium silicates, tantalum oxide, calcium phosphate monobasic, and filler and thickening agents (http://www.technomedics.no/Produkter/Endo/obturasjon/images/pdf/bcsealer/Bioceramic%20brosjyre.pdf). Both RRM and RRP are bioceramics, which are a combination of calcium silicate and calcium phosphate.

Physical properties

RRM and RRP are premixed, ready-to-use, bright white materials composed of nanosphere particles. The fine particle size allows the materials to enter dentinal tubules and act with moisture inside the tubules for final setting as well as provide a mechanical seal (Damas *et al.* 2011; Hirschman *et al.* 2012). RRP, like BA and white ProRoot MTA, showed bioactivity after placement in PBS. In a period of two months, all the materials tested showed a precipitation of apatite aggregate over the materials' surfaces (Shokouhinejad *et al.* 2012a). The manufacturer has claimed that EndoSequence RRM is a highly radiopaque and alkaline material that has ideal working (more than 30 min) and setting time and 70–90Mpa strength (http://www.brasselerusa.com/brass/assets/File/B_3248_ES%20RRM%20NPR.pdf). In an *in vitro* study, intracanal placement of EndoSequence RRM provided a significantly lower pH change on the surface of the simulated resorption defect compared to white ProRoot MTA (Hansen *et al.* 2011).

Antibacterial activities

Both forms of RRP and RRM as well as white ProRoot MTA showed similar antibacterial activity against different clinical strains of *E. faecalis* (Lovato & Sedgley 2011).

Sealing ability

The results of a bacterial leakage study that used *E. faecalis* showed no significant difference on sealing ability between EndoSequence Bioceramic Root-end Repair and white ProRoot MTA (Nair *et al.* 2011).

Biocompatibility

Cell culture studies

EndoSequence RRM showed similar cytotoxicity to both white ProRoot MTA and white AMTA in an adult human dermal fibroblast cell culture study. However, RRP showed significantly lower cell viability compared to the RRM, white ProRoot MTA and white AMTA during the first 24 hours (Damas *et al.* 2011). In contrast, another investigation on human gingival fibroblasts reported similar cell viability associated with gray ProRoot MTA, RRP, and RRM (Ma *et al.* 2011). In a human osteoblast-like cell study, EndoSequence RRM and RRP as well as ProRoot MTA showed no significant difference in cell growth and morphology. In the same study, all materials tested were capable of expressing cytokines (IL-1β, IL-6, IL-8) in the cell culture. However, gray ProRoot MTA induces significantly higher expression of IL-6 compared to both RRP and RRM after 48 hours (Ciasca *et al.* 2012). In another investigation on human dermal fibroblast cell culture, similar cell viability was found between RRP and white AMTA after 5 days, whereas at 8 days RRP showed less cytotoxicity than white AMTA (Hirschman *et al.* 2012).

An investigation on osteoblast like cells showed that EndoSequence RRM decreased both cell's bioactivity and alkaline phosphatase activity, whereas white ProRoot MTA had no effect on either (Modareszadeh *et al.* 2012). No significant difference was reported between set and freshly mixed white and gray ProRoot MTA and EndoSequence RRM in a cell culture study using L929 mouse fibroblast cells (Alanezi *et al.* 2010).

EndoSequence BC Sealer

EndoSequence BC Sealer is a premixed, ready-to-use root canal sealer that can be employed for both single cone and lateral condensation techniques of permanent root canal obturation (http://www.technomedics.no/Produkter/Endo/obturasjon/images/pdf/bcsealer/Bioceramic%20brosjyre.pdf).

Chemical composition

According to the manufacturer's safety data sheet, EndoSequence BC Sealer is composed of zirconium oxide, calcium silicates, calcium phosphate monobasic, CH, and filling and thickening agents (http://www.technomedics.no/Produkter/Endo/obturasjon/images/pdf/bcsealer/Bioceramic%20brosjyre.pdf).

Physical properties

EndoSequence BC Sealer has an alkaline pH (Candeiro *et al.* 2012); however, it could not completely be removed from the root canal by using conventional retreatment techniques (Hess *et al.* 2011). Candeiro and associates (2012) reported that Endosequence BC Sealer has had radiopacity and flow according to ISO 6876/2001 recommendations. In addition, the material releases calcium ions higher than AH Plus.

Biocompatibility

EndoSequence BC Sealer remained moderately cytotoxic over five weeks during a cell culture investigation on mouse osteoblast cells (Loushine *et al.* 2011). In contrast to the results of Loushine and associates (2011), results of a cell culture study on L929 mouse fibroblasts showed that EndoSequence BC Sealer induced significantly lower cytotoxicity compared to AH Plus and Tubliseal root canal sealers (Zoufan *et al.* 2011).

In conclusion, EndoSequence Root Repair Material is an alkaline, bioactive radiopaque material with fine particle sizes. However, so far, investigations on EndoSequence RRM have been confined to laboratory studies and, therefore, *in vivo* and human investigations are highly recommended.

PROROOT ENDO SEALER

ProRoot Endo Sealer (Dentsply Tulsa Dental Specialties, Tulsa, OK, USA) is a calcium silicate powder that is mixed with a liquid-to-powder ratio of 1:2.

Chemical composition

The powder is mainly composed of tricalcium silicate, dicalcium silicate, calcium sulfate (as a setting retardant), bismuth oxide (as a radiopacifier), and a small amount of tricalcium aluminate. The liquid is composed of water and a viscous water-soluble polymer.

Physical properties

The sealer showed significantly higher dislocation resistance compared to AH Plus and Pulp Canal Sealer, particularly after storage in a simulated body fluid (Huffman *et al.* 2009). Sealing ability of ProRoot Endo Sealer was reported to be better than that of a ZOE-based sealer (Pulp Canal Sealer) and comparable to that of an epoxy-based sealer (AH Plus) after immersion in phosphate-containing fluid (Weller *et al.* 2008). ProRoot Endo Sealer showed bioactivity in synthetic tissue fluid (Weller *et al.* 2008; Huffman *et al.* 2009).

In conclusion, more laboratory, *in vivo*, and clinical investigations should be performed for further evaluation of this material.

MTA PLUS

Chemical composition

The manufacturers have claimed that MTA Plus (Prevest-Denpro, Jammu City, India) and (Avalon Biomed Inc., Bradenton, FL, USA) is composed of ingredients similar to those found in ProRoot MTA and AMTA, but with a finer particle size.

Two formulations have been introduced to the market with water or a hydrosoluble gel for decreasing washout property (Formosa *et al.* 2013).

Physical properties

The results of an investigation have shown that both formulations of MTA Plus (with either water or hydrosoluble gel) has a significantly lower washout compared to AMTA. Anti-washout formulations of MTA Plus (adding hydrosoluble gel to MTA) reduce the loss of the material in a modified washout test (Formosa *et al.* 2013). Effect of MTA Plus on hardness of dentin resulted in a decrease of dentin flexural strength, presumably through the partial degradation of collagen fibrils after three months of storage (Leiendecker *et al.* 2012; Sawyer *et al.* 2012).

In conclusion, despite encouraging results of early investigations, more laboratory, *in vivo*, and clinical investigations are needed for further analysis of the material's efficacy.

ORTHO MTA

Ortho MTA (BioMTA, Seoul, Korea) is a recently introduced material for root canal filling. The manufacturer claims that the material is bioactive and improves sealing ability by both mechanical and chemical bonds between the material and the dentinal wall of the root canal. The material particle size is less than $2\,\mu m$, allowing it to penetrate dentinal tubules and provide leakage resistance in root canal filling (http://www.biomta.com).

Chemical composition

The amount of arsenic in ProRoot MTA is 1.16 ppm (meeting ISO specification 9917–1 requirement of less than 2 ppm), but the element was not detected in Ortho MTA. Neither ProRoot MTA nor Ortho MTA has hexavalent chromium or lead in their compositions. Ortho MTA contains significantly less chromium than ProRoot MTA (Chang *et al.* 2011). Ortho MTA has significantly lower amounts of cadmium, copper, iron, manganese, and nickel than white ProRoot MTA, but significantly higher levels of zinc (Kum *et al.* 2013).

Biocompatibility

Cell culture studies

A recent investigation on MG-63 cell viability using ProRoot MTA and Ortho MTA showed that at 24 hours there was no significant difference between the materials. However, at 4 days and 7 days, Ortho MTA showed significantly lower cell viability compared to the ProRoot MTA (Lee B.N. *et al.* 2012). Ortho MTA enhances the expression of dentin sialophosphoprotein in MDPC 23 cell culture (Lee W. *et al.* 2012).

In conclusion, despite lower amounts of trace elements in the material composition compared to ProRoot MTA, *in vivo* and clinical investigations on the material's ability to seal, induct, and conduct hard tissue is recommended.

MTA BIO

Chemical composition

MTA Bio (Angelus; Londrina, or Angelus Solucoes Odontologicas, PR, Brazil) is composed of 80% PC and 20% bismuth oxide (Gonçalves *et al.* 2010; Borges *et al.* 2011). The material is claimed to be produced in the laboratory to avoid the presence of arsenic in the material's composition (Vivan *et al.* 2010).

However, De-Deus and associates have shown that the material has 8.6 ± 0.85 ppm type III arsenic in its composition, which is higher than the amount in white and gray ProRoot MTA and white and gray AMTA (De-Deus *et al.* 2009a). It has been shown, however, that the amount of arsenic ion release was not significantly different compared to white ProRoot MTA (Gonçalves *et al.* 2010).

Physical properties

MTA Bio's initial and final setting time was reported to be 11 min and 23.33 mi, respectively (Vivan *et al.* 2010). The material's solubility is similar to that of AMTA. MTA Bio produces an alkaline pH value similar to white ProRoot MTA (Gonçalves *et al.* 2010). The pH value of MTA Bio in storage solution was reported to be significantly higher than light-cured MTA (Vivan *et al.* 2010). The material has significantly less radiopacity than AMTA; conversely, it has significantly higher radiopacity compared to light-cured MTA (Vivan *et al.* 2009) and gray and white PC (Borges *et al.* 2011). The radiopacity of MTA Bio is equal to 3.93 ± 0.22 mm Al. No significant difference was found between MTA Bio's radiopacity and either white or gray ProRoot MTA. MTA Bio fulfills the requirement of ANSI/ADA specification 57/2000 (Borges *et al.* 2011) and ISO 6876/2001 (Camilleri *et al.* 2011a) for radiopacity of endodontic sealing materials. Push-out bond strength of MTA Bio was not significantly different than that of ProRoot MTA and AMTA when the materials were stored in PBS, whereas all types of MTA showed significantly higher pushout bond strength than PC (Reyes-Carmona 2010). One of the physical properties of each dental material is its electrical conductivity in a medium that is in direct relation to the concentration of ions. That proportion of ions is in direct relation to the solubility of the material. MTA Bio showed no significant difference in electrical conductivity compared to PC and white ProRoot MTA (Gonçalves *et al.* 2010). MTA Bio had a higher level of calcium ion release compared to AMTA 24 hours and 168 hours following setting (Vivan *et al.* 2010). Meanwhile, MTA Bio showed significantly higher levels of calcium ion release compared to white ProRoot MTA (Gonçalves *et al.* 2010).

Biocompatibility

Cell culture studies

MTA Bio has more porous and less homogeneous surfaces compared to white AMTA. No significant difference on odontoblast-like cell culture was reported between MTA Bio and white AMTA as well as the control (Lessa *et al.* 2010).

Subcutaneous implantation

An *in vivo* investigation showed that the material is bioactive and produces intratubular mineralization similar to AMTA and significantly better than PC.

A subcutaneous reaction showed that the material, like AMTA, produces biomineralization at 30- and 60-day intervals (Dreger *et al.* 2012).

In conclusion, MTA Bio is an alkaline, bioactive, nontoxic material with low initial and final setting time. Despite promising results on the material's bioactivity and cell viability, more laboratory, *in vivo*, and clinical investigations should be performed for further evaluation of the material.

MTA SEALER (MTAS)

Chemical compositions and physical properties

Two different sealers have been introduced as MTA sealer. First, an MTA sealer introduced by Camilleri and associates (2011a) consists of a mixture of 80% white PC (Aalborg White, Aalborg, Denmark) and 20% bismuth oxide (Fischer Scientific, Leicester, UK) This MTA sealer is a bioactive material that releases calcium in PBS and has the potential to form calcium phosphate crystals over the sealer. The sealing ability of the material is similar to that of pulp canal sealer.

The second MTA sealer is from Brazil and is composed of PC, zirconium oxide (radiopacifying agent), calcium chloride, and a resinous vehicle. The sealer is mixed in a powder-to-liquid ratio of 5:3 by weight. The material's initial and final setting time was reported to be 535 ± 29.5 min and 982.5 ± 53.46 min, respectively. The material's alkaline pH up to 48 hours following setting was higher than that of white AMTA. The amount of calcium release was higher than that of white AMTA up to 28 days after mixing (Massi *et al.* 2011). Subcutaneous reaction to the MTAS showed a response similar to that of white AMTA and PC (Viola *et al.* 2012).

More laboratory, *in vivo*, and clinical investigations are needed for evaluating the material's safety and efficacy.

FLUORIDE-DOPED MTA CEMENT

Fluoride-doped MTA (FMTA) is a novel root canal sealer.

Chemical composition

The material contains sodium fluoride mixed into white PC, anhydrite, and bismuth oxide. The presence of sodium fluoride in the composition improves its retention and induces expansion properties (Gandolfi & Prati 2010). Addition of sodium fluoride and calcium chloride to the MTA improves the material's calcium release, bioactivity, and formation of fluoroapatite in an environment containing phosphorus.

Physical properties

The FMTA had an alkaline pH during the 28 days of an investigation (Gandolfi *et al.* 2011).

Sealing ability

Sealing ability of FMTA mixed with articaine anesthetic solution (2.8 powder-to-liquid ratio by weight) during a period of up to 6 months was reported to be comparable to AH Plus root canal sealer in conjunction with warm gutta-percha in a fluid filtration test (Gandolfi & Prati 2010).

Future laboratory and clinical investigations are needed to ensure the efficacy of this material.

CAPASIO

Chemical composition and physical properties

Capasio (Primus Consulting, Bradenton, FL) is a novel calcium silicate that is claimed to employ different calcium cements and novel setting reactions to obtain shorter working time as well as higher resistance to acid (as acid in infected sites can prevent the setting of MTA) (Porter *et al.* 2010). The material is a calcium-phosphor-aluminosilicate-based cement that is presented in powder and liquid form. The powder contains bismuth oxide as a radiopacifier and hydroxyapatite (Washington *et al.* 2011). Capasio has an alkaline pH after setting, superior handling characteristics, and better washout resistance properties compared to white ProRoot MTA. Its setting time is 2.5 h. The material's radiopacity is lower than that of white ProRoot MTA. However, it fulfills the requirement of ISO 6876/2001. The material's compressive strength is slightly higher than that of white ProRoot MTA. The material seems adhesive after setting compared to white ProRoot MTA. The material's pH is lower than that of white ProRoot MTA (Porter *et al.* 2010). Capasio is a bioactive material, and the presence of apatite crystals was observed when the material, like white ProRoot MTA, was placed in a synthetic tissue fluid. SEM observation showed that Capasio penetrated significantly better into dentinal tubules compared to ProRoot MTA (Bird *et al.* 2012). No osteoblast growth was observed in the presence of Capasio in a cell culture study (Washington *et al.* 2011).

In conclusion, despite some encouraging physical properties, the biocompatibility of the material is in question.

GENEREX A

Chemical composition and physical properties

Generex-A (Dentsply Tulsa Dental Specialties, Tulsa, OK), is a calcium silicate–based material formulated with finer powder components than white ProRoot MTA. Because of the material's mixing gel, its handling has been improved and its working time has been shortened (Porter *et al.* 2010). The material contains hydroxyapatite and bismuth oxide (Washington *et al.* 2011). The material has an alkaline pH after setting (but lower than white ProRoot MTA) and a higher washout resistance compared to white ProRoot MTA. Its setting time is 75 min. The material's radiopacity is lower than that of white ProRoot MTA. However, it fulfills the requirements for ISO 6876/2001. Generex A has higher compressive strength compared to white ProRoot MTA (Porter *et al.* 2010).

Biocompatibility

Cell culture study

The material, like white ProRoot MTA, supported osteoblast growth in a cell culture study. A recently introduced material, Generex B, showed initial osteoblast cell growth, whereas no osteoblast growth was observed at three days, followed by few cells present at 6 days (Washington *et al.* 2011).

In conclusion, more laboratory and clinical investigations are needed for proper analysis of the efficacy of the material.

CERAMICRETE-D

Chemical composition and physical properties

Ceramicrete-D (Tulsa Dental Specialties/Argonne National Laboratory, Argonne, IL) is a self-setting material composed of hydroxyapatite powder, phosphosilicate ceramic, and cerium oxide radiopaque filler (Tay & Loushine 2007), though it may also contain bismuth oxide as a radiopacifier (Washington *et al.* 2011). The pH of the material is reported differently in two separate studies. Tay & Loushine (2007) reported an alkaline pH for the material, whereas Porter and associates (Porter *et al.* 2010) reported a very acidic pH value (2.2). The radiopacity of Ceramicrete-D is similar to that of root dentin (Tay & Loushine 2007) and fulfills the requirement of ISO 6876/2001, though it is lower than that of white ProRoot MTA. The material's handling and washout resistance properties are superior to those of white ProRoot MTA. Its setting time is 150 minutes. Ceramicrete-D's compressive strength is significantly lower than that of white ProRoot MTA (Porter *et al.* 2010).

It has been claimed that the material has the potential for bioactivity in presence of phosphate-containing fluids. It also has significantly better sealing ability compared to white ProRoot MTA (Tay & Loushine 2007). The biocompatibility of Ceramicrete-D is, however, questioned because no osteoblast cell growth has been observed in the presence of the material (Washington *et al.* 2011).

In conclusion, it seems that the biocompatibility of Ceramicrete-D is in doubt.

NANO-MODIFIED MTA (NMTA)

Chemical composition and physical properties

A nano-modification of WMTA, NMTA (Kamal Asgar Research Center, US patent #13/211.880) has a similar composition to white ProRoot MTA. However, it has been claimed that with a finer particle size, it may provide a faster and better hydration process compared to original MTA. In addition, the material has a small amount of strontium in its composition in order to be resistant to acidic environments. In both acidic and neutral pH values the surface microhardness of NMTA was significantly higher than that of white ProRoot MTA. NMTA has a 6 ± 1 min setting time, with significantly higher microhardness and more surface area as well as lower porosity over the surface compared to white ProRoot MTA. The push-out bond strength of NMTA has been reported to be significantly higher than that of white AMTA and BA (Saghiri *et al.* 2013).

In conclusion, as the material has not been introduced to the market and only a limited number of physical properties have been investigated, further laboratory, *in vivo*, and clinical investigations are needed.

LIGHT-CURED MTA

Chemical composition and physical properties

Light-cured MTA (Bisco, Itasca, IL) is an experimental material that contains AeroSil (8.0%), resin (42.5%), MTA material (44.5%), and barium sulfate (5.0%) (Gomes-Filho *et al.* 2008).

Light-cured MTA has significantly higher initial and final setting times compared to MTA Bio (Vivan *et al.* 2010). The material had significantly lower radiopacity than AMTA, MTA Bio, and Clinker PC and did not meet the criteria of ISO 6876/2001 (Vivan *et al.* 2009).

Biocompatibility

Subcutaneous implantation

Despite producing more intense chronic inflammatory subcutaneous reactions at 30 days compared to AMTA, the material has a similar subcutaneous reaction at 60 days. However, in contrast to AMTA, the light-cured MTA failed to produce calcification up to 60 days following implantation (Gomes-Filho *et al.* 2008). After placing light-cured MTA into the socket of freshly extracted teeth a bone reaction similar to that of AMTA was observed (Gomes-Filho *et al.* 2010, 2011).

A novel light-cured MTA named Theracal (Bisco Inc, Schamburg, IL, USA) contains type III Portland cement, a radiopaque component, a hydrophilic thickening agent (fumed silica), and resin introduced as pulp capping material. The material showed an alkaline pH in the storage fluid, lower solubility, and a higher calcium release than ProRoot MTA and Dycal. In contrast, Theracal uptakes significantly less water compared to white ProRoot MTA. The material's radiopacity is lower than that of white ProRoot MTA and did not fulfill the requirement of ISO 6876/2001 (Gandolfi *et al.* 2012).

More investigations are needed in order to evaluate the material's efficacy in various clinical applications.

CALCIUM SILICATE (CS)

Chemical composition and physical properties

CS is an experimental root canal sealer that contains a powder composed of tricalcium silicate, dicalcium silicate, calcium sulfate (as a setting retardant), bismuth oxide (as a radiopacifier), a small amount of tricalcium aluminate, and a liquid component comprised of a viscous aqueous solution of a water-soluble polymer. It has been claimed that the sealer produces CH and releases calcium and hydroxyl ions when set, resulting in the formation of apatite structures over the material's surface in a synthetic tissue fluid. A cell culture study revealed that the set form of the material has minimal cytotoxicity after one week and is less cytotoxic than AH Plus. The material showed alkaline phosphatase activity similar to that of white ProRoot MTA (Bryan *et al.* 2010).

ENDOCEM

Endocem (Maruchi,Wonju, Korea) is a newly introduced MTA lookalike material (Choi *et al.* 2013).

Chemical composition and physical properties

The manufacturer has claim that the material composed of CaO (46.7%), Al_2O_3 (5.43%), SiO_2 (12.8%), MgO (3.03%), Fe_2O_3 (2.32%), SO_3 (2.36%), TiO_2 (0.21%), H_2O/CO_2 (14.5%), and Bi_2O_3 (11%) as wt%. The initial and final setting time of Endocem was 120 ± 30 and 240 ± 30 s, respectively. These setting times were significantly lower than ProRoot MTA. Endocem showed higher washout resistance compared to ProRoot MTA. The fast setting properties of Endocem is because of the presence of small particles pozzolan cement (Choi *et al.* 2013).

Biocompatibility

Cell culture study

Both Endocem and ProRoot MTA showed similar cell growth and morphology with no significant difference on MG63 cell culture. Based on Alizarin red S staining, the presence of mineralized nodules in the cells was significantly increased when Endocem and ProRoot MTA were added to the cell culture. Moreover, the presence of mRNA of osteopontin, and bone sialoprotein were increased in the presence of ProRoot MTA and Endocem in the same cell culture (Choi *et al.* 2013).

In conclusion, Endocem is a newly introduced MTA lookalike material that needs extensive investigations on various physical properties, antibacterial activity, biocompatibility, *in vivo*, and clinical applications.

OTHER EXPERIMENTAL MTA LOOKALIKE MIXTURES

There is a limited history in the literature of other materials, such as Aureoseal MTA (Giovanni Ogna and Figli, Muggiò, Milano, Italy) (Taschieri *et al.* 2010).

CONCLUSION

Despite the presence of a number of calcium silicate–based cements (MTA lookalike materials) in the market, most have not been comprehensively investigated. Future *in vivo* and in vitro studies regarding their efficacy, safety, and biocompatibility are needed.

REFERENCES

Abbasipour, F., Akheshteh, V., Rastqar, A., *et al.* (2012) Comparison the cellular effects of mineral trioxide aggregate and calcium enriched mixture on neuronal cells: An electrophysiological approach. *Iranian Endodontic Journal* **7**, 79–87.

Akbari, M., Rouhani, A., Samiee, S., *et al.* (2012) Effect of dentin bonding agent on the prevention of tooth discoloration produced by mineral trioxide aggregate. *International Journal of Dentistry* **563**, 203.

Al-Hezaimi, K., Salameh, Z., Al-Fouzan, K., *et al.* (2011a) Histomorphometric and micro-computed tomography analysis of pulpal response to three different pulp capping materials. *Journal of Endodontics* **374**, 507–12.

Al-Hezaimi, K., Al-Tayar, B.A., Bajuaifer, Y.S., *et al.* (2011b) A hybrid approach to direct pulp capping by using emdogain with a capping material. *Journal of Endodontics* **37**, 667–72.

Alanezi, A.Z., Jiang, J., Safavi, K.E., *et al.* (2010) Cytotoxicity evaluation of endosequence root repair material. *Oral Surgery Oral Medicine Oral Pathology Oral Radiology Endodontics* **109**, e122–5.

Amin, S.A., Seyam, R.S., El-Samman, M.A. (2012) The effect of prior calcium hydroxide intracanal placement on the bond strength of two calcium silicate-based and an epoxy resin-based endodontic sealer. *Journal of Endodontics* **38**, 696–9.

Amini Ghazvini, S., Abdo Tabrizi, M., Kobarfard, F., *et al.* (2009) Ion release and pH of a new endodontic cement, MTA and Portland cement. *Iranian Endodontic Journal* **4**, 74–8.

Asgary, S. (2009) Autogenous transplantation of mandibular third molar to replace vertical root fractured tooth. *Iranian Endodontic Journal* **4**, 117–21.

Asgary, S. (2010) Furcal perforation repair using calcium enriched mixture cement. *Journal of Conservative Dentistry* **13**, 156–8.

Asgary, S. (2011) Management of a hopeless mandibular molar: A case report. *Iranian Endodontic Journal* **6**, 35–8.

Asgary, S., Ahmadyar, M. (2012) One-visit endodontic retreatment of combined external/internal root resorption using a calcium-enriched mixture. *General Dentistry* **60**, e244–8.

Asgary, S., Eghbal, M.J. (2007) Root canal obturation of an open apex root with calcium enriched mixture. *International Journal of Case Reports and Images* **3**, 50–2.

Asgary, S., Eghbal, M.J. (2010) The effect of pulpotomy using a Calcium-Enriched Mixture cement versus one-visit root canal therapy on postoperative pain relief in irreversible pulpitis: a randomized clinical trial. *Odontology* **98**, 126–33.

Asgary, S., Eghbal, M.J. (2012) Root canal obturation of an open apex root with calcium enriched mixture. *International Journal of Case Reports and Images* **3**, 50–2.

Asgary, S., Eghbal, M.J. (2013) Treatment outcomes of pulpotomy in permanent molars with irreversible pulpitis using biomaterials: A multi-center randomized controlled trial. *Acta Odontologica Scandinavica* **71**, 130–6.

Asgary, S., Ehsani, S. (2009) Permanent molar pulpotomy with a new endodontic cement: A case series. *Journal of Conservative Dentistry* **12**, 31–6.

Asgary, S., Kamrani, F.A. (2008) Antibacterial effects of five different root canal sealing materials. *Journal of Oral Science* **50**, 469–74.

Asgary, S., Parirokh, M., Eghbal, M.J., *et al.* (2004) A comparative study of mineral trioxide aggregate and white Portland cements using x-ray analysis. *Australian Endodontic Journal* **30**, 86–9.

Asgary, S., Parirokh, M., Eghbal, M., *et al.* (2005) Chemical differences between white and grey mineral trioxide aggregate. *Journal of Endodontics* **31**, 101–3.

Asgary, S., Eghbal, M.J., Parirokh, M., *et al.* (2006a) Sealing ability of three commercial mineral trioxide aggregates and an experimental root-end filling material. *Iranian Endodontic Journal* **1**, 101–5.

Asgary, S., Parirokh, M., Eghbal, M.J., *et al.* (2006b) SEM evaluation of pulp reaction to different pulp capping materials in dog's teeth. *Iranian Endodontic Journal* **1**, 117–22.

Asgary, S., Akbari Kamrani, F., Taheri, S. (2007) Evaluation of antimicrobial effect of mineral trioxide aggregate, calcium hydroxide, and CEM cement. *Iranian Endodontic Journal* **2**, 105–9.

Asgary, S., Eghbal, M.J., Parirokh, M. (2008a) Sealing ability of a novel endodontic cement as a root-end filling material. *Journal of Biomedical Material Research Part A* **87**, 706–9.

Asgary, S., Eghbal, M.J., Parirokh, M., *et al.* (2008b) A comparative study of histologic response to different pulp capping materials and a novel endodontic cement. *Oral Surgery Oral Medicine Oral Pathology Oral Radiology Endodontics* **106**, 609–14.

Asgary, S., Eghbal, M.J., Parirokh, M., *et al.* (2009a) Effect of two storage solutions on surface topography of two root-end fillings. *Australian Endodontic Journal* **35**, 147–52.

Asgary, S., Eghbal, M.J., Parirokh, M., *et al.* (2009b) Comparison of mineral trioxide aggregate's composition with Portland cements and a new endodontic cement. *Journal of Endodontics* **35**, 243–50.

Asgary, S., Eghbal, M.J., Ehsani, S. (2010) Periradicular regeneration after endodontic surgery with calcium-enriched mixture cement in dogs. *Journal of Endodontics* **36**, 837–41.

Asgary, S., Nosrat, A., Seifi, A. (2011a) Management of inflammatory external root resorption using Calcium Enriched Mixture cement. *Journal of Endodontics* **37**, 411–3.

Asgary, S., Kheirieh, S., Soheilipour, E. (2011b) Particle size of a new endodontic cement compared to MTA and Portland cement. *Biointerface Research in Applied Chemistry* **1**, 83–8.

Asgary, S., Moosavi, S.H., Yadegari, Z., *et al.* (2012) Cytotoxic effect of MTA and CEM cement in human gingival fibroblast cells. Scanning electronic microscope evaluation. *The New York State Dental Journal* **78**, 51–4.

Asgary, S., Eghbal, M.J., Ghoddusi, J., *et al.* (2013) One-year results of vital pulp therapy in permanent molars with irreversible pulpitis: an ongoing multicenter, randomized, non-inferiority clinical trial. *Clinical Oral Investigation* **17**, 431–9.

Asgary, S., Shahabi, S., Jafarzadeh, T., *et al.* (2008c) The properties of a new endodontic material. *Journal of Endodontics* **34**, 990–3.

Assmann, E., Scarparo, R.K., Böttcher, D.E., *et al.* (2012) Dentin bond strength of two mineral trioxide aggregate-based and one epoxy resin-based sealers. *Journal of Endodontics* **38**, 219–21.

Bidar, M., Disfani, R., Gharagozlo, S., *et al.* (2011) Effect of previous calcium hydroxide dressing on the sealing properties of the new endodontic cement apical barrier. *European Journal of Dentistry* **5**, 260–4.

Bin, C.V., Valera, M.C., Camargo, S.E., *et al.* (2012) Cytotoxicity and genotoxicity of root canal sealers based on mineral trioxide aggregate. *Journal of Endodontics* **38**, 495–500.

Bird, D.C., Komabayashi, T., Guo, L., *et al.* (2012) In vitro evaluation of dentinal tubule penetration and biomineralization ability of a new root-end filling material. *Journal of Endodontics* **38**, 1093–6.

Borges, A.H., Pedro, .FL., Miranda, C.E., et al. (2010) Comparative study of physico-chemical properties of MTA-based and Portland cements. *Acta Odontológica Latinoamericana* **23**, 175–81.

Borges, A.H., Pedro, F.L., Semanoff-Segundo, A., *et al.* (2011) Radiopacity evaluation of Portland and MTA-based cements by digital radiographic system. *Journal of Applied Oral Science* **19**, 228–32.

Borges, R.P., Sousa-Neto, M.D., Versiani, M.A., *et al.* (2012) Changes in the surface of four calcium silicate-containing endodontic materials and an epoxy resin-based sealer after a solubility test. *International Endodontic Journal* **45**, 419–28.

Bortoluzzi, E.A., Arau´jo, G.S., Guerreiro Tanomaru, J.M., *et al.* (2007) Marginal gingiva discoloration by gray MTA: a case report. *Journal of Endodontics* **33**, 325–7.

Bryan, T.E., Khechen, K., Brackett, M.G., *et al.* (2010) In vitro osteogenic potential of an experimental calcium silicate-based root canal sealer. *Journal of Endodontics* **36**, 1163–9.

Camilleri, J. (2008) Characterization and chemical activity of Portland cement and two experimental cements with potential for use in dentistry. *International Endodontic Journal* **41**, 791–9.

Camilleri, J. (2010) Evaluation of the physical properties of an endodontic Portland cement incorporating alternative radiopacifiers used as root-end filling material. *International Endodontic Journal* **43**, 231–40.

Camilleri, J. (2011) Evaluation of the effect of intrinsic material properties and ambient conditions on the dimensional stability of white mineral trioxide aggregate and Portland cement. *Journal of Endodontics* **37**, 239–45.

Camilleri, J., Gandolfi, M.G., Siboni, F., *et al.* (2011a) Dynamic sealing ability of MTA root canal sealer. *International Endodontic Journal* **44**, 9–20.

Camilleri, J., Cutajar, A., Mallia, B. (2011b) Hydration characteristics of zirconium oxide replaced Portland cement for use as a root-end filling material. *Dental Materials* **27**, 845–54.

Camilleri, J., Kralj, P., Veber, M., *et al.* (2012) Characterization and analyses of acid-extractable and leached trace elements in dental cements. *International Endodontic Journal* **45**, 737–43.

Candeiro, G.T., Correia, F.C., Duarte, M.A., *et al.* (2012) Evaluation of radiopacity, pH, release of calcium ions, and flow of a bioceramic root canal sealer. *Journal of Endodontics* **38**, 842–5.

Carvalho, F.B., Gonçalves, P.S., Lima, R.K., *et al.* (2013) Use of cone-beam tomography and digital subtraction radiography for diagnosis and evaluation of traumatized teeth treated with endodontic surgery and MTA. A case report. *Dental Traumatology* **29**, 404–9.

Chang, S.W., Shon, W.J., Lee, W., *et al.* (2010) Analysis of heavy metal contents in gray and white MTA and 2 kinds of Portland cement: a preliminary study. *Oral Surgery Oral Medicine Oral Pathology Oral Radiology Endodontics* **109**, 642–6.

Chang, S.W., Baek, S.H., Yang, H.C., *et al.* (2011) Heavy metal analysis of ortho MTA and ProRoot MTA. *Journal of Endodontics* **37**, 1673–6.

Chedella, S.C., Berzins, D.W. (2010) A differential scanning calorimetry study of the setting reaction of MTA. *International Endodontic Journal* **43**, 509–18.

Choi, Y., Park, S.J., Lee, S.H., *et al.* (2013) Biological effects and washout resistance of a newly developed fast-setting pozzolan cement. *Journal of Endodontics* **39**, 467–72.

Ciasca, M., Aminoshariae, A., Jin, G., *et al.* (2012) A comparison of the cytotoxicity and proinflammatory cytokine production of EndoSequence root repair material and

ProRoot mineral trioxide aggregate in human osteoblast cell culture using reverse-transcriptase polymerase chain reaction. *Journal of Endodontics* **38**, 486–9.

Cutajar, A., Mallia, B., Abela, S., *et al.* (2011) Replacement of radiopacifier in mineral trioxide aggregate; characterization and determination of physical properties. *Dental Materials* **27**, 879–91.

D'Antò, V., Di Caprio, M.P., Ametrano, G., *et al.* (2010) Effect of mineral trioxide aggregate on mesenchymal stem cells. *Journal of Endodontics* **36**, 1839–43.

da Silva, G.F., Guerreiro-Tanomaru, J.M., Sasso-Cerri, E., *et al.* (2011) Histological and histomorphometrical evaluation of furcation perforations filled with MTA, CPM and ZOE. *International Endodontic Journal* **44**, 100–10.

Damas, B.A., Wheater, M.A., Bringas, J.S., *et al.* (2011) Cytotoxicity comparison of mineral trioxide aggregates and EndoSequence bioceramic root repair materials. *Journal of Endodontics* **37**, 372–5.

Dammaschke, T., Gerth, H.U., Züchner, H., *et al.* (2005) Chemical and physical surface and bulk material characterization of white ProRoot MTA and two Portland cements. *Dental Materials* **21**, 731–8.

De-Deus, G., de Souza, M.C., Sergio Fidel, R.A., *et al.* (2009a) Negligible expression of arsenic in some commercially available brands of Portland cement and mineral trioxide aggregate. *Journal of Endodontics* **35**, 887–90.

De-Deus, G., Canabarro, A., Alves, G., *et al.* (2009b) Optimal cytocompatibility of a bioceramic nanoparticulate cement in primary human mesenchymal cells. *Journal of Endodontics* **35**, 1387–90.

De-Deus, G., Canabarro, A., Alves, G.G., *et al.* (2012) Cytocompatibility of the ready-to-use bioceramic putty repair cement iRoot BP Plus with primary human osteoblasts. *International Endodontic Journal* **45**, 508–13.

de Vasconcelos, B.C., Bernardes, R.A., Cruz, S.M., *et al.* (2009) Evaluation of pH and calcium ion release of new root-end filling materials. *Oral Surgery Oral Medicine Oral Pathology Oral Radiology Endodontics* **108**, 135–9.

dos Santos, C.L., Saito, C.T., Luvizzuto, E.R., *et al.* (2011) Influence of a parafunctional oral habit on root fracture development after trauma to an immature tooth. *Journal of Craniofacial Surgery* **22**, 1304–6.

Dreger, L.A., Felippe, W.T., Reyes-Carmona, J.F., *et al.* (2012) Mineral trioxide aggregate and Portland cement promote biomineralization in vivo. *Journal of Endodontics* **38**, 324–9.

El Sayed, M., Saeed, M. (2012) In vitro comparative study of sealing ability of Diadent BioAggregate and other root-end filling materials. *Journal of Conservative Dentistry* **15**, 249–52.

Fallahinejad Ghajari, M., Asgharian Jeddi, T., Iri, S., *et al.* (2010) Direct pulp-capping with calcium enriched mixture in primary molar teeth: a randomized clinical trial. *Iranian Endodontic Journal* **1**, 1–4.

Fayazi, S., Ostad, S.N., Razmi, H. (2011) Effect of ProRoot MTA, Portland cement, and amalgam on the expression of fibronectin, collagen I, and TGFβ by human periodontal ligament fibroblasts in vitro. *Indian Journal of Dental Research* **22**, 190–4.

Formosa, L.M., Mallia, B., Bull, T., *et al.* (2012) The microstructure and surface morphology of radiopaque tricalcium silicate cement exposed to different curing conditions. *Dental Materials* **28**, 584–95.

Formosa, L.M., Mallia, B., Camilleri, J. (2013) A quantitative method for determining the antiwashout characteristics of cement-based dental materials including mineral trioxide aggregate. *International Endodontic Journal* **46**, 179–86.

Gandolfi, M.G., Prati, C. (2010) MTA and F-doped MTA cements used as sealers with warm gutta-percha. Long-term study of sealing ability. *International Endodontic Journal* **43**, 889–901.

Gandolfi, M.G., Taddei, P., Tinti, A., *et al.* (2010) Kinetics of apatite formation on a calcium-silicate cement for root-end filling during ageing in physiological-like phosphate solutions. *Clinical Oral Investigation* **14**, 659–68.

Gandolfi, M.G., Taddei, P., Siboni, F, *et al.* (2011) Fluoride-containing nanoporous calcium-silicate MTA cements for endodontics and oral surgery: early fluorapatite formation in a phosphate-containing solution. *International Endodontic Journal* **44**, 938–49.

Gandolfi, M.G., Siboni, F., Prati, C. (2012) Chemical-physical properties of TheraCal, a novel light-curable MTA-like material for pulp capping. *International Endodontic Journal* **45**, 571–9.

Ghoddusi, J., Tavakkol Afshari, J., Donyavi, Z., *et al.* (2008) Cytotoxic effect of a new endodontic cement and mineral trioxide aggregate on L929 line culture. *Iranian Endodontic Journal* **3**, 17–23.

Ghorbani, Z., Kheirieh, S., Shadman, B., *et al.* (2009) Microleakage of CEM cement in two different media. *Iranian Endodontic Journal* **4**, 87–90.

Gomes-Filho, J.E., de Faria, M.D., Bernabé, P.F., *et al.* (2008) Mineral trioxide aggregate but not light-cure mineral trioxide aggregate stimulated mineralization. *Journal of Endodontics* **34**, 62–5.

Gomes-Filho, J.E., Watanabe, S., Bernabé, P.F., *et al.* (2009a) A mineral trioxide aggregate sealer stimulated mineralization. *Journal of Endodontics* **35**, 256–60.

Gomes-Filho, J.E., Rodrigues, G., Watanabe, S., *et al.* (2009b) Evaluation of the tissue reaction to fast endodontic cement (CER) and Angelus MTA. *Journal of Endodontics* **35**, 1377–80.

Gomes-Filho, J.E., Watanabe, S., Gomes, A.C., *et al.* (2009c) Evaluation of the effects of endodontic materials on fibroblast viability and cytokine production. *Journal of Endodontics* **35**, 1577–9.

Gomes-Filho, J.E., de Moraes Costa, M.T., Cintra, L.T., *et al.* (2010) Evaluation of alveolar socket response to Angelus MTA and experimental light-cure MTA. *Oral Surgery Oral Medicine Oral Pathology Oral Radiology Endodontics* **110**, e93–7.

Gomes-Filho, J.E., de Moraes Costa, M.M., Cintra, L.T., *et al.* (2011) Evaluation of rat alveolar bone response to Angelus MTA or experimental light-cured mineral trioxide aggregate using fluorochromes. *Journal of Endodontics* **37**, 250–4.

Gomes-Filho, J.E., Watanabe, S., Lodi, C.S., *et al.* (2012) Rat tissue reaction to MTA FILLAPEX(®). *Dental Traumatology* **28**, 452–6.

Gonçalves, J.L., Viapiana, R., Miranda, C.E., *et al.* (2010) Evaluation of physico-chemical properties of Portland cements and MTA. *Brazilian Oral Research* **24**, 277–83.

Grech, L., Mallia, B., Camilleri, J. (2013) Characterization of set IRM, Biodentine, Bioaggregate and a prototype calcium silicate cement for use as root-end filling materials. *International Endodontic Journal* **46**, 632–41.

Han, L., Okiji, T. (2011) Uptake of calcium and silicon released from calcium silicate-based endodontic materials into root canal dentine. *International Endodontic Journal* **44**, 1081–7.

Hansen, S.W., Marshall, J.G., Sedgley, C.M. (2011) Comparison of intracanal EndoSequence Root Repair Material and ProRoot MTA to induce pH changes in simulated root resorption defects over 4 weeks in matched pairs of human teeth. *Journal of Endodontics* **37**, 502–6.

Hashem, A.A., Wanees Amin, S.A. (2012) The effect of acidity on dislodgment resistance of mineral trioxide aggregate and bioaggregate in furcation perforations: an in vitro comparative study. *Journal of Endodontics* **38**, 245–9.

Hasheminia, M., Loriaei Nejad, S., Asgary, S. (2010) Sealing ability of MTA and a new endodontic cement as root-end fillings of human teeth in dry, saliva or blood-contaminated conditions. *Iranian Endodontic Journal* **5**, 151–6.

Hess, D., Solomon, E., Spears, R., *et al.* (2011) Retreatability of a bioceramic root canal sealing material. *Journal of Endodontics* **37**, 1547–9.

Hirschman, W.R., Wheater, M.A., Bringas, J.S., *et al.* (2012) Cytotoxicity comparison of three current direct pulp-capping agents with a new bioceramic root repair putty. *Journal of Endodontics* **38**, 385–8.

http://www.biomta.com (accessed 31 January 2014).

http://www.technomedics.no/Produkter/Endo/obturasjon/images/pdf/bcsealer/Bioceramic %20brosjyre.pdf. (accessed 3 February 2014)

http://www.ibioceramix.com/iRootSP.html (accessed 31 January 2014).

http://www.ibioceramix.com/products.html (accessed 31 January 2014).

Huffman, B.P., Mai, S., Pinna, L., *et al.* (2009) Dislocation resistance of ProRoot Endo Sealer, a calcium silicate-based root canal sealer, from radicular dentine. *International Endodontic Journal* **42**, 34–46.

Hungaro Duarte, M.A., Minotti, P.G., Rodrigues, C.T., *et al.* (2012) Effect of different radiopacifying agents on the physicochemical properties of white Portland cement and white mineral trioxide aggregate. *Journal of Endodontics* **38**, 394–7.

Ioannidis, K., Mistakidis, I., Beltes, P., *et al.* (2013) Spectrophotometric analysis of coronal discolouration induced by grey and white MTA. *International Endodontic Journal* **46**, 137–44.

Kangarlou, A., Sofiabadi, S., Yadegari, Z., *et al.* (2009) Antifungal effect of Calcium Enriched Mixture (CEM) cement against *Candida albicans*. *Iranian Endodontic Journal* **4**, 101–5.

Kangarlou, A., Sofiabadi, S., Asgary, S., *et al.* (2012) Assessment of antifungal activity of Proroot mineral trioxide aggregate and mineral trioxide aggregate-Angelus. *Dental Research Journal (Isfahan)* **9**, 256–60.

Kazem, M., Eghbal, M.J., Asgary, S. (2010) Comparison of bacterial and dye microleakage of different root-end filling materials. *Iranian Endodontic Journal* **5**, 17–22.

Krastl, G., Allgayer, N., Lenherr, P., *et al.* (2013) Tooth discoloration induced by endodontic materials: a literature review. *Dental Traumatology* **29**, 2–7.

Kum, K.Y., Zhu, Q., Safavi, K., *et al.* (2013) Analysis of six heavy metals in Ortho mineral trioxide aggregate and ProRoot mineral trioxide aggregate by inductively coupled plasma–optical emission spectrometry. *Australian Endodontic Journal* **39**, 126–30.

Kvinnsland, S.R., Bårdsen, A., Fristad, I. (2010) Apexogenesis after initial root canal treatment of an immature maxillary incisor - a case report. *International Endodontic Journal* **43**, 76–83.

Laurent, P., Camps, J., About, I. (2012) Biodentine(TM) induces TGF-β1 release from human pulp cells and early dental pulp mineralization. *International Endodontic Journal* **45**, 439–48.

Leal, F., De-Deus, G., Brandão, C., *et al.* (2011) Comparison of the root-end seal provided by bioceramic repair cements and White MTA. *International Endodontic Journal* **44**, 662–8.

Lee, B.N., Son, H.J., Noh, H.J. *et al.* (2012) Cytotoxicity of newly developed ortho MTA root-end filling materials. *Journal of Endodontics* **38**, 1627–30.

Lee, W., Oh, J.H., Park, J.C., *et al.* (2012) Performance of electrospun poly(ε-caprolactone) fiber meshes used with mineral trioxide aggregates in a pulp capping procedure. *Acta Biomaterialia* **8**, 2986–95.

Leiendecker, A.P., Qi, Y.P., Sawyer, A.N., *et al.* (2012) Effects of calcium silicate-based materials on collagen matrix integrity of mineralized dentin. *Journal of Endodontics* **38**, 829–33.

Lenherr, P., Allgayer, N., Weiger, R., *et al.* (2012) Tooth discoloration induced by endodontic materials: a laboratory study. *International Endodontic Journal* **45**, 942–9.

Lenzi, R., Trope, M. (2012) Revitalization procedures in two traumatized incisors with different biological outcomes. *Journal of Endodontics* **38**, 411–4.

Lessa, F.C., Aranha, A.M., Hebling, J., *et al.* (2010) Cytotoxic effects of White-MTA and MTA-Bio cements on odontoblast-like cells (MDPC-23). *Brazilian Dental Journal* **21**, 24–31.

Loushine, B.A., Bryan, T.E., Looney, S.W., *et al.* (2011) Setting properties and cytotoxicity evaluation of a premixed bioceramic root canal sealer. *Journal of Endodontics* **37**, 673–7.

Lovato, K.F., Sedgley, C.M. (2011) Antibacterial activity of endosequence root repair material and proroot MTA against clinical isolates of *Enterococcus faecalis*. *Journal of Endodontics* **37**, 1542–6.

Ma, J., Shen, Y., Stojicic, S., *et al.* (2011) Biocompatibility of two novel root repair materials. *Journal of Endodontics* **37**, 793–8.

Malekafzali Ardekani, B., Shekarchi, F., Asgar,y S. (2011) Treatment outcomes of pulpotomy in primary molars using two endodontic biomaterials: A 2-year randomized clinical trial. *European Journal of Paediatric Dentistry*, **12**:189–193.

Marão, H.F., Panzarini, S.R., Aranega, A.M., *et al.* (2012) Periapical tissue reactions to calcium hydroxide and MTA after external root resorption as a sequela of delayed tooth replantation. *Dental Traumatology* **28**, 306–13.

Massi, S., Tanomaru-Filho, M., Silva, G.F., *et al.* (2011) pH, calcium ion release, and setting time of an experimental mineral trioxide aggregate-based root canal sealer. *Journal of Endodontics* **37**, 844–6.

Milani, A.S., Rahimi, S., Borna, Z., *et al.* (2012) Fracture resistance of immature teeth filled with mineral trioxide aggregate or calcium-enriched mixture cement: An ex vivo study. *Dental Research Journal (Isfahan)* **9**, 299–304.

Min, K.S., Kim, H.I., Park, H.J., *et al.* (2007) Human pulp cells response to Portland cement in vitro. *Journal of Endodontics* **33**, 163–6.

Modareszadeh, M.R., Di Fiore, P.M., Tipton, D.A., *et al.* (2012) Cytotoxicity and alkaline phosphatase activity evaluation of endosequence root repair material. *Journal of Endodontics* **38**, 1101–5.

Monteiro Bramante, C., Demarchi, A.C., de Moraes, I.G., *et al.* (2008) Presence of arsenic in different types of MTA and white and gray Portland cement. *Oral Surgery Oral Medicine Oral Pathology Oral Radiology Endodontics* **106**, 909–13.

Moore, A., Howley, M.F., O'Connell, A.C. (2011) Treatment of open apex teeth using two types of white mineral trioxide aggregate after initial dressing with calcium hydroxide in children. *Dental Traumatology* **27**, 166–73.

Morgental, R.D., Vier-Pelisser, F.V., Oliveira, S.D., *et al.* (2011) Antibacterial activity of two MTA-based root canal sealers. *International Endodontic Journal* **44**, 1128–33.

Mozayeni, M.A., Salem Milani, A., Alim Marvasti, L., *et al.* (2012) Cytotoxicity of calcium enriched mixture (CEM) cement compared with MTA and IRM. *Australian Endodontic Journal* **38**, 70–5.

Nagas, E., Uyanik, M.O., Eymirli, A., *et al.* (2012) Dentin moisture conditions affect the adhesion of root canal sealers. *Journal of Endodontics* **38**, 240–4.

Nair, U., Ghattas, S., Saber, M., *et al.* (2011) A comparative evaluation of the sealing ability of 2 root-end filling materials: an in vitro leakage study using *Enterococcus faecalis*. *Oral Surgery Oral Medicine Oral Pathology Oral Radiology Endodontics* **112**, e74–7.

Nekoofar, M.H., Aseeley, Z., Dummer, P.M. (2010) The effect of various mixing techniques on the surface microhardness of mineral trioxide aggregate. *International Endodontic Journal* **43**, 312–20.

Nosrat, A., Asgary, S. (2010a) Apexogenesis of a symptomatic molar with Calcium Enriched Mixture: a case report. *International Endodontic Journal* **43**, 940–4.

Nosrat, A., Asgary, S. (2010b) Apexogenesis treatment with a new endodontic cement: a case report. *Journal of Endodontics* **36**, 912–4.

Nosrat, A., Asgary, S., Eghbal, M.J., *et al.* (2011a) Calcium-enriched mixture cement as artificial apical barrier: A case series. *Journal of Conservative Dentistry* **14**, 427–31.

Nosrat, A., Asgary, S., Seifi, A. (2011b) Regenerative endodontic treatment (revitalization) for necrotic immature permanent molars: A review and report of two cases using a new biomaterial. *Journal of Endodontics* **37**, 562–7.

Nosrat, A., Asgary, S., Homayounfar, N. (2012) Periapical healing after direct pulp capping with calcium-enriched mixture cement: A case report. *Operative Dentistry* **37**, 571–5.

Nosrat, A., Seifi, A., Asgary, S. (2013) Pulpotomy in caries-exposed immature permanent molars using calcium-enriched mixture cement or mineral trioxide aggregate: a randomized clinical trial. *International Journal of Paediatric Dentistry* **23**, 56–63.

Oliveira, I.R., Pandolfelli, V.C., Jacobovitz, M. (2010) Chemical, physical and mechanical properties of a novel calcium aluminate endodontic cement. *International Endodontic Journal* **43**, 1069–76.

Orosco, F.A., Bramante, C.M., Garcia, R.B., *et al.* (2008) Sealing ability of grar MTA AngelusTM, CPM TM and MBPc used as apical plugs. *Journal of Applied Oral Sciences* **16**, 50–4.

Orosco, F.A., Bramante, C.M., Garcia, R.B., *et al.* (2010) Sealing ability, marginal adaptation and their correlation using three root-end filling materials as apical plugs. *Journal of Applied Oral Sciences* **18**, 127–34.

Oskoee, S.S., Kimyai, S., Bahari, M., *et al.* (2011) Comparison of shear bond strength of calcium-enriched mixture cement and mineral trioxide aggregate to composite resin. *Journal of Contemporary Dental Practice* **12**, 457–62.

Parirokh, M., Torabinejad, M. (2010a) Mineral trioxide aggregate: a comprehensive literature review- Part I: Chemical, Physical, and antibacterial properties. *Journal of Endodontics* **36**, 16–27.

Parirokh, M., Torabinejad, M. (2010b) Mineral trioxide aggregate: a comprehensive literature review- Part III: Clinical applications, drawbacks, and mechanism of action. *Journal of Endodontics* **36**, 400–12.

Parirokh, M., Asgary, S., Eghbal, M.J., *et al.* (2005) A comparative study of white and grey mineral trioxide aggregate as pulp capping agent. *Dental Traumatology* **21**, 150–4.

Parirokh, M., Asgary, S., Eghbal, M.J., *et al.* (2007) The long-term effect of saline and phosphate buffer solution on MTA: an SEM and EPMA Investigation. *Iranian Endodontic Journal* **3**, 81–6.

Parirokh, M., Askarifard, S., Mansouri, S., *et al.* (2009) Effect of phosphate buffer saline on coronal leakage of mineral trioxide aggregate. *Journal of Oral Science* **51**, 187–92.

Parirokh, M., Mirsoltani, B., Raoof, M., *et al.* (2011) Comparative study of subcutaneous tissue responses to a novel root-end filling material and white and grey mineral trioxide aggregate. *International Endodontic Journal* **44**, 283–9.

Park, J.W., Hong, S.H., Kim, J.H., *et al.* (2010) X-ray diffraction analysis of white ProRoot MTA and Diadent BioAggregate. *Oral Surgery Oral Medicine Oral Pathology Oral Radiology Endodontics* **109**, 155–8.

Porter, M.L., Bertó, A., Primus, C.M., *et al.* (2010) Physical and chemical properties of new-generation endodontic materials. *Journal of Endodontics* **36**, 524–8.

Rahimi, S., Mokhtari, H., Shahi, S., *et al.* (2012) Osseous reaction to implantation of two endodontic cements: mineral trioxide aggregate (MTA) and calcium enriched mixture (CEM). *Medicina Oral, Patología Oral y Cirugía Bucal* **17**, e907–11.

Rekab, M.S., Ayoubi, H.R. (2010) Evaluation of the apical sealability of mineral trioxide aggregate and portland cement as root canal filling cements: an in vitro study. *Journal of Dentistry (Tehran)* **7**, 205–13.

Reyes-Carmona, J.F., Felippe, M.S., Felippe, W.T. (2010) The biomineralization ability of mineral trioxide aggregate and Portland cement on dentin enhances the push-out strength. *Journal of Endodontics* **36**, 286–91.

Saghiri, M.A., Asgar, K., Lotfi, M., *et al.* (2012) Nanomodification of mineral trioxide aggregate for enhanced physiochemical properties. *International Endodontic Journal* **45**, 979–88.

Saghiri, M.A., Garcia-Godoy, F., Gutmann, J.L., *et al.* (2013) Push-out bond strength of a nano-modified mineral trioxide aggregate. *Dental Traumatology* **29**, 323–7.

Sağsen, B., Ustün, Y., Demirbuga, S., *et al.* (2011) Push-out bond strength of two new calcium silicate-based endodontic sealers to root canal dentine. *International Endodontic Journal* **44**, 1088–91.

Sağsen, B., Ustün, Y., Pala, K., *et al.* (2012) Resistance to fracture of roots filled with different sealers. *Dental Materials Journal* **31**, 528–32.

Sahebi, S., Nabavizadeh, M., Dolatkhah, V., *et al.* (2012) Short term effect of calcium hydroxide, mineral trioxide aggregate and calcium-enriched mixture cement on the strength of bovine root dentin. *Iranian Endodontic Journal* **7**, 68–73.

Sakai, V.T., Moretti, A.B., Oliveira, T.M., *et al.* (2009) Pulpotomy of human primary molars with MTA and Portland cement: a randomised controlled trial. *British Dental Journal* 207,E5.

Salles, L.P., Gomes-Cornélio, A.L., Guimarães, F.C. *et al.* (2012) Mineral trioxide aggregate-based endodontic sealer stimulates hydroxyapatite nucleation in human osteoblast-like cell culture. *Journal of Endodontics* **38**, 971–6.

Samara, A., Sarri, Y., Stravopodis, D., *et al.* (2011) A comparative study of the effects of three root-end filling materials on proliferation and adherence of human periodontal ligament fibroblasts. *Journal of Endodontics* **37**, 865–70.

Samiee, S., Eghbal, M.J., Parirokh, M., *et al.* (2010) Repair of furcal perforation using a new endodontic cement. *Clinical Oral Investigation* **14**, 653–8.

Santos, A.D., Moraes, J.C., Araújo, E.B., *et al.* (2005) Physico-chemical properties of MTA and a novel experimental cement. *International Endodontic Journal* **38**, 443–7.

Santos, A.D., Araújo, E.B., Yukimitu, K., *et al.* (2008) Setting time and thermal expansion of two endodontic cements. *Oral Surgery Oral Medicine Oral Pathology Oral Radiology Endodontics* **106**, e77–9.

Sawyer, A.N., Nikonov, S.Y., Pancio, A.K., *et al.* (2012) Effects of calcium silicate-based materials on the flexural properties of dentin. *Journal of Endodontics* **38**, 680–3.

Scarparo, R.K., Haddad, D., Acasigua, G.A., *et al.* (2010) Mineral trioxide aggregate-based sealer: analysis of tissue reactions to a new endodontic material. *Journal of Endodontics* **36**, 1174–8.

Scelza, M.Z., Linhares, A.B., da Silva, L.E., *et al.* (2012) A multiparametric assay to compare the cytotoxicity of endodontic sealers with primary human osteoblasts. *International Endodontic Journal* **45**, 12–8.

Schembri, M., Peplow, G., Camilleri, J. (2010) Analyses of heavy metals in mineral trioxide aggregate and Portland cement. *Journal of Endodontics* **36**, 1210–5.

Shahi, S., Rahimi, S., Hasan, M., *et al.* (2009) Sealing ability of mineral trioxide aggregate and Portland cement for furcal perforation repair: a protein leakage study. *Journal of Oral Science* **51**, 601–6.

Shahi, S., Rahimi, S., Yavari, H.R., *et al.* (2010) Effect of mineral trioxide aggregates and Portland cements on inflammatory cells. *Journal of Endodontics* **36**, 899–903.

Shahi, S., Yavari, H.R., Rahimi, S., *et al.* (2011) Comparison of the sealing ability of mineral trioxide aggregate and Portland cement used as root-end filling materials. *Journal of Oral Science* **53**, 517–22.

Shetty, P., Xavier, A.M. (2011) Management of a talon cusp using mineral trioxide aggregate. *International Endodontic Journal* **44**, 1061–8.

Shokouhinejad, N., Gorjestani, H., Nasseh, A.A., *et al.* (2013) Push-out bond strength of gutta-percha with a new bioceramic sealer in the presence or absence of smear layer. *Australian Endodontic Journal* **39**, 102–6.

Shokouhinejad, N., Nekoofar, M.H., Razmi, H., *et al.* (2012a) Bioactivity of EndoSequence Root repair material and bioaggregate. *International Endodontic Journal* **45**, 1127–34.

Shokouhinejad, N., Razmi, H., Fekrazad, R., *et al.* (2012b) Push-out bond strength of two root-end filling materials in root-end cavities prepared by Er,Cr:YSGG laser or ultrasonic. *Australian Endodontic Journal* **38**, 113–7.

Silva, E.J., Herrera, D.R., Almeida, J.F., *et al.* (2012) Evaluation of cytotoxicity and up-regulation of gelatinases in fibroblast cells by three root repair materials. *International Endodontic Journal* **45**, 815–20.

Silva, E.J.L., Rosa, T.P., Herrera, D.R., *et al.* (2013) Evaluation of cytotoxicity and physico-chemical properties of calcium silicate-based endodontic sealer MTA Fillapex. *Journal of Endodontics* **39**, 274–7.

Soheilipour, E., Kheirieh, S., Madani, M., *et al.* (2009) Particle size of a new endodontic cement compared to Root MTA and calcium hydroxide. *Iranian Endodontic Journal* **4**, 112–6.

Tabarsi, B., Parirokh, M., Eghbal, M.J., *et al.* (2010) A comparative study of dental pulp response to several pulpotomy agents. *International Endodontic Journal* **43**, 565–71.

Tabarsi, B., Pourghasem, M., Moghaddamnia, A., *et al.* (2012) Comparison of skin test reactivity of two endodontic biomaterials in rabbits. *Pakistan Journal of Biological Sciences* **15**, 250–4.

Tanalp, J., Dikbas, I., Malkondu, O., *et al.* (2012) Comparison of the fracture resistance of simulated immature permanent teeth using various canal filling materials and fiber posts. *Dental Traumatology* **28**, 457–64.

Tanomaru-Filho, M., Chaves Faleiros, F.B., Saçaki, J.N., *et al.* (2009) Evaluation of pH and calcium ion release of root-end filling materials containing calcium hydroxide or mineral trioxide aggregate. *Journal of Endodontics* **35**, 1418–21.

Taschieri, S., Tamse, A., Del Fabbro, M., *et al.* (2010) A new surgical technique for preservation of endodontically treated teeth with coronally located vertical root fractures: a prospective case series. *Oral Surgery Oral Medicine Oral Pathology Oral Radiology Endodontics* **110**, e45–52.

Tavares, C.O., Bottcher, D.E., Assmann, E., *et al.* (2013) Tissue reactions to a new mineral trioxide aggregate–containing endodontic sealer. *Journal of Endodontics* **39**, 653–7.

Tay, K.C., Loushine, B.A., Oxford, C., *et al.* (2007) In vitro evaluation of a Ceramicrete-based root-end filling material. *Journal of Endodontics* **33**, 1438–43.

Torabinejad, M., Parirokh, M. (2010) Mineral trioxide aggregate: a comprehensive literature review- Part II: Sealing ability and biocompatibility properties. *Journal of Endodontics* **36**, 190–202.

Torabzadeh, H., Aslanzadeh, S., Asgary, S. (2012) Radiopacity of various dental biomaterials. *Research Journal of Biological Science* **7**, 152–8.

Tuna, E.B., Dinçol, M.E., Gençay, K., *et al.* (2011) Fracture resistance of immature teeth filled with BioAggregate, mineral trioxide aggregate and calcium hydroxide. *Dental Traumatology* **27**. 174–8.

Ulusoy, Ö.İ., Nayır, Y., Darendeliler-Yaman, S. (2011) Effect of different root canal sealers on fracture strength of simulated immature roots. *Oral Surgery Oral Medicine Oral Pathology Oral Radiology Endodontics* **112**, 544–7.

Vallés, M., Mercadé, M., Duran-Sindreu, F., *et al.* (2013) Color stability of white mineral trioxide aggregate. *Clinical Oral Investigation* **17**, 1155–9.

Vier-Pelisser, F.V., Pelisser, A., Recuero, L.C., *et al.* (2012) Use of cone beam computed tomography in the diagnosis, planning and follow up of a type III dens invaginatus case. *International Endodontic Journal* **45**, 198–208.

Viola, N.V., Guerreiro-Tanomaru, J.M., da Silva, G.F., *et al.* (2012) Biocompatibility of an experimental MTA sealer implanted in the rat subcutaneous: quantitative and immunohistochemical evaluation. *Journal of Biomedical Material Research B Applied Biomaterials* **100B**, 1773–81.

Vivan, R.R., Ordinola-Zapata, R., Bramante, C.M., *et al.* (2009) Evaluation of the radiopacity of some commercial and experimental root-end filling materials. *Oral Surgery Oral Medicine Oral Pathology Oral Radiology Endodontics* **108**, e35–8.

Vivan, R.R., Zapata, R.O., Zeferino, M.A., *et al.* (2010) Evaluation of the physical and chemical properties of two commercial and three experimental root-end filling materials. *Oral Surgery Oral Medicine Oral Pathology Oral Radiology Endodontics* **110**, 250–6.

Wälivaara, D.Å., Abrahamsson, P., Isaksson, S., *et al.* (2012) Periapical tissue response after use of intermediate restorative material, gutta-percha, reinforced zinc oxide cement, and mineral trioxide aggregate as retrograde root-end filling materials: a histologic study in dogs. *Journal of Oral & Maxillofacial Surgery* **70**, 2041–7.

Washington, J.T., Schneiderman, E., Spears, R., *et al.* (2011) Biocompatibility and osteogenic potential of new generation endodontic materials established by using primary osteoblasts. *Journal of Endodontics* **37**, 1166–70.

Weller, R.N., Tay, K.C., Garrett, L.V., *et al.* (2008) Microscopic appearance and apical seal of root canals filled with gutta-percha and ProRoot Endo Sealer after immersion in a phosphate-containing fluid. *International Endodontic Journal* **41**, 977–86.

Yan, P., Yuan, Z., Jiang, H., *et al.* (2010) Effect of bioaggregate on differentiation of human periodontal ligament fibroblasts. *International Endodontic Journal* **43**, 1116–21.

Yavari, H.R., Samiei, M., Shahi, S., *et al.* (2012) Microleakage comparison of four dental materials as intra-orifice barriers in endodontically treated teeth. *Iranian Endodontic Journal* **7**, 25–30.

Yilmaz, H.G., Kalender, A., Cengiz, E. (2010) Use of mineral trioxide aggregate in the treatment of invasive cervical resorption: a case report. *Journal of Endodontics* **36**, 160–3.

Yuan, Z., Peng, B., Jiang, H., *et al.* (2010) Effect of bioaggregate on mineral-associated gene expression in osteoblast cells. *Journal of Endodontics* **36**, 1145–8.

Zarrabi, M.H., Javidi, M., Jafarian, A.H., *et al.* (2010) Histologic assessment of human pulp response to capping with mineral trioxide aggregate and a novel endodontic cement. *Journal of Endodontics* **36**, 1778–81.

Zarrabi, M.H., Javidi, M., Jafarian, A.H., *et al.* (2011) Immunohistochemical expression of fibronectin and tenascin in human tooth pulp capped with mineral trioxide aggregate and a novel endodontic cement. *Journal of Endodontics* **37**, 1613–8.

Zeferino, E.G., Bueno, C.E., Oyama, L.M., *et al.* (2010) Ex vivo assessment of genotoxicity and cytotoxicity in murine fibroblasts exposed to white MTA or white Portland cement with 15% bismuth oxide. *International Endodontic Journal* **43**, 843–8.

Zhang, H., Pappen, F.G., Haapasalo, M. (2009a) Dentin enhances the antibacterial effect of mineral trioxide aggregate and bioaggregate. *Journal of Endodontics* **35**, 221–4.

Zhang, H., Shen, Y., Ruse, N.D., *et al.* (2009b) Antibacterial activity of endodontic sealers by modified direct contact test against *Enterococcus faecalis*. *Journal of Endodontics* **35**, 1051–5.

Zhang, W., Li, Z., Peng, B. (2010) Ex vivo cytotoxicity of a new calcium silicate-based canal filling material. *International Endodontic Journal* **43**, 769–74.

Zmener, O., Martinez Lalis, R., Pameijer, C.H., *et al.* (2012) Reaction of rat subcutaneous connective tissue to a mineral trioxide aggregate-based and a zinc oxide and eugenol sealer. *Journal of Endodontics* **38**, 1233–8.

Zoufan, K., Jiang, J., Komabayashi, T., *et al.* (2011) Cytotoxicity evaluation of Gutta Flow and Endo Sequence BC sealers. *Oral Surgery Oral Medicine Oral Pathology Oral Radiology Endodontics* **112**, 657–61.

Index

Note: Page numbers in *italics* refer to Figures; those in **bold** to Tables

Mineral Trioxide Aggregate: Properties and Clinical Applications, First Edition.
Edited by Mahmoud Torabinejad.
© 2014 John Wiley & Sons, Inc. Published 2014 by John Wiley & Sons, Inc.